Manual of Oculoplasty

Manual of Oculoplasty

Ruchi Goel MS DNB FAICO (Oculoplasty)
Professor
Maulana Azad Medical College and
Guru Nanak Eye Center
New Delhi, India

Foreword
Gangadhara Sundar

JAYPEE BROTHERS MEDICAL PUBLISHERS
The Health Sciences Publisher
New Delhi | London | Panama

Jaypee Brothers Medical Publishers (P) Ltd

Headquarters

Jaypee Brothers Medical Publishers (P) Ltd
4838/24, Ansari Road, Daryaganj
New Delhi 110 002, India
Phone: +91-11-43574357
Fax: +91-11-43574314
Email: jaypee@jaypeebrothers.com

Overseas Offices

J.P. Medical Ltd
83 Victoria Street, London
SW1H 0HW (UK)
Phone: +44 20 3170 8910
Fax: +44 (0)20 3008 6180
Email: info@jpmedpub.com

Jaypee-Highlights Medical Publishers Inc
City of Knowledge, Bld. 235, 2nd Floor
Clayton, Panama City, Panama
Phone: +1 507-301-0496
Fax: +1 507-301-0499
Email: cservice@jphmedical.com

Jaypee Brothers Medical Publishers (P) Ltd
Bhotahity, Kathmandu, Nepal
Phone: +977-9741283608
Email: kathmandu@jaypeebrothers.com

Website: www.jaypeebrothers.com
Website: www.jaypeedigital.com

Manual of Oculoplasty

First Edition: **2019,** Reprint: 2023

ISBN 978-93-5270-992-2

Printed in India

Dedicated to

My Mother, Dr Prakash Sangal
My Husband, Dr Amit Goel
My Son, Saumaya Goel
And my teacher, Professor KPS Malik
Who always bring the best out of me!

Contributors

AK Grover MD MNAMS FRCS (Glasgow) FIMSA FICO
Chairman
Department of Ophthalmology
Sir Ganga Ram Hospital and Vision Eye Center
New Delhi, India

Abhilasha Sanoria MS
Consultant
Lions Eye Hospital
Guna, Madhya Pradesh, India

Akshay Gopinathan Nair DNB
Consultant
Ophthalmic Plastic Surgery and Ocular Oncology Services
Advanced Eye Hospital and Institute
Aditya Jyot Eye Hospital
Mumbai, Maharashtra, India

Amit Goel MS FNB
Associate Professor
ESI Medical College
New Delhi, India

Amrita Sawhney DNB MNAMS FAICO (Oculoplasty)
Associate Consultant
Sir Ganga Ram Hospital
New Delhi, India

Bita Esmaeli MD FACS
Director
Ophthalmic Plastic and Orbital Surgery Fellowship Program
Department of Plastic Surgery
MD Anderson Cancer Center
Houston, Texas 77030, USA

Deepika Kapoor DNB FICO
Senior Fellow
Sri Sankaradeva Nethralaya
Guwahati, Assam, India

Gangadhara Sundar DO FRCSEd FAMS Diplomate (The American Board of Ophthalmology)
Head of Orbit and Oculofacial Surgery
Department of Ophthalmology
National University Hospital, Singapore
Assistant Professor
Department of Ophthalmology
National University Hospital, Singapore

Ishita Anand DNB MNAMS
Clinical Assistant
Sir Ganga Ram Hospital
New Delhi, India

Kanika Jain
Resident
PGIMER and Dr RML Hospital
New Delhi, India

Kasturi Bhattacharjee MS DNB FRCSEd
Senior Consultant
Sri Sankaradeva Nethralaya
Guwahati, Assam, India

KPS Malik MS MNAMS
Visiting Professor
All India Institute of Medical Sciences (AIIMS)
Rishikesh, Uttarakhand, India

Mohammad Javed Ali MD PhD FRCS
Head
Govindram Seksaria Institute of Dacryology (GSID)
LV Prasad Eye Institute, Hyderabad, Telangana, India
Visiting Professor
Friedrich Alexander University
Nuremberg, Germany
Adjunct Associate Professor
University of Rochester, New York
Alexander Von Humboldt Scientist
FAU University, Nuremberg, Germany

Mohit Chhabra MS
Senior Resident
Maulana Azad Medical College and
Guru Nanak Eye Centre
New Delhi, India

Neha Rathie MS
Consultant
Healing Touch Eye Centre
New Delhi, India

Raj Anand MS
Consultant
Eye 7 Hospital
New Delhi, India

Raksha Rao MS
Consultant
Orbit, Oculoplasty and Ocular Oncology
Chaithanya Eye Hospital and Research Institute
Thiruvananthapuram, Kerala, India

RK Saran MD (Pathology) DNB (Pathology) MBA (Health care)
Director-Professor
GIPMER (GB Pant Hospital)
New Delhi, India

Ruchi Goel MS DNB FAICO (Oculoplasty)
Professor
Maulana Azad Medical College and
Guru Nanak Eye Center
New Delhi, India

Samir Serasiya DNB FICO
Senior Fellow
Sri Sankaradeva Nethralaya
Guwahati, Assam, India

Samreen Khanam MS
Senior Resident
Maulana Azad Medical College and
Guru Nanak Eye Centre
New Delhi, India

Santosh G Honavar MD FACS
Senior Consultant
National Retinoblastoma Foundation
Ocular Oncology Service, Centre for Sight
Hyderabad, Telangana, India

Saurabh Kamal MS DNB
Director
Eye HUB Vision Care
Faridabad, Haryana, India

Shaloo Bageja DNB MNAMS
Senior Consultant
Sir Ganga Ram Hospital
New Delhi, India

Shweta Raghav MS
Senior Resident
Guru Nanak Eye Centre
Maulana Azad Medical College
New Delhi, India

Sima Das MS
Head
Oculoplasty and Ocular Oncology Services
Dr Shroff's Charity Eye Hospital
New Delhi, India

Smriti Bansal MS
Consultant
Oculoplasty and Ocular Oncology Services
Dr Shroff's Charity Eye Hospital
New Delhi, India

Smriti Nagpal Gupta MS DNB FICO FRCS(Glasgow)
Consultant
Oculoplasty and Anterior Segment
ICare Eye Hospital and Postgraduate Institute
Noida, Gautam Budh Nagar, India

Sumit Kumar MS
Senior Resident
Maulana Azad Medical College and
Guru Nanak Eye Centre
New Delhi, India

Sushil Kumar MS
Director and Head
Guru Nanak Eye Centre
New Delhi, India

Swapnil Jadhav DO DNB
Trainee
Sir Ganga Ram Hospital
New Delhi, India

Swati Singh MS
Consultant
LJ Eye Institute
Ambala, Haryana, India

Taru Dewan MS FRCSEd
Professor
PGIMER and Dr Ram Manohar Lal Hospital
New Delhi, India

Foreword

A parent or a teacher has only his lifetime; a good book can teach forever.

—*Louis L'Amour*

It is with the greatest pleasure that I write and share my thoughts on this excellent undertaking of Dr Ruchi Goel and her team of able and competent oculoplastic surgeons.

The field of oculoplastic surgery has numerous manuals, atlases and comprehensive textbooks from all around the world. However, given the fact that it is a constantly evolving field with newer concepts, approaches and thresholds for intervention, a comprehensive manual addressing all aspects of orbit and oculofacial surgery—basics such as applied anatomy, instrumentation, histopathology, etc. to clinical conditions in eyelid, lacrimal, and orbital surgery was much needed.

Primarily aimed at postgraduates in ophthalmology, this all-encompassing manual, which is easily readable, will serve as an extremely useful review and reference not only for residents in ophthalmology and fellows in ophthalmic plastic and reconstructive surgery but also for general ophthalmologists and junior consultants in oculoplastics, facial plastics and craniomaxillofacial surgery who are involved in multidisciplinary management of these complex conditions.

Dr Ruchi Goel, with her immense expertise in clinical acumen, surgical skills, and teaching career, has brought together an experienced group of seasoned and accomplished oculoplastic surgeons with experience and international repute who have compiled solid principles and practical pearls for effective diagnosis and management of common as well as rare yet serious vision threatening or disfiguring conditions.

The manual is well-illustrated with schematics, clinical photographs, imaging and intraoperative photographs, which complement the text and make it an easy-to-read for all.

I have no doubt that this manual will have not just have a regional but also a global reach and once again compliment Dr Goel on this arduous yet rewarding endeavor.

Gangadhara Sundar DO FRCSEd FAMS
Diplomate, The American Board of Ophthalmology
Head of Orbit and Oculofacial Surgery
Department of Ophthalmology
National University Hospital, Singapore
Assistant Professor
Department of Ophthalmology
National University Hospital, Singapore

Preface

The genesis of this project dates to my days of postgraduation when I would struggle to make notes from different books for the lid, orbit and lacrimal system. The literature though rich in reference books, yet a simplified book covering all the subjects in oculoplasty was lacking.

The *Manual of Oculoplasty* is a compilation of all the topics that a postgraduate student is expected to know in oculoplasty. It is also a good read for postgraduate teachers, fellows and practitioners for planning management of their patients. The references have been deliberately kept to a minimum to reduce the number of pages and thereby the cost.

The book is divided into seven sections with the first three sections dedicated to orbit, lids and lacrimal system followed by those on instruments, histopathology slides, and university questions.

Each section has basic chapters on anatomy, physiology and examination techniques followed by surgical techniques illustrated in detail with diagrams. Numerous flowcharts and tables have been added to ease revision. The build-up is from a brief history to recent classifications and advances wherever appropriate.

The book thus will serve as a useful manual for a quick reference and for preparation of the postgraduate/fellowship exit examination.

I would like to acknowledge the help rendered by Director-Professor, Sushil Kumar and all the residents of our unit in compilation of this book.

Ruchi Goel

Contents

Section 4: Tumors

Orbit

Surgical Anatomy of Orbit

Shaloo Bageja, Ishita Anand, Swapnil Jadhav

INTRODUCTION

A comprehensive knowledge of the orbit and periorbital area aids in diagnosis and management of disorders in this region.

The two orbital cavities are situated on either side of the sagittal plane of the skull between the cranium and the skeleton of the face.

RELATIONS OF ORBIT

- *Superiorly*—anterior cranial fossa and frontal sinus
- *Laterally*—temporal fossa (anteriorly); middle cranial fossa (posteriorly)
- *Inferiorly*—maxillary sinus
- *Medially*—ethmoid sinus and anterior part of sphenoid sinus.

Due to the close proximity of these structures, any infection can spread across these regions. For instance, an infection of the ethmoid sinuses can easily invade the orbit through the thin lamina papyracea.

EMBRYOLOGY

Orbital Walls

- The orbital walls are derived from the cranial neural crest cells which expand to form the frontonasal process and maxillary process
- Inferior, medial, and lateral walls develop from the lateral nasal process and maxillary process
- Orbital roof is formed from capsule of forebrain
- Ossification of the orbital bones can be either enchondral or membranous

- First bone to develop is maxillary bone, around 6 weeks of intrauterine life. It develops from elements in the region of the canine tooth. Secondary ossification centers are in the orbitonasal and premaxillary regions
- Other orbital bones develop at around 7 weeks of intrauterine development
- Frontal, zygomatic, maxillary, and palatine bones have intermembranous origin
- Sphenoid bone has both enchondral and membranous origin
  - Lesser wing of sphenoid—develops at 7 weeks of intrauterine development. It has enchondral origin
  - Greater wing of sphenoid—develops at 10 weeks, has intermembranous origin
  - Both wings join at 16 weeks of age.
- Ossification completes at birth, except the orbital apex
- In the early stages of development, human eyes are directed in opposite direction. With facial development, angle between optic stalk decreases and is about 68° in adults.

Size, Shape, and Volume of Orbit

Orbit is shaped like a quadrilateral pyramid, with the base anteriorly and apex directed posteriorly. The orbits are aligned such that medial walls are parallel to each other and lateral walls are perpendicular to each other. The angle between medial and lateral wall is 45°. The axis between visual axis and orbital axis is 23°.

The average dimensions of the orbit are as follows (Figs. 1A and B):
- Height of orbital margin—40 mm
- Width of orbital margin—35 mm
- Interorbital distance—25 mm

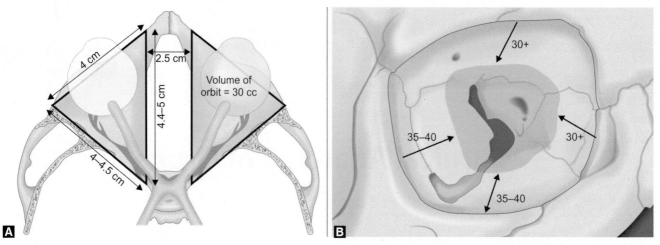

Figs. 1A and B: (A) Dimensions of the orbit; (B) Depth of Safe limit for intraorbital dissection of orbital walls during surgery.

- Volume of orbit—30 cm³
- Depth of orbit—40–50 mm
- It is approximately 1 cm shorter from the lateral orbital rim to apex
- The widest circumference of the orbit is 1.5 cm inside the orbital rim at the level of lacrimal recess.

OSTEOLOGY

The orbit is composed of seven bones: frontal, lacrimal bone, zygoma, maxilla, ethmoid, sphenoid, and palatine bone (Fig. 2).

Superior Wall or Roof

- Formed by:
  - Orbital plate of frontal bone
  - Lesser wing of sphenoid
- Concave in shape
- Separates orbit from anterior cranial fossa
- Optic foramina in lesser wing of sphenoid:
  - Transmits optic nerve and ophthalmic artery from middle cranial fossa.
- The medial aspect has fovea for trochlea, 4 mm behind the orbital margin
- The lateral most aspect accommodates fossa for lacrimal gland, behind the zygomatic process of frontal bone
- The superior orbital rim has a notch at the junction of medial one-third and lateral two-thirds:
  - Transmits supraorbital nerve and vessels-supplies forehead.

Medial Orbital Wall

Composed of four bones, from anterior to posterior:
1. Frontal process of maxilla
2. Lacrimal bone

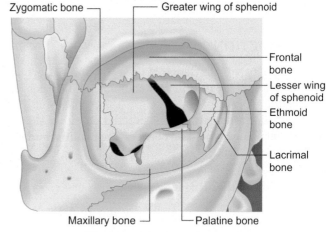

Fig. 2: Seven bones of the orbit.

3. Orbital plate of ethmoid
4. Body of sphenoid.

Orbital plate of ethmoid is the largest part of medial orbital wall. It is very thin (papyraceous). It separates orbit from ethmoid sinuses.

The *frontoethmoidal suture line* marks the approximate level of ethmoidal sinus roof, hence any dissection above this line should be avoided as it will expose the cranial cavity.

Anterior and posterior ethmoid foramina are present behind the medial orbital rim at the junction of medial wall and roof. They transmit anterior and posterior ethmoidal arteries (branches of ophthalmic artery) and ethmoidal nerves (branches of nasociliary nerve). The anterior ethmoidal foramen is located at a distance of 24 mm from the anterior lacrimal crest, while the posterior ethmoidal foramen is located at a distance of 36 mm from the anterior lacrimal crest (Fig. 3).

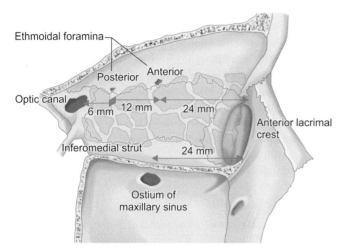

Fig. 3: Relations of anterior and posterior ethmoidal foramina.

Lacrimal fossa is a depression in the inferomedial orbital rim. It is formed by maxillary (anterior part) and the lacrimal bone (posterior part). It is bounded by two projections, i.e. anterior lacrimal crest of maxillary bone and posterior lacrimal crest of lacrimal bone. Lacrimal bone is thin whereas the maxillary bone is quite thick. If maxillary bone is predominant in the lacrimal fossa, then osteotomy becomes quite difficult during dacryocystorhinostomy (DCR) surgery.

Nasolacrimal canal lies in the inferomedial part of orbit through which nasolacrimal duct traverses.

The *nasolacrimal duct* is 3–4 mm in diameter, it passes backward, downward, and laterally to open into the inferior meatus under the inferior turbinate.

Sutura longitudinalis imperfecta of Weber lies in the frontal process of maxilla just anterior to the lacrimal fossa. This suture runs parallel to the anterior lacrimal crest. Small branches of infraorbital artery pass through this groove to supply the nasal mucosa. The presence of these vessels should be anticipated in any lacrimal sac surgery to avoid intraoperative bleeding.

Disruption of medial wall leading to nasoorbitoethmoidal fracture (NOE fracture) or any lateral displacement of the walls leads to hypertelorism.

Any trauma to frontal process of maxilla where medial canthal ligament is attached, leads to telecanthus.

Lateral Wall

- Formed by:
  - Greater wing of sphenoid (posteriorly)
  - Zygoma (anteriorly)
- Thickest bone
- Greater wing of sphenoid separates orbit from middle cranial fossa. Congenital absence of this bone in cases

like neurofibromatosis results in pulsatile proptosis due to orbital encephalocele
- Whitnall's tubercle:
  - 4–5 mm behind the lateral orbital rim
  - 1 cm inferior to frontozygomatic suture
  - Attachments:
    - Lateral canthal tendon
    - Lateral horn of levator aponeurosis
    - Lateral rectus check ligament
    - Suspensory ligament of lower lid (Lockwood's ligament)
    - Lacrimal gland fascia
    - Orbital septum.
- The frontal process of zygomatic bone and zygomatic process of frontal bone are thick bones and thus protect globe during injury
- Posterior part of this lateral wall is thin (about 1 mm), composed of orbital plate of greater wing of sphenoid and posterior zygomatic bone
- The superior orbital fissure (between lateral and superior walls of orbit) and the inferior orbital fissure (between lateral and inferior walls of orbit) transmit important structures
- Zygomaticosphenoid suture is an important landmark for lateral orbitotomy. Superiorly the bony incision is usually made just above the frontozygomatic suture. The lateral wall removal is completed by fracturing the bone at the zygomaticosphenoid suture
- The recurrent meningeal branches of the ophthalmic artery (internal carotid supply) exit the orbit via the frontosphenoid suture to anastomose with the middle meningeal artery (external carotid supply)
- The zygomaticofacial and zygomaticotemporal neurovascular structures leave the orbit via their respective foramina.

Orbital Floor

- Triangular in shape and shortest of all the walls
- Formed by:
  - Orbital plate of maxilla
  - Zygoma
  - Palatine.
- Separated from lateral wall by inferior orbital fissure
- Inferior orbital fissure weakens the floor. Blow out fractures usually occur medial to it
- Medially, it is bounded by maxilla ethmoidal strut. It is important to preserve this during orbital decompression surgery to avoid hypoglobus and postoperative diplopia
- Infraorbital groove becomes a canal anteriorly, through this groove passes the infraorbital nerve and artery (maxillary division of trigeminal nerve and the terminal

branch of internal maxillary artery). They exit through the infraorbital foramen to supply the lower eye lid, cheek, upper lip, and upper anterior gingiva
- The infraorbital foramen is located about 6-10 mm below the infraorbital rim
- The inferior oblique muscle arises anteromedially, immediately lateral to the nasolacrimal canal.

FISSURES AND CANAL

Various important nerves and vessels are transmitted through fissures and canals in the orbit (Fig. 4).

Superior Orbital Fissure

- Location—between greater and lesser wing of sphenoid. It lies between roof and lateral walls of orbit (Fig. 5).
- Also known as sphenoidal fissure
- It is 22 mm long, largest communication between orbit and middle cranial fossa

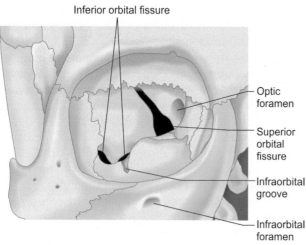

Fig. 4: Orbital fissures and foramina.

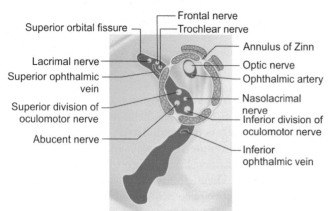

Fig. 5: Superior orbital fissure.

- It usually narrows laterally and widens medially, below the optic foramen
- Its tip is about 30-40 mm from frontozygomatic suture
- Its medial part is separated from optic foramen by posterior part of lesser wing of sphenoid
- The annulus of Zinn, a tight fibrous ring, divides the superior orbital fissure into intraconal and extraconal spaces.

Structures passing through upper part:
- Lacrimal nerve
- Frontal nerve
- Trochlear nerve
- Superior ophthalmic vein.

Structures passing through annulus of Zinn:
- Superior division of 3rd nerve
- Nasociliary nerve
- Sympathetic root of cervical ganglion
- Inferior division of 3rd nerve
- 6th nerve
- Sympathetic fibers.

Structures passing through lower part, outside the annulus of Zinn:
Inferior ophthalmic vein.

Inferior Orbital Fissure

- Location—lies between lateral wall and floor of the orbit. It is about 1 cm posterior to the inferolateral orbital rim
- It is also known as sphenomaxillary fissure
- It is about 20 mm long
- The orbit communicates with the pterygopalatine and infratemporal fossa
- Structure passing:
  - Maxillary division of the trigeminal nerve
  - Zygomatic nerve
  - Branches from the sphenopalatine ganglion
  - Branches of the inferior ophthalmic vein leading to the pterygoid plexus
- The maxillary division of trigeminal nerve and the terminal branch of internal maxillary artery enter the infraorbital groove and canal to become the infraorbital nerve and artery.

Optic Foramen

- The foramen is present in the lesser wing of sphenoid lies medial to the superior orbital fissure and is separated from it by a bony optic strut
- Conveys the optic nerve and ophthalmic artery
- The optic foramen is about 6.5 mm in diameter
- Optic canal attains its adult size by 3 years of age. It is supposed to be bilaterally symmetrical. Any variation

in size between two sides should be considered pathological
- In adults the optic canal is 8–10 mm long and 5–7 mm wide
- Any trauma to optic canal, can result in injury to optic nerve.

ORBITAL SOFT TISSUES

- Orbital septum
- Periorbita
- Orbital fat
- Extraocular muscles
- Lacrimal system.

Orbital Septum

- It is anterior soft tissue boundary. It is extension of periorbita (Fig. 6)
- It originates from arcus marginalis. It extends from tarsus to orbital rim
- It acts as a physical barrier, separates the orbital contents from eyelids
- It is covered anteriorly by preseptal orbicularis muscle and skin.

Periorbita

- It is periosteal lining of the orbital walls
- It is firmly attached at the suture lines, the foramina, the fissures, the arcus marginalis, and the posterior lacrimal crest
- Posteriorly, the periorbita is continuous with the optic nerve sheath where the dura is fused to the optic canal

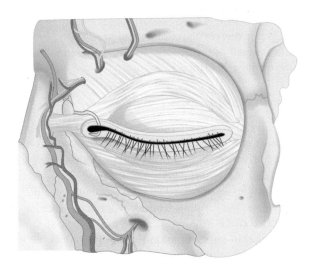

Fig. 6: Extension of orbital septum.

- Periorbita thickens on the orbital surface of the optic canal and the medial aspect of the superior orbital fissure and gives rise to the tendinous attachments of the four rectus muscles, the levator superioris, and the superior oblique muscle. This tendinous ring is called the annulus of Zinn.

Tenon's Capsule

- Also known as fascia bulbi or bulbar sheath
- It is dense, elastic, and vascular connective tissue that surrounds the globe
- It begins from perilimbal area and extends posteriorly along the globe till optic nerve and fuses with dural sheath and sclera
- It is separated from sclera by periscleral lymph space which is in continuation with subdural and subarachnoid space.

Orbital Fat

- Acts as a cushion to orbital structures
- In upper eyelid it lies anterior to levator complex and posterior to orbital septum
- It is divided into compartments by connective tissue septa
- Infratrochlear nerve and medial palpebral artery branch of the ophthalmic artery course through the medial fat pad
- In lower eyelid, medial fat pad is separated from central pad of fat by inferior oblique muscle.

Extraocular Muscles

Each orbit contains six extraocular muscles that function together to move the eye:
- *Rectus muscles (4)*—superior, inferior, lateral, and medial recti muscle
- *Oblique muscles (2)*—superior and inferior
- *Other muscles*—the levator palpebrae and Müller's muscle (Fig. 7).

Recti Muscles

The rectus muscles originate at the annulus of Zinn, a fibrous tendon that encircles the optic foramen. The annulus of Zinn is divided into the superior Lockwood tendon and the inferior tendon of Zinn. The inferior tendon gives origin to parts of medial and lateral recti and entire inferior rectus muscle. The superior tendon gives origin to part of medial and lateral recti and all of the superior rectus muscle. The attachments of superior and medial recti muscles are close to the dural sheath of optic nerve. Thus causing pain during

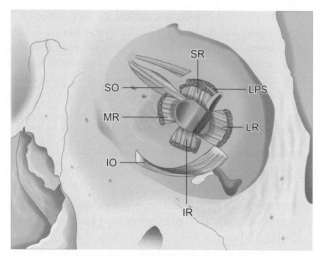

Fig. 7: Origin of extraocular muscles.
(SR: superior rectus; IR: inferior rectus; SO: superior oblique; IO: inferior oblique; LR: lateral rectus; MR medial rectus; LPS: levator palpebrae superioris)

extreme eye movements in retrobulbar neuritis. The recti are inserted 6–8 mm posterior to the limbus into the sclera.

Actions:
- Medial rectus—Adduction
- Lateral rectus—Abduction
- Superior rectus—Elevation, adduction, intorsion
- Inferior rectus—Depression, adduction, extorsion.

Oblique Muscles

The superior and inferior oblique muscles originate separately from the posterior orbital wall.

The *superior oblique* muscle arises from the sphenoid bone superomedial to the optic canal. It courses in the forward direction lying above the medial rectus, and through a cartilaginous pulley (the trochlea) attached to the frontal bone. Thereafter, the tendon passes posterolaterally, running inferior to the tendon of the superior rectus to insert into the posterior sclera.

The *inferior oblique* muscle arises from the maxilla at the anteromedial floor of the orbit, passes in a posterolateral direction, immediately inferior to the inferior rectus to insert into the posterior sclera.

Actions:
- Inferior oblique—extorsion, elevation, abduction
- Superior oblique—intorsion, depression, abduction.

Nerve supply: The superior oblique muscle is supplied by the trochlear nerve, the lateral rectus by the abducent nerve, and all the other extraocular muscles are supplied by the oculomotor nerve.

Levator Palpebrae Superioris

It is a striated muscle. It helps in elevation of the eyelid.

Origin

Levator palpebrae superioris (LPS) arises from the under surface of lesser wing of sphenoid just above and in front of optic foramen, and usually it is blended with the origin of superior rectus muscle. From this attachment this ribbon-like muscle passes forward below the roof on top of the superior rectus muscle.

Insertion

Levator palpebrae superioris inserts into the skin of the upper eyelid and upper tarsal plate.

Nerve Supply

It is innervated by the superior division of 3rd cranial nerve.

Müller's Muscle

It is a smooth muscle which acts as an eyelid elevator.

Origin

It arises from the inferior aspect of LPS.

Insertion

Inserted into the upper edge of tarsal plate.

Nerve Supply

It is innervated by sympathetic fibers.

SURGICAL SPACES (FIG. 8)

- Subperiosteal space
- Peripheral orbital space
- Muscular cone.

Subperisoteal Space

- It lies between orbital bones and periorbita
- It is limited anteriorly by strong adhesions between periorbita and orbital margins.

Extraconal Space

- It is bounded peripherally by periorbita and centrally by four recti muscles and their intermuscular septa, anteriorly by orbital septum and posteriorly by:
  - Peripheral orbital fat
  - Muscles—superior and inferior oblique, LPS
  - Nerves—lacrimal, frontal, trochlear, anterior and posterior ethmoidal
  - Vessels—superior and inferior ophthalmic veins
  - Lacrimal gland
  - Lacrimal sac.

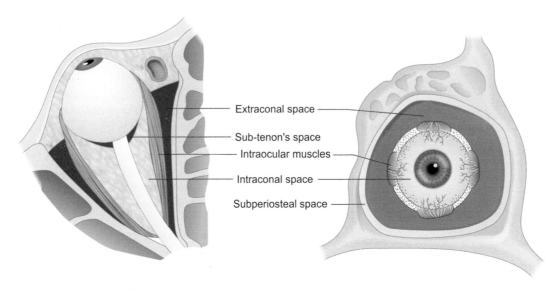

Fig. 8: Surgical spaces of orbit (in sagittal and coronal sections).

Intraconal Space

- Bounded anteriorly by Tenon's capsule, peripherally by four recti and intermuscular septa and posteriorly continuous with peripheral space
- Contents:
  - Central orbital fat
  - Nerves—optic nerve, oculomotor, abducens, nasociliary, ciliary ganglion
  - Vessels—ophthalmic artery, superior ophthalmic vein.

Sub-Tenon's Space

It lies between sclera and Tenon's capsule.

LACRIMAL APPARATUS

Lacrimal apparatus comprises of lacrimal gland and its excretory passage.

Lacrimal Gland

The lacrimal gland lies in the superotemporal orbit, in lacrimal fossa of the frontal bone. It measures about 20 mm by 12 mm. It is divided into larger orbital and smaller palpebral part by levator aponeurosis. The gland is composed of numerous secretory units known as acini which progressively drain in to small and larger ducts. About 2–6 ducts from the orbital lobe pass through the palpebral lobe joining with the ducts from the palpebral lobe to form 6–12 tubules to empty into the superolateral conjunctiva. Hence, damage to the palpebral lobe may block drainage

from the entire gland. About 20–40 accessory lacrimal glands of Krause are located in the superior conjunctival fornix, about half this number is located over the lower fornix.

Nerve Supply

Nerve supply is innervated by branches from 5th and 7th cranial nerves, sympathetic supply to lacrimal gland is via the nerves from the superior cervical ganglion. The parasympathetic fibers are supplied via the 6th nerve. Sensory supply is via the branches of trigeminal nerve.

Vessels

- *Arterial supply*—lacrimal artery branch of ophthalmic artery
- *Venous drainage*—ophthalmic veins
- *Lymphatic drainage*—preauricular lymph nodes.

Lacrimal Excretory System

The lacrimal excretory system begins with punctum, about 0.3 mm in size. It lies at the medial end of each eyelids, at the junction of ciliated and nonciliated part. The punctal opening widens into ampulla, makes a sharp turn to drain into the canaliculi. The canaliculi measures 0.5–1 mm in diameter and courses parallel to the lid margins. It has two parts—vertical 2 mm in size and horizontal about 8 mm in length. The superior canaliculus is slightly shorter than the inferior canaliculus. In 90% of individuals the superior and inferior canaliculi merge into a common canaliculi before draining into lacrimal sac. There is a valve at the junction

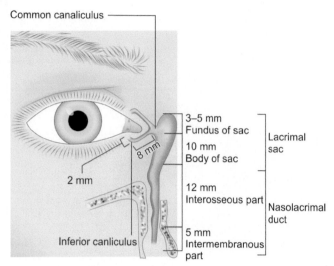

Fig. 9: Lacrimal excretory system.

of common canaliculus and lacrimal sac known as the Rosenmuller valve. The lacrimal sac resides in the lacrimal fossa. It measures about 12–15 mm vertically and 4–8 mm anteroposteriorly. It opens into nasolacrimal duct, which is about 15 mm in length. It has interosseous and meatal part. It is directed downward, backward, and laterally and opens in inferior meatus. Valve of Hasner is found at the lower end of the nasolacrimal duct at the level of inferior meatus of nose. Imperforate Hasner's valve in new born infants results in congenital nasolacrimal obstruction (Fig. 9).

Vessels

- *Arterial supply*—palpebral branch of ophthalmic artery, angular and infraorbital arteries, and nasal branch of sphenopalatine
- *Venous*—angular and infraorbital vessels above and nasal veins below
- *Lymphatic drainage*—submandibular and deep cervical nodes.

Nerve Supply

Infratrochlear and anterior superior alveolar nerves.

ORBITAL NERVES

Orbit contains seven nerves. It comprises of:
- *Component of central nervous system*—Optic nerve
- *Motor nerves*—Oculomotor, trochlear, and abducens nerves
- *Sensory nerve*—Ophthalmic division of trigeminal nerve (V1) and some contribution from maxillary division (V2)
- *Autonomic center*—Ciliary ganglion.

Optic Nerve

Optic nerve is the second cranial nerve
- It is about 4 cm in length
- Parts:
  - Intraocular—1 mm
  - Intraorbital—30 mm
  - Intracanalicular—5 mm
  - Intracranial—10 mm
- *Intraocular*: The nerve fibers start from axons of ganglion cell layer of retina, converge on the optic disc, and pierce the layers of the eye. It is 1.5 mm in diameter and expands to 3 mm behind sclera as it receives myelin sheaths
- *Intraorbital*: Extends from back of eye to optic foramina
  - Its course is tortuous
  - The entire intraorbital optic nerve is surrounded by meningeal and arachnoidal sheaths in continuation with the respective intracranial layers
  - The optic nerve lies within the muscular cone
  - Relations:
    - Long and short ciliary nerves and arteries surround the optic nerve before they enter the eyeball
    - Ophthalmic artery, superior ophthalmic vein and nasociliary nerve crosses the nerve superiorly from lateral to medial side
    - Between optic nerve and lateral rectus muscle lies ciliary ganglion, nasociliary nerve, divisions of oculomotor nerve, and abducent and sympathetic nerve.
  - Nerve passes through the optic canal to enter the middle cranial fossa.
- *Intracanalicular*:
  - Ophthalmic artery crosses inferiorly from medial to lateral side
  - Sphenoid and posterior ethmoidal sinuses lie medially to it, thus results in retrobulbar neuritis following infection.
- *Intracranial*—Lies above cavernous sinus and combines with opposite nerve to form optic chiasma.

Motor Nerves

- Oculomotor nerve (III)
- Abducens nerve (VI)
- Trochlear nerve (IV).

Oculomotor Nerve (Fig. 10)

- The oculomotor nerve divides in the cavernous sinus into superior and inferior divisions that enter the orbit through the annulus of Zinn. Within this ring,

nasociliary nerve lies between two branches, while abducens nerve on the outside
- The two branches enter the muscular cone and diverges
- The superior division moves up on the lateral side of optic nerve. It supplies the LPS and superior rectus muscles
- The inferior division is located inferiorly and outside the optic nerve and then splits to supply the medial rectus, inferior rectus, and the inferior oblique
- The branch to inferior oblique travels along the lateral border of inferior rectus and enters the inferior oblique
- From the branch to inferior oblique a small branch arises which goes to ciliary ganglion to form its parasympathetic root. After synapses the fibers of third nerve combine with sympathetic fibers to constitute short ciliary nerve which supplies ciliary muscle and iris sphincter.

Trochlear Nerve (Fig. 11)

- The trochlear nerve enters the orbit just outside the annulus of Zinn, having crossed superior to the oculomotor nerve in the lateral wall of the cavernous sinus
- It travels forward in the orbit crossing from lateral to medial above the origin of LPS to enter the lateral border

of superior oblique at the junction of the posterior third and anterior two-thirds.

Abducens Nerve (Fig. 12)

- The abductor nerve starts in the medial part of the superior orbital fissure inside the annulus of Zinn and outside the branches of the oculomotor nerve
- It travels along the medial surface of lateral rectus piercing the muscle at the junction of the posterior third and anterior two-thirds.

Sensory Nerves (Fig. 13)

- The trigeminal nerve supplies sensory innervation to the orbit and surrounding structures. It originates at the lateral and ventral portion of the pons
- Most of the supply is from ophthalmic division (V1) of trigeminal nerve with some contribution from maxillary division (V2)
- The ophthalmic division extends from the trigeminal ganglion and passes through the cavernous sinus to the orbit via the superior orbital fissure.

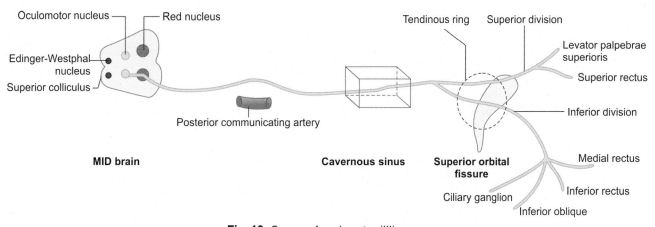

Fig. 10: Course of oculomotor (III) nerve.

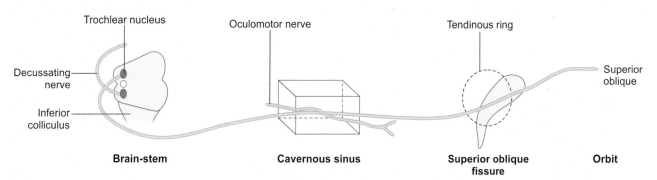

Fig. 11: Course of trochlear (IV) nerve.

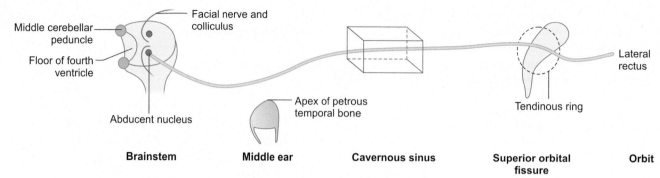

Fig. 12: Course of abducens (VI) nerve.

- Before entering the orbit through superior orbital fissure it divides into lacrimal, frontal, and nasociliary branches
- The lacrimal and frontal nerves enter the fissure outside the annulus of Zinn and travel forward in the superior orbit
- The lacrimal nerve, the smallest branch of ophthalmic nerve, travels along the superior border of the lateral rectus and supplies the postganglionic secretomotor fibers to the lacrimal gland, and sensory fibers to surrounding conjunctiva and upper eyelid. The parasympathetic fibers travel from the lacrimal nucleus in the pons to the greater superficial petrosal nerve via the nervus intermedius, to the vidian nerve, to the sphenopalatine ganglion, to the zygomatic branch of the maxillary nerve, to the zygomaticotemporal nerve, and to the lacrimal nerve, to innervate the lacrimal gland
- The frontal nerve, largest division of ophthalmic nerve, divides into the supraorbital and supratrochlear nerves. The supraorbital nerve moves anteriorly above LPS, leaves the orbit through the supraorbital notch, and supplies the forehead, scalp, upper eyelid, and frontal sinus. The supratrochlear nerve, medial one, runs anteriorly above the trochlea and supplies medial part of the forehead and upper eyelid
- The nasociliary branch enters the orbit through the annulus of Zinn. It crosses the optic nerve and passes forward between the superior oblique and medial rectus muscles. Its branches into the anterior and posterior ethmoidal nerves, two or three long posterior ciliary nerves to the globe, short ciliary nerves which pass through the ciliary ganglion, and do not synapse. It terminates as the infratrochlear nerve which supplies the medial canthus and the tip of the nose. The ethmoidal nerves contribute branches to the nasal cavity and external nose. The long ciliary nerves carry sympathetics from the superior cervical ganglion responsible for dilatation of the pupil

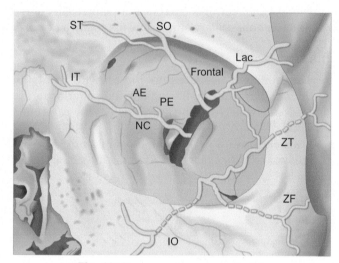

Fig. 13: Sensory nerve supply of orbit.
(ST: supratrochlear nerve; SO: supraorbital nerve; Lac: lacrimal nerve; ZT: zygomaticotemporal nerve; ZF: zygomaticofacial nerve; IO: infraorbital nerve; NC: nasociliary nerve; AE: anterior ethmoidal nerve; PE: posterior ethmoidal nerve; IT: infratrochlear nerve)

- The maxillary division of the trigeminal nerve leaves the middle cranial fossa through the foramen rotundum and enters the pterygopalatine fossa
- Within fossa after giving off sphenopalatine, posterior superior alveolar, and zygomatic branches, the main part of nerve passes through the inferior orbital fissure to enter the infraorbital sulcus as the infraorbital nerve. It exits at the infraorbital foramen and supplies the lower lid skin, conjunctiva, cheek, and the upper lip
- Within the infraorbital canal, the infraorbital nerve gives off the anterior superior alveolar branch supplying the upper front teeth
- The zygomatic branch of V_2 passes through the inferior orbital fissure and divides into zygomaticotemporal and zygomaticofacial branches that supply the skin overlying the lateral orbit and zygoma. The zygomaticotemporal branch also gives secretomotor fibers to the lacrimal nerve that supplies lacrimal gland.

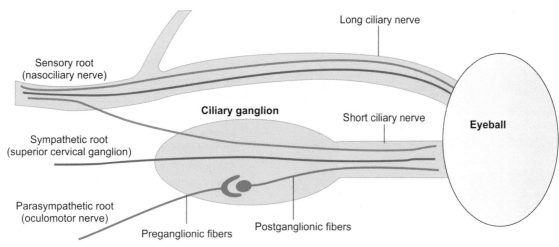

Fig. 14: Ciliary ganglion.

Ciliary Ganglion (Fig. 14)

- It is peripheral parasympathetic ganglion
- It is located near the orbital apex
- Lies between the optic nerve and lateral rectus
- It has three roots:
  1. *Motor or parasympathetic root*—comes from the inferior branch of the third cranial nerve (by the inferior oblique branch). Its fibers mainly innervate the ciliary muscle and, to a lesser extent, the sphincter of the iris.
  2. *Sympathetic root*—a branch of the carotid plexus which enters the orbit via the common tendinous ring
  3. *Sensory root*—a long and fine fiber which rejoins the nasociliary nerve where it enters the orbit. This supplies the eye and the cornea.
- Filamentous branches of the ganglion, 8–10 in number, are called the short ciliary nerves and they move forward around the optic nerve, together with ciliary arteries and the long ciliary nerves.

VASCULAR SUPPLY OF ORBIT

Arterial Supply (Fig. 15)

- Ophthalmic artery, first main branch of internal carotid artery, provides the main arterial supply to the orbit, with some contributions from maxillary and middle meningeal artery, branches of external carotid artery
- The ophthalmic artery originates from the internal carotid medial to the anterior clinoid process, as it exits the cavernous sinus. The ophthalmic artery courses on the inferior aspect of the optic nerve and enters the orbit through the optic canal

- At the entrance, it lies lateral to optic nerve and medial to ciliary ganglion. Then accompanied by the nasociliary nerve, it turns medially, crossing the optic nerve superiorly and below the superior rectus muscle. It then moves forward between superior oblique muscle and the medial rectus muscle. It terminates by splitting into two different arteries, the supratrochlear artery and the angular artery
- Branches are divided into three groups—ocular, orbital, and extraorbital
  - Ocular branches:
    - Central retinal artery
    - Ciliary arteries
    - Collateral branches to optic nerve
  - Orbital branches:
    - Lacrimal artery
    - Muscular arteries
    - Periosteal branches
  - Extraorbital branches:
    - Posterior and anterior ethmoid arteries
    - Supraorbital artery
    - Medial palpebral artery
    - Dorsal nasal artery
    - Supratrochlear artery.

Ocular Branches (Fig. 16)

Central Retinal Artery

- First and smallest branch of ophthalmic artery
- End artery
- *Course*: It runs beneath the optic nerve, then at about 10–15 mm behind the posterior part of eyeball it pierces the dural and arachnoid sheath of the optic nerve and enters the eyeball through lamina cribrosa

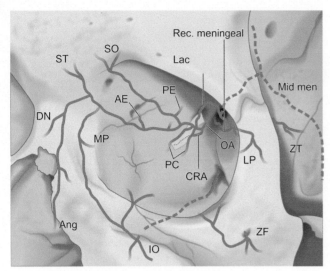

Fig. 15: Arterial supply of orbit.
(OA: ophthalmic artery; CRA: central retinal artery; PC: posterior ciliary artery; Lac: lacrimal artery; LP: lateral palpebral artery; IO: infraorbital artery; ZT: zygomaticotemporal artery; ZF: zygomaticofacial artery; Mid men: middle meningeal artery; Rec meningeal: recurrent meningeal artery; Ang: angular artery; MP: medial palpebral artery; DN: dorsal nasal artery; ST: supratrochlear artery; SO: supraorbital artery; AE: anterior ethmoidal artery; PE: posterior ethmoidal artery)

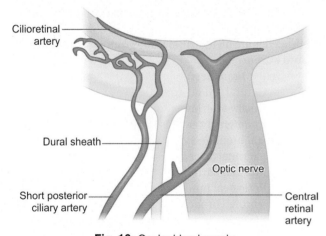

Fig. 16: Ocular blood supply.

- It continues till papilla and then gives the terminal branches.

Ciliary Arteries

- Three types—long posterior ciliary artery, short posterior ciliary artery, and anterior posterior ciliary artery
- Long posterior ciliary arteries:
  - Commonly two in number
  - Arise in the ophthalmic artery at the point at which it crosses over the optic nerve. These enter the sclera not far from where the optic nerve entry point

- It runs in the epichoroidal space till the ciliary body, where it divides into upper and lower branches and encircle iris
  - Anastomose with artery ciliary arteries to form major arterial circle of iris
- Short posterior ciliary arteries:
  - Seven in number
  - Moves in forward direction around the optic nerve and pierce sclera and supply choroid
  - At equator it anastomoses with long posterior ciliary artery, anterior ciliary artery, and major arterial circle of iris.
- Anterior ciliary arteries:
  - Seven in number
  - Arise from muscular branches and pass in front, over the tendons of the rectus muscles.

Cilioretinal Artery

- Present in 15–20%
- Enters from lateral aspect of optic nerve
- Supplies retina between disk and macula.

Orbital Branches

Lacrimal Artery

- Arises near the optic canal above and lateral to optic nerve. It travels superolaterally above the lateral rectus muscle to supply lacrimal gland
- Branches:
  - Lateral palpebral artery supplies upper and lower eyelid and anastomoses with medial palpebral artery
  - Zygomatic artery which passes through zygomatic facial and zygomatic temporal foramina
  - Muscular branch to lateral rectus
  - Recurrent meningeal anastomoses with the middle meningeal artery.

Muscular Branches

- Supply the extraocular muscles
- Accompany oculomotor nerve along their course.

Extraorbital Branches

Supraorbital Artery

- Runs between levator muscle and periorbita
- Leaves orbit through superior orbital foramen along with the nerve
- It anastomoses with supratrochlear and superficial temporal arteries.

Supratrochlear Artery

- It is the terminal branch
- Pierces the orbital septum above superior oblique pulley.

Ethmoidal Arteries

Anterior Ethmoidal Artery

- Enters anterior ethmoidal canal
- Supplies anterior and middle ethmoidal cells, frontal sinus, meninges, anterior nasal mucosa, and skin of nose.

Posterior Ethmoidal Artery

- Runs between medial rectus and superior oblique muscle to enter posterior ethmoidal canal
- It supplies posterior ethmoidal sinuses, dura of anterior cranial fossa, and upper nasal mucosa.

Medial Palpebral Artery

- It arises below the superior oblique pulley
- Descends behind the lacrimal sac
- It pierces the orbital septum and forms peripheral and marginal arterial arches; runs between the orbicularis oculi and tarsal plate.

Lateral Palpebral Artery

- Branches from lacrimal artery
- Supplies eyelid
- Anastomoses with medial palpebral artery.

Dorsal Nasal Artery

- Terminal branch
- Pierces the orbital septum and passes above the medial palpebral ligament and descends to nose
- Supplies lacrimal sac and anastomose with facial artery.

Infraorbital Artery

- A terminal branch of the maxillary artery
- It courses through the inferior orbital fissure into the infraorbital sulcus where it gives off branches to the orbital fat and muscular branches to the inferior rectus and inferior oblique muscles prior to entering the infraorbital canal to exit at the infraorbital foramen
- It anastomoses with the angular artery and the inferior palpebral vessels.

Venous Drainage (Fig. 17)

The venous drainage of the orbit is through the valve less superior and inferior ophthalmic veins.

Superior Ophthalmic Vein

- Larger of the two
- It is formed superomedially near the trochlea by the union of the angular, supraorbital, and supratrochlear veins
- It communicates with central retinal vein, receive inferior ophthalmic vein and two vorticose veins from upper part of eyeball
- Leaves the orbit through superior orbital fissure and drains into the cavernous sinus (Fig. 18).

Inferior Ophthalmic Vein

- It is usually formed anteriorly as a plexus within the inferomedial orbital fat
- It also communicates with the pterygoid plexus via the inferior orbital fissure and facial vein
- Receives muscular branches and inferior vorticose veins

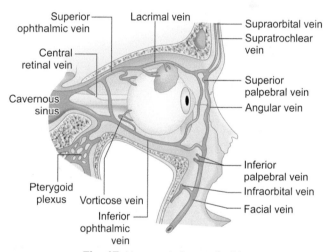

Fig. 17: Venous drainage of orbit.

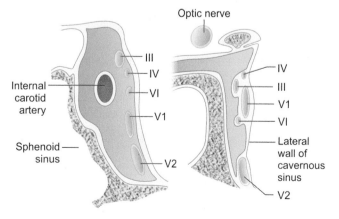

Fig. 18: Cavernous sinus.

- It courses posteriorly along the inferior rectus and usually drains into the superior ophthalmic vein.

SUGGESTED READING

1. Cornelius CP, Mayer P, Ehrenfeld M, et al. The orbits—Anatomical features in view of innovative surgical methods. Facial Plast Surg. 2014;30(5):487-508.
2. Martins C, Costa e Silva IE, Campero A, et al. (2011). Microsurgical anatomy of the orbit: The rule of seven. Hindawi Publishing Corporation, Anatomy Research International. [online] Available from https://www.hindawi.com/journals/ari/2011/468727/abs/. [Accessed January, 2019].
3. Patanaik VVG, Bala S, Sangla RK. Anatomy of the bony orbit-some applied aspects. J Anat Soc India. 2001;50(1):59-67.
4. René C. Update on orbital anatomy. Eye (Lond). 2006;20(10):1119-29.
5. Rootman J, Stewart B, Goldberg RA. Orbital anatomy. In: Orbital Surgery: A Conceptual Approach, 1st edition. Philadelphia, New York: Lippincott-Raven; 1995. pp. 75-150.
6. Turvey TA, Golden BA. Orbital anatomy for the surgeon. Oral Maxillofac Surg Clin North Am. 2012;24(4):525-36.

Evaluation of Orbital Disorders

Mohit Chhabra, Ruchi Goel

INTRODUCTION

Orbital disorders are somewhat different from intraocular disorders which are usually amenable to direct visualization. Owing to this inaccessibility of orbital contents to direct examination, a different clinical skill set along with rational and relevant imaging and diagnostic modalities are required to localize the pathology and predict the most probable cause and extent of disease. Despite this, certainty of diagnosis is by no means guaranteed and many a times a definitive decision depends on a close watch on clinical evolution of the disease, and its response to therapy.

Orbital disorders can be classified into five basic clinical patterns:
1. Inflammatory disorders
2. Mass effect causing axial or abaxial proptosis
3. Bony structural abnormalities
4. Vascular lesions
5. Functional disorders of neuromuscular structures

The evaluation begins with a detailed history which is of paramount importance in orbital diseases.

HISTORY

A good clinical history helps in guiding examination, investigations, and therapy. The demographic details of the patients are extremely important to reach appropriate differential diagnoses.

The usual symptom complex of orbital diseases includes one or more of the following—pain, proptosis, enophthalmos, diminution of vision, diplopia, epiphora, congestion and a significant cosmetic blemish.

A detailed evaluation of these complaints should include:
- Age of onset, duration, progression and previous photographs to establish timeline
- Systemic disease and therapeutic history (e.g. thyroid disorders)
- Prior injury or surgery
- Family history
- Personal history such as smoking that may aggravate thyroid orbitopathy; weight gain (hypothyroidism) or weight loss (hyperthyroidism).

Age of onset serves as an important guide to differential diagnosis while most congenital and developmental anomalies present at an early age, metastatic diseases and malignancies such as leukemia present at a much later age (Table 1).

Pain is usually a symptom of inflammation, infection, emphysema, hemorrhage, invasive malignancies or metastatic tumors.

Duration of symptoms is necessary to ascertain probable pathology. The rate of progression may vary from days to weeks in cases of cellulitis, hemorrhage, fulminant neoplasms, thrombophlebitis or metastatic tumors. Conditions occurring over months to years include dermoid cysts, benign lacrimal tumors, hemangioma, lymphoma or osteoma. Lymphangioma may have an acute presentation following upper respiratory infection. A dermoid cyst may also present in emergency following trauma, leading to rupture of cyst.

Poor vision in orbital diseases may be due to a variety of reasons and must be evaluated extensively for proper therapy and prognosis.

A plethora of signs also provide clues to diagnosis (Table 2).

Involvement of one or both the orbits may occur.

TABLE 1: Common causes of proptosis according to age.

Age group	Common causes of proptosis
Infants	Dermoid cyst, teratoma, capillary hemangioma, teratoma, microphthalmia with cyst, orbital extension of retinoblastoma, histiocytosis, orbital cellulitis
Children	Dermoid cyst, teratoma, microphthalmia with cyst, lymphangioma, Rhabdomyosarcoma, chloroma, neuroblastoma, optic nerve glioma, histiocytosis, parasitic cysts, hematoma, orbital cellulitis
Adults	Thyroid orbitopathy, cavernous hemangioma, pseudotumor, lacrimal gland tumor, orbital varix, schwannoma, lymphoma, metastasis, optic nerve meningioma, orbital cellulitis

TABLE 2: Signs in orbital pathology.

Signs	Probable pathology
S-shaped deformity of lid	Lacrimal gland enlargement, plexiform neurofibroma
Injection around insertion of recti	Thyroid orbitopathy
Opticociliary shunt vessels on the disc	Meningioma, metastases, inflammatory tumor
Corkscrew conjunctival vessels	Arteriovenous fistula
Vascular anomaly of eyelid skin	Varix, lymphatic malformation, hemangioma
Lid retraction	Thyroid eye disease
Ecchymosis of eyelid skin	Leukemia, metastatic neuroblastoma
Frozen globe	Orbital malignancy or zygomycosis
Salmon colored mass on conjunctiva	Lymphoma
Café au lait spots	NF1
Facial asymmetry	Fibrous dysplasia, neurofibromatosis

CAUSES OF BILATERAL PROPTOSIS

- Thyroid orbitopathy
- Dacryoadenitis due to sarcoidosis and tuberculosis
- Lymphoma
- Leukemia
- Metastatic carcinoma
- Metastatic neuroblastoma
- Histiocytosis.

Thyroid orbitopathy is the most common cause of proptosis in adults. Other endocrine disorders causing proptosis are:
- Diabetes mellitus
- Pituitary adenomata
- Cushings syndrome
- Acromegaly.

PHYSICAL EXAMINATION

Due to its intimate relation to surrounding structures, diseases of the orbit are bound to matters, of much wider than just ocular interests. Apart from anatomical proximity, intimacy of venous drainage with surrounding structures makes it an important focus in this region. Hence, examination must not be limited to the eye and orbit but should also encompass nose, paranasal sinuses, face, and cranium. Of course, general medical examination also requires adequate attention as many diseases are linked to systemic disorders, e.g. in cases of thyroid disorders, abnormalities of pulse, rhythm, blood pressure and temperature should be evaluated along with an examination of the neck.

General examination of the orbit includes inspection, palpation, auscultation, transillumination and several special methods of examination specific to the orbit.

INSPECTION

- Globe displacement is the most common manifestation of an orbital anomaly that may be caused by a tumor, vascular disease, inflammation or a traumatic event. The usual terms that describe this displacement include:
  - *Proptosis or exophthalmos*: Forward displacement of the globe (exophthalmos refers to dynamic rather than passive mechanical factors)
  - *Enophthalmos*: Retrodisplacement of globe within the bony confines of the eye socket
  - *Exorbitism*: Angle between the lateral walls greater than 90°
  - *Hypertelorism*: Wider than normal separation between medial orbital walls
  - *Telecanthus*: Increase in distance between medial canthi
  - *Hyperglobus*: Vertical upward displacement of globe
  - *Hypoglobus*: Vertical downward displacement of globe
  - *Orbital Dystopia*: Abnormal displacement of entire orbital cones and their contents types:
    1. *Vertical:* Orbits do not lie on the same horizontal plane
    2. *Horizontal/transverse dystopia:* Orbits are displaced laterally or medially

Proptosis needs to be differentiated from pseudo-proptosis.
Causes of pseudoproptosis:
- High myopia

- Buphthalmos
- Staphyloma
- Eyelid retraction
- Shallow orbit as in Crouzon syndrome
- Progressive facial hemiatrophy as in Parry–Romberg syndrome

The detection of proptosis can be done by two methods:

1. *Naffziger's method*: The patient sits in front of the examiner with the head slightly thrown back and looking downward. The surgeon raises the upper lids with the index fingers and compares the apex of the cornea. As the patient bends his head forward the two corneas should disappear at the same time (Fig. 1).

2. *Worm's eye view*: The examination is performed from below with the patient's head tilted back (Fig. 2). The direction of any displacement gives valuable diagnostic information regarding site of disease.
   - *Downward and outward*: Medial side or roof of orbit, e.g. ethmoidal or frontal mucocele, meningocele, and dermoid
   - *Downward and inward*: Lacrimal gland neoplasia and dermoid
   - *Upward*: Lesion in the maxillary antrum, lacrimal sac tumor

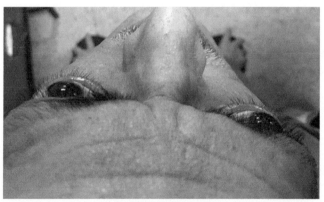

Fig. 1: Naffziger's view.

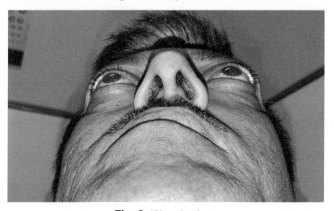

Fig. 2: Worm's view.

- *Axial proptosis*: Lesion within the muscle cone or apex of the orbit. Axial proptosis may occur in intraconal cavernous hemangioma, optic nerve glioma, optic nerve sheath meningioma, thyroid orbitopathy, etc.
- Periocular changes in color, abnormal vasculature, erythema, frank induration or ulceration should be noted. Any limitation of extraocular movements may point to restrictive or paretic pathologies of orbital structures.
- Intermittent proptosis that becomes prominent on Valsalva maneuver or by asking patient to bend forward is suggestive of orbital varix.

Palpation

It should be done to confirm findings of inspection.

- Orbital rim and anterior portion of the orbital cavity should be felt and compared to the other side in case of any suspected mass, erosion or irregularity. Though very deep palpation is not possible in the orbital space, it is desirable to feel as deeply as possible to explore the mass. The skin temperature of the surrounding area should also be noted
- Presence of tenderness should be noted, especially of the bony structures
- Retropulsion should be elicited by pushing the globe through the upper eyelid and feeling the resistance or compressibility of the mass. Vascular lesions are usually compressible while retrobulbar tumors or thyroid ophthalmopathy give a resistance to retropulsion
- Reducibility should be checked to differentiate between vascular lesions and others
- Orbital thrill or pulsation should be felt by placing two fingers over the orbit through closed lids. A *true pulsation* causes the fingers to move up and separate while a *transmitted pulsation* causes the fingers to move up but not separate.
  True pulsation is felt in caroticocavernous fistula, while transmitted pulsation is felt in neurofibromatosis due to sphenoid wing dysplasia, meningoencephalocele (children), and large mucoceles that have eroded the bony walls of both orbit and intracranial vault (adults).
- Infra or supraorbital anesthesia or paresthesia may result from perineural spread of malignant tumors like adenoid cystic carcinoma of the lacrimal glands.

Auscultation

Whenever a pulsation is evident, an auscultation must be done to look for an audible bruit as in case of AV malformations. A stethoscope should be used over the eyeball or temporal area.

Transillumination

A penlight must be used for this test and the findings vary depending upon the opacity of the mass relative to the surrounding tissue.

- A fluid filled cystic lesion gives a bright transillumination (Fig. 3)
- Lipoma causes the area to light up equally as the surrounding area
- Solid tumors and aneurysms create a dark transillumination due to their shadow effect
- Alternatively, transillumination can also be interpreted as *positive or negative* based on the above findings.

Ophthalmological Examination

- Conjunctiva when examined may reveal dilated tortuous vessels, corkscrew-shaped episcleral vessels, hyperemia or a subconjunctival mass as an extension of a deeper orbital mass
- Cornea should be examined for signs of exposure keratopathy
- Tests for dry eye should be performed especially in thyroid eye disease
- Sclera and iris should be seen for signs of inflammation
- Presence of a relative afferent pupillary defect in many cases is the first clue of optic nerve involvement
- Measurement of ductions in degrees
- *Visual fields*: The defects may not be as distinct as those caused by intracranial lesions. All orbital lesions if large enough will cause irregular quadrantic contractions or relative scotomas due to direct pressure on the eye. A central scotoma disproportionately greater than the amount of proptosis suggests optic nerve glioma. The defects in meningioma are more irregular in contour and density and effect the peripheral field much sooner than central field.

In children, confrontation testing may reveal gross defects in the peripheral field.

- Intraocular pressure should be measured in all gazes (differential tonometry), especially in cases of suspected thyroid ophthalmopathy. A difference of greater than 6 mm Hg is significant (*Brailey's sign*) (Figs. 4A and B) In children, rise in intraocular pressure in proptosed eye may indicate an associated neurofibromatosis.
- Lens and vitreous are usually unaffected except for intraocular tumors
- Fundus examination must be done to look for venous engorgement, tortuosity, choroidal folds, papilledema, or optic atrophy. In cases of cavernous sinus thrombosis, there may be retinal edema, exudates, and venous engorgement.

SPECIAL METHODS OF EXAMINATION

Several methods require mention such as exophthalmometry, orbitonometry and several imaging techniques (*See* Chapter 3).

Exophthalmometry

Proptosis is measured by protrusion of the apex of the cornea in front of the outer orbital margin while the eye looks straight ahead.

- *Normal value*: 10–20 mm
- *Average values*:
  - *Male*: 17 mm
  - *Female*: 16 mm
  - *Children*: 14.5 mm.

Absolute reading of more than 21 mm or difference of more than 2 mm between the two eyes is considered abnormal. Anything less than 14 mm should be considered as enophthalmos and may be encountered in metastatic disease or trauma.

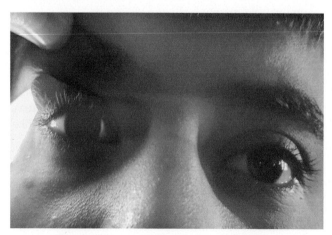

Fig. 3: Transillumination of an upper lid mass.

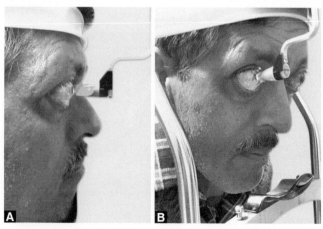

Figs. 4A and B: Differential tonometry in a case of thyroid ophthalmopathy in primary gaze (A) and in upgaze (B).

Three types of measurements have been described:
1. Absolute exophthalmometry (result compared with normal value)
2. Comparative exophthalmometry (result compared over a period of time)
3. Relative exophthalmometry (results of the two eyes are compared).

The first attempt at exophthalmometry was made in 1865 by Cohn who produced an instrument used to measure the distance between the orbital rim and the corneal apex from the side. Since that time, many instruments of varying mechanisms have been devised.

- *Hertel's exophthalmometer (1905)*: This is a binocular instrument, allowing the examiner, with the aid of mirrors, to see the two eyes superimposed upon a measuring scale and measuring the distance between the lateral orbital rim and the corneal apex. A difference of greater than 2 mm is significant. The procedure is not possible in uncooperative patients with poor fixation, in presence of lateral orbital rim fractures and abaxial proptosis
  - Patient and examiner must be at the same eye level to remove parallax
  - The footplates of the instrument are placed on the orbital notch (deepest point on the rim) with the patient's eye closed
  - The baseline reading of the separation of the two prisms should be carefully noted and all future measurements must be done on that baseline reading
  - The patient is asked to look straight. The red lines should overlap and the millimeter marking corresponding to the corneal apex should be noted (Fig. 5).

Sources of error: Parallax, compression of soft tissues at the lateral orbital rim can produce error of 0.5–1.0 mm.

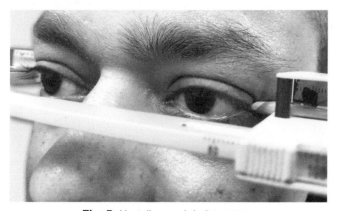

Fig. 5: Hertel's exophthalmometry.

- Other attempts at exophthalmometry were made by Luedde, Naugle, Davanger (right angled 45° prism to see the cornea), Zehender (introduction of mirror), Coccius (plunger sliding on the measuring scale placed on lids) and Gormaz (plunger placed on the anesthetized cornea)

  Luedde's exophthalmometer is the simplest and consists of a simple thick transparent ruler with a groove to rest on the lateral rim. It is more accurate than Hertel's in cases of facial asymmetry.
- Stereo photographic methods of exophthalmometry introduced by Lobeck and Ollers provide for more accurate measurements
- Radiographic exophthalmometry employs superimposing the lateral radiograph with a radiopaque contact lens with a central dot placed on the cornea. The nasion-clinoid distance and the cornea-clinoid distance are measured.

Despite many advancements in exophthalmometry, vertical or horizontal globe dystopia is usually not counted for and may require a special instrument known as the ocular topometer (Watson, 1967) which can measure a displacement in any direction. It consists of a horizontal plastic plate with sliding scales for measurement.

A simpler method employed routinely involves the use of a perspex ruler.

- With the upper edge of the ruler corresponding with the outer canthi, vertical deviation may be measured
- Horizontal deviations are measured from a mark on the bridge of the nose to the nasal limbus (Figs. 6A to D).

Orbitonometry (Piezometry)

Though not done routinely nowadays, it deserves mention to stress upon the importance of orbital compressibility in many disorders.

The compressibility of orbital contents depends partly upon orbital volume and partly on tissue consistency.

From the clinical viewpoint, orbitonometry may be an adjunct but cannot be used as a criterion for diagnosis that still depends upon assessment of clinical signs and symptoms.

LABORATORY TESTS

- Total and differential leukocyte count, absolute eosinophil count peripheral smear—useful in leukemia, lymphoma and parasitic infestation
- Thyroid function tests—T3, T4, TSH. Additional tests include thyrotropin-releasing hormone, anti-thyroglobulin and antimicrosomal antibodies
- Angiotensin converting enzyme—sarcoidosis

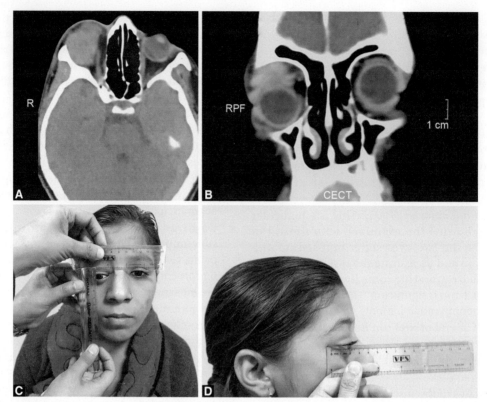

Figs. 6A to D: (A) Axial view of CT orbit showing a mass in the lateral extraconal compartment encroaching the intraconal compartment and causing excavation of lateral wall of the orbit and proptosis; (B) Coronal view CT scan showing inferior displacement of globe by the superiorly located mass; (C) Measurement of vertical displacement of the globe. The horizontal displacement is estimated by measuring the distance from a mark on the center of bridge of the nose to the nasal limbus or corneal reflex (the contralateral eye is occluded in presence of squint); (D) Measurement of proptosis with plastic ruler.

(*Note***:** Either cut the end of the ruler to start with zero or subtract no marking zone from your reading).

- Antinuclear cytoplasmic antibody (C-ANCA)—Wegener's granulomatosis
- Other tests like bone marrow studies, chest X-ray abdominal, and chest CT scan are performed whenever indicated.

Orbital Imaging

Ruchi Goel, Sushil Kumar

INTRODUCTION

The advent of computed tomography (CT) and magnetic resonance imaging (MRI) have taken over the role of plain film radiography. The fine structures within the orbit require more attention to imaging protocol than other regions of the body to ensure optimal diagnostic information.[1] Standardized ultrasonography, a noninvasive modality, is still being used for quickly examining children without sedation, for follow-up examinations, and studying the kinetic properties of lesions. However, for orbital apex lesions CT and MRI are superior.

COMPUTED TOMOGRAPHY

Principle

A narrow collimated X-ray beam passes through thin slices of tissues at multiple angles and is received by detectors. The attenuation of X-ray as they pass through the tissues depends on their density. Tissues like water that are less dense, allow more X-rays to pass through resulting in a darker region on the final image. More dense tissues, such as bone, attenuate the X-rays to a greater extent resulting in a lighter or white area on the final image.[2] The variations in radio absorbency are analyzed by a computer and then images are generated.[3] The high contrast between the orbital structures, i.e. bone, muscle, and fat, provides excellent visualization.[4]

The location, extent, and configuration of the lesion and its effect on adjacent structures is visualized well in the two-dimensional CT. This helps in planning an appropriate surgical approach to minimize morbidity. Eight slices are required to perform an orbital scan which extend from the maxillary sinus below to inferior part of frontal lobe above, and include the optic chiasm and pituitary area. Its spatial resolution is 0.5 mm. Spatial resolution of a CT depends on slice thickness; thinner the slice, higher the resolution. The radiation dose per imaging plane is 5 cGy.[5] The posteroanterior and lateral chest radiograph administers a dose approximately 5 mGy. The slice thickness can vary from 1 mm to 10 mm. Thin slices are good for spatial resolution, but require higher radiation dose, a greater number of slices, and eventually longer examination time. Usually, 2–3 mm cuts are sufficient for the ocular region. For optic nerve lesions, thinner cuts of 1 mm are used. In the routine CT scan of the orbit axial and coronal sections are taken. Axial scan is done in supine position and coronal in prone position. The axial section is obtained parallel to infraorbital meatal line and coronal is perpendicular to infraorbital meatal line.[6] Axial scan shows both globes, the horizontal rectus muscle, optic nerve, other soft tissue, and bony structures. Coronal scan anteriorly shows globe with relation to recti muscles. Reformatted sagittal views along the axis of the inferior rectus muscle are useful for studying orbital floor blow-out fracture. A 30° inclination to the orbito-meatal line depicts the optic canal and the entire anterior visual pathway. "Windows" provide more specific anatomic details. The process of choosing the number of gray shades for a display is referred to as "selecting a window". The width of the window directly depends on the number of gray shades. The number at which the window setting is centered is called window level.[7] For examination of bone details, a bone window setting is used allowing greater detail of bone densities, but with loss of detail for tissue densities. Bone window settings are valuable for the evaluation of lesions suspected of eroding, remolding, or displacing adjacent bony orbital walls. The CT unit is called a Hounsfield unit. The values for air, water, and dense bone are –1,000, 0, and +1,000, respectively.

Three dimensional CT is required for complex orbital fractures where CT information is reformatted into three-dimensional projections of the bony orbital wall.

Suspected orbital diseases associated with paranasal sinus disease, thyroid orbitopathy, foreign bodies, hemorrhage, or orbital trauma are evaluated using noncontrast CT, while the visualization of tumors that are well supplied with blood vessels (e.g. meningioma) or whose blood vessels leak is improved by the use of intravenous contrast enhancing agents.

MAGNETIC RESONANCE IMAGING

Principle

Magnetic resonance imaging is a noninvasive procedure that does not require X-rays.[8,9] The spinning proton nuclei within biological tissues orient themselves on application of a magnetic field. When an external radiofrequency (RF) pulse is applied to the system at a specific frequency, energy is absorbed by the atomic nuclei changing their orientations. On switching off the RF pulse, the nuclei flip back to their original magnetized position. The time taken for this realignment is called relaxation time. T1 or longitudinal relaxation time is the net bulk magnetization to realign itself along the original axis. T2 or transverse relaxation is an indirect measure of the effect the nuclei have on each other.

The various body tissues have different relaxation times. A tissue may be best visualized on either T1 or T2 weighted image. Coronal, sagittal, and axial scans can be directly obtained. A surface coil is used for ophthalmic purpose to enhance spatial resolution. High signal is produced by tissues with high proton density and low proton flow. Low signal is produced by bone, sclera, sinus air, and faster proton flow like in flowing blood. In T1 image fat is bright and vitreous is back, and is reverse in T2 image. T1 image provides more spatial resolution therefore more anatomic details are visible whereas T2 gives more contrast resolution.

Unlike CT scanning, which depends on the density of tissue (i.e. hyperdense, isodense, or hypodense) to induce the attenuation of signal, MRI is expressed in terms of signal intensity (i.e. hyperintense, isointense, or hypointense). MRI in particular has proven valuable in delineating orbital structures including blood vessels, nerves, and connective tissue septae.[9] MR imaging is superior in differentiating fat prolapse from muscle entrapment in blow-out fractures. Both CT and MR imaging can identify and localize foreign bodies consisting of glass, plastic, and wood. CT scans may miss dry wood and small plastic objects; MR imaging would visualize these better.[10] As with CT, MRI with intravenous contrast material is better in detection of pathology. Iodinated contrast is used in CT and paramagnetic material called gadolinium is used in MRI. The gadolinium paramagnetic metal ion enhances the local magnetic field and increases signal intensity. Contrast enhanced MRI is useful in the study of orbital lesions such as cavernous hemangioma, A-V malformations, myositis, metastasis, and lesions extending into the cavernous sinus.

Merits of MRI over CT scan are:
- Procurement of images in any plane without the need of patient repositioning
- Greater resolution of soft tissue with less artifact from dense bone
- Superior visualization of the orbital apex
- Excellent safety profile of Gadolinium.

Side effects that have been reported include hypotension and a transient elevation of serum bilirubin and iron levels. Severe allergic reactions are rare. There are a few contraindications for MRI. These include intraocular metallic foreign bodies, ferromagnetic cerebral aneurysm clips, and cardiac pacemaker.[4] Relative contraindications include metallic heart valves, claustrophobic patients, severely obese patients, and uncooperative patients.

ULTRASONOGRAPHY

The orbital examination includes:
- Assessment of soft tissues
- Evaluation of extraocular muscles
- Examination of retrobulbar optic nerve using transocular (examination through the globe) or paraocular (examination next to the globe) approach.

Once an orbital mass lesion is detected a topographic, quantitative, and a kinetic echography is performed to form a provisional diagnosis (Flowchart 1).

Topographic Echography
- *Location:* Position and meridians
- Shape
- Borders
- *Contour abnormalities:* Bone-excavation, defects, or hyperostosis; globe-indentation, or flattening.

Quantitative Echography
- *Internal reflectivity:* Spike height
- *Internal structure:* Histologic architecture
- *Sound attenuation:* Absorption or shadowing.

Flowchart 1: Flowchart for diagnosis of orbital lesions on B scan.

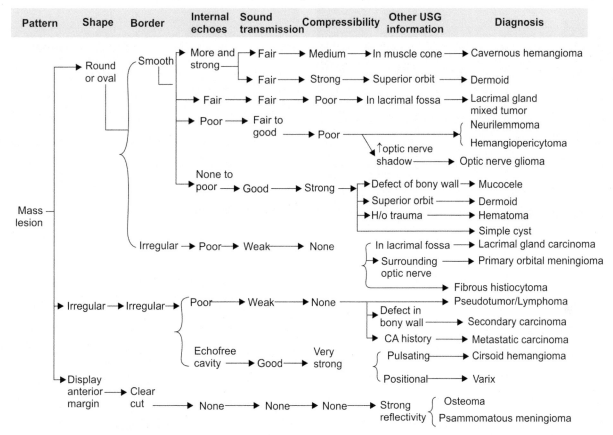

Kinetic Echography

- *Consistency*: Soft vs. Hard
- *Vascularity*: Blood flow
- Mobility of lesion or its contents.

For topographic echography, the patient fixates toward the lesion and the probe is placed on the globe opposite to the lesion and moved from limbus to the fornix. Quantitative echography correlates with the histological structure of the lesion. The spike height on A scan and signal brightness on B scan measures the reflectivity. A fall in spike height on A scan and echodensity on B scan either within or posterior to the lesion occurs due to sound attenuation because of scattering, reflection, or absorption of sound energy. The angle kappa by Ossoinig is the angle between an imaginary line drawn through the peaks of the internal spikes and the horizontal baseline on an A scan. Greater the attenuation, steeper the angle; therefore substances such as bone, calcium, and foreign bodies that produce strong sound attenuation result in steeper angle kappa.

Kinetic echography is employed for dynamic assessment of motion within a lesion. Vascularity is detected by presence of fast, spontaneous flickering motion in the internal lesion echoes with the eye and probe stationary.

Mobility is checked by observing the B scan as the patient blinks or during a saccade. Shifting fluid is seen in lymphangiomas with hemorrhage, hematomas, and cysts.

A continuous convection like motion occurs in cholesterol within a hematic cyst and after movements are seen with membranes within the globe or septa within a lymphangioma.

Common Orbital Pathologies

Trauma

Computed tomography is the imaging modality of choice in evaluating patients with orbital trauma. Orbital floor fractures are common in the thinner posterior part of the floor.[11] A downward curvature of the orbital floor with bony discontinuity, and displacement of fragments into the maxillary sinus may be seen on CT scan. Prolapse of orbital fat or inferior rectus, as well as opacification of maxillary sinus with or without fluid level may be seen and a "tear drop" shape pointing toward the fracture, indicating muscle sheath tethering (Fig. 1). In medial wall fractures, orbital

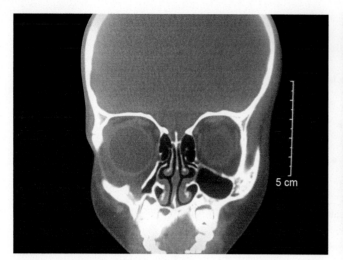

Fig. 1: Coronal CT scan showing fracture floor and lateral wall of right orbit with herniation of orbital contents into the maxillary sinus.

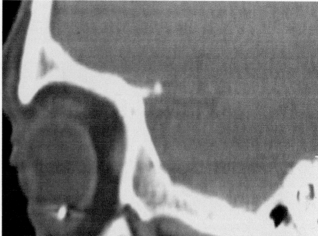

Fig. 2: Sagittal CT scan showing intraocular foreign body.

emphysema is also seen in addition to bony discontinuity. Optic canal fractures may be suspected in severe head injuries associated with impaired vision. Presence of blood within the ethmoid sinus seen as soft tissue density on the CT, can be a helpful clue to detect optic canal fracture. CT in retained foreign body determines its location (extraocular or intraocular) and its relationship to the surrounding ocular structures. Both coronal and axial scans are required for exact localization. Metal foreign bodies up to 0.5 mm can be detected (Figs. 2 and 3). Stone, plastic, or wood foreign bodies of more than or equal to 1.5 mm can be picked up by CT scan.

Magnetic resonance imaging is especially useful in staging the orbital hematoma. The iron atoms of hemoglobin have a different magnetic effect depending on the physical and oxidative state of hemoglobin (Table 1).[12]

On ultrasonography, intraocular foreign bodies are seen as echodense spots with a 100% reflectivity on A scan spike irrespective of the nature of the foreign body. Exact sizing and localization can also be done on ultrasonography. Shadowing effect is usually seen in foreign bodies (Figs. 4 and 5). Dense blood clot and lens fragment need to be differentiated from the foreign bodies. Persistence of signals even on decreasing the gain on the machine by 10 db and presence of shadowing are characteristic features of foreign bodies that are not seen with lens fragments. However, foreign bodies less than 0.2 mm in size and those in the orbit obscured by hemorrhage are best picked up by CT scan. *Spherical foreign body,* like gunshot pellets, have an anterior and posterior surface in between which occur multiple internal reverberations/echoes. These echoes are seen as echogenic opacities with a wedge-shaped trail of spikes. The trail disappears on decreasing the overall gain of machine but the initial echodense spot remains unchanged.

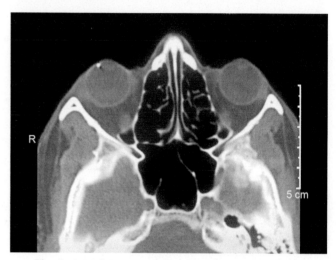

Fig. 3: Axial CT scan showing intraocular foreign body.

Orbital Cellulitis

A CT aids in detection of the underlying cause of orbital cellulitis. A paranasal sinus pathology appears as an opacification or air-fluid level within the sinus. CT scan facilitates in differentiation of preseptal from postseptal orbital cellulitis.[4] In preseptal cellulitis, the orbital septum acts as a barrier between inflamed adnexal tissue anteriorly and normal appearing postseptal structures posteriorly (Table 2).[13] As the infection spreads posterior to the orbital septum, small stippled densities appear within the orbital fat (best seen with wide window settings). More discrete densities eventually develop in the form of secondary thickening of extraocular muscles, particularly the medial rectus. A frank orbital subperiosteal abscess results in a typical ring enhancement on contrast study (Figs. 6 and 7).

TABLE 1: Staging of orbital hematoma.

Stage	Hyperacute	Acute	Subacute	Subacute-chronic	Chronic
Time	Few hours	1–3 days	3–7 days	7 days-weeks	Months-years
Type	Fresh blood	Early clot	Before cell lysis	After cell lysis	Organized
Content	Oxy Hb	Deoxy Hb	Intracellular MethHb	Extracellular Meth Hb	Hemosiderin
T1	Low-high	Low-Iso	High	High	Low
T2	High	Low	Low	High	Low

TABLE 2: Staging of orbital cellulitis.

S. no.	Stage	Features
1	Inflammatory edema	Eyelid swelling and erythema.
2	Preseptal cellulitis	Eyelid swelling and erythema associated with inflammatory soft tissue thickening anterior to orbital septum
3	Postseptal cellulitis	Edema of orbital contents, proptosis, chemosis and decreased extraocular muscle movements. Visual loss +/–
4	Subperiosteal abscess	Collection between periorbita and involved sinus. Globe proptotic and displaced by abscess, Visual loss
5	Orbital abscess	Marked proptosis, ophthalmoplegia, visual loss associated with abscess formation within the orbital fat or muscle
6	Cavernous sinus thrombosis	Proptosis, ophthalmoplegia with development of similar signs on contralateral side associated with cranial nerve palsies III, IV, V, VI; visual loss

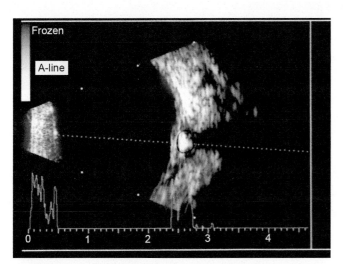

Fig. 4: Intraretinal foreign body with acoustic shadowing.

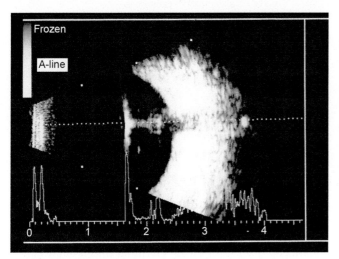

Fig. 5: Intravitreal foreign body with acoustic shadowing.

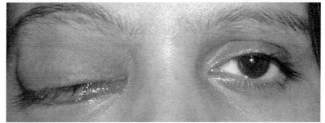
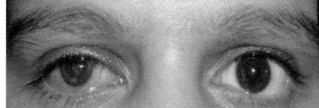

Fig. 6: Clinical picture showing right orbital cellulitis pre- and post-treatment.

Cystic Lesions of the Orbit

Cystic lesions characteristically have a smooth contour, round to oval shape, sharp outline, and absence of internal vascularity. The commonly found cystic lesions in the orbit are dermoid cyst, epidermoid cyst, dermolipoma, epithelial inclusion cyst, hematic cyst, microphthalmos with cyst, congenital cystic eye, teratoma, lacrimal ductal cyst, and mucocele.

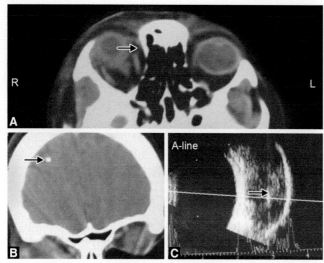

Figs. 7A to C: (A) Axial CT scan showing right orbital cellulitis along with cysticercosis cyst; (B) Coronal scan showing cysticercosis cyst in the brain; (C) B scan showing cysticercosis cyst in the orbit.

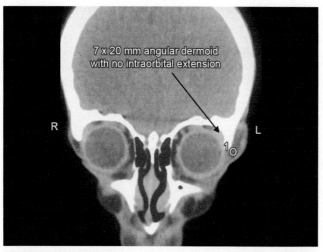

Fig. 8: Coronal CT scan showing external angular dermoid cyst.

Dermoid cyst is the most common orbital cyst which appears usually in the superotemporal or superonasal quadrant (Fig. 8). It can be superficial or deep and are thin walled, uniocular masses with homogenously decreased attenuation. Deeper cysts may erode the adjacent bony wall. The contents of the dermoid cyst such as keratin, sebaceous materials, hair follicles, and inflammatory cells influence the internal reflectivity on A scan (Fig. 9). Differentiation is not possible from epidermoid cyst on echography. Histopathologically, the epidermoid cyst wall does not contain adenexal structures. Epidermoid and dermoid cysts appear as radiolucent cystic lesions with a hypodense to isodense lumen. Dermoids may demonstrate fat-density, fluid-fluid levels, and intralesional calcification.[14] They

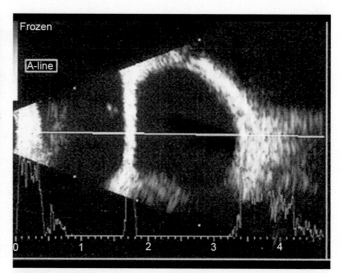

Fig. 9: Transocular scan of a dermoid cyst indenting the globe.

TABLE 3: CT and MR features of orbital cysts.

Cyst	CT features	MR features
Epidermoid	• Nonenhancing mass, +/− bone erosion • No calcification • Minimal enhancement of capsule	• Hypointense on T1 • Hyperintense on T2
Dermoid	• Nonenhancing mass, +/− bone erosion • Scalloping with sclerosis of adjacent bone • Calcification if present is characteristic • Hypodensity if present is characteristic • Fat-fluid level is present	
Congenital cystic eye	Nonenhancing low density mass	
Parasitic cyst	• Cystic lesion within or near the extraocular muscle • Some degree of enhancement around the cyst wall • Scolex can be identified • Diffuse myositis may be present	

(CT: computerized tomography; MR: magnetic resonance)

usually do not enhance with contrast, except for rim enhancement in some cases. Dermoid tumors may cause bone molding and erosion from compression atrophy, which is best seen on coronal views (Table 3).[15]

Microophthalmia with Cyst

Persistence of a small hiatus in closure of the embryonic fissure may result in a miniature eye with a cystic appendage (Fig. 10).

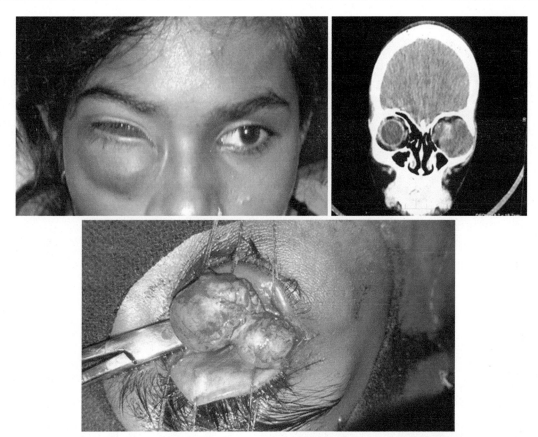

Fig. 10: Clinical picture, coronal CT scan and dissected specimen of microphthalmia with cyst.

Graves' Ophthalmopathy

Graves' ophthalmopathy is characterized by unilateral or bilateral involvement of single or multiple muscles. CT shows fusiform muscle enlargement with smooth muscle borders, especially posteriorly.[16] The tendons are usually not involved and orbital fat is normal, but preseptal edema may be seen (Figs. 11 and 12). The muscle involvement from the most common to least common—inferior rectus, medial rectus, superior rectus/levator complex, and lateral rectus. The differential diagnosis of extraocular muscle disorders is given in Table 4.[17]

The normal values of extraocular muscles are shown in Table 5.[18]

Nonspecific Orbital Inflammation or Orbital Pseudotumor

Pseudotumor has a varied CT findings from a well-defined mass or resemblance to malignancy. Contrast enhancement may occur in some of the cases. There may be enlargement of lacrimal gland, or thickening of the posterior scleral rim, with surrounding soft tissue involvement. Myositis usually involves a diffuse (occasionally irregular) enlargement of

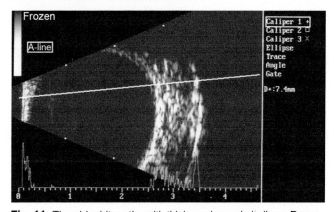

Fig. 11: Thyroid orbitopathy with thickened muscle belly on B scan.

one or more muscles that conforms to the shape of the globe and the surrounding structures. Bony changes are absent and tendinous insertion is involved. Infiltrations within the orbital fat, perioptic area or sclerouveal thickening is highly suggestive of an inflammatory process.[19,20] Sclerosing orbital pseudotumor may look like a lacrimal gland tumor.

On B scan, the small densely packed cells with regular internal structure result in low–medium internal reflectivity, weak sound attenuation, and variable borders or shape (Fig. 13).

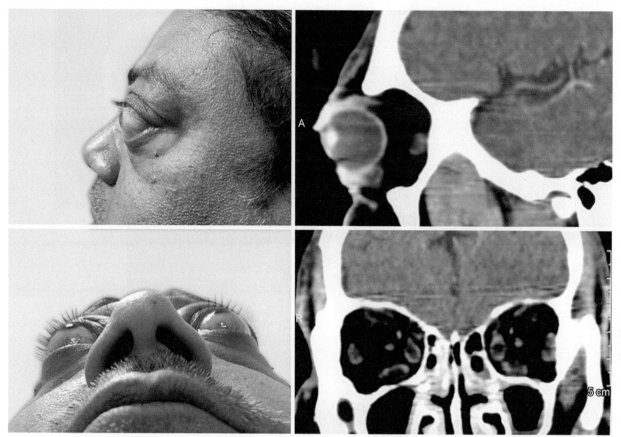

Fig. 12: Clinical picture and CT scan showing proptosis and thickened belly of extraocular muscles in thyroid eye disease.

TABLE 4: Differential diagnosis of extraocular muscle enlargement.

Disorder	Reflectivity	Internal structure	Insertions
Thyroid ophthalmopathy	Medium-high	Irregular	Normal
Myositis	Low	Regular	Thickened
Tumors	Low-medium	Regular	Normal
Venous congestion	Medium-high	Variable	Normal
Hematoma	Low-medium	Regular	Variable

TABLE 5: Values of extraocular muscle thickness as measured by ultrasonography.

Muscle	Normal range (mm)	Difference between contralateral muscles
Superior rectus/ levator complex	3.9–6.8	0.8
Lateral rectus	2.2–3.8	0.4
Inferior rectus	1.6–3.6	0.4
Medial rectus (thickest)	2.3–4.7	0.5
Sum of all muscles	11.9–16.9	1.2

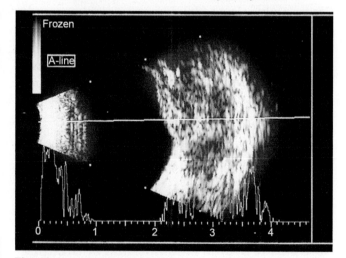

Fig. 13: Pseudotumor of orbit seen as a well circumscribed mass with low to medium internal reflectivity, indenting the globe with moderate sound attenuation.

Vascular Tumors

A *capillary hemangioma* usually appears as a well demarcated, homogenous, high density, lobulated, and contrast enhancing, extraconal mass occupying the periorbital soft tissue and anterior orbit. On B scan it appears as irregular, poorly outlined with high internal reflectivity, irregular internal structure, and variable sound attenuation.

Cavernous hemangioma on CT scan shows a well-demarcated, encapsulated lesion, round or oval in shape, occasionally lobulated (Fig. 14). There is usually no nerve or muscle attachments to the lesions.[21] They have homogenous enhancement with contrast, which increases in density with intratumoral accumulation of dye on later scans. Calcified phleboliths may occasionally be seen. On T1 image, they appear isointense or slightly more intense as compared to the muscles. The lesions show marked signal intensity on T2 weighted image. On B scan, these round or oval, well-outlined tumors show high internal reflectivity, regular internal structure, moderate sound attenuation, and absence of vascularity (Fig. 15).

Lymphangiomas on the other hand appear as irregular, poorly circumscribed, and heterogenous masses. Hemorrhage is common and appears as fluid-filled cystic spaces. Enhancement after contrast is variable. MRI characteristics include increased signal on T1-weighted images and marked signal intensity on T2-weighted images (Figs. 16 and 17).

On B scan, the multiple lymph filled spaces are low reflective with endothelium lined walls that are highly reflective resulting an irregular structure and large dilated lymphatic spaces. The borders are indistinct like capillary hemangioma but internal vascularity is lacking (Figs. 18 and 19).

Orbital varices may be seen as a single lesion or several round or tubular images, occasionally associated with calcification.[19,20] The CT appearance may be normal in the axial sections, but abnormal in the coronal sections because

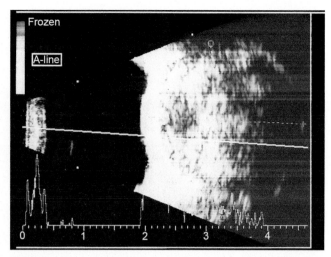

Fig. 15: Cavernous hemangioma appearing as a well circumscribed mass with multiple interfaces, moderate to high internal reflectivity, marked attenuation and producing hyperopia due to globe indentation.

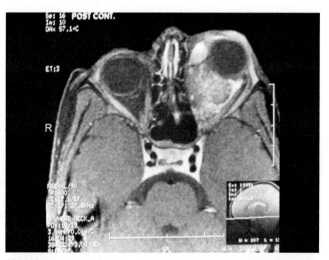

Fig. 16: Postcontrast T1-weighted image showing lymphangioma.

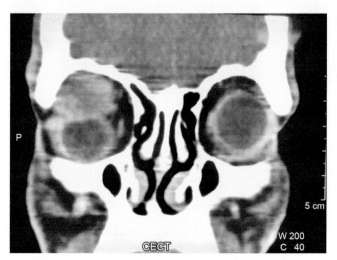

Fig. 14: Coronal CT showing cavernous hemangioma.

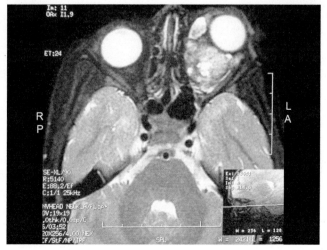

Fig. 17: T2-weighted image of lymphangioma.

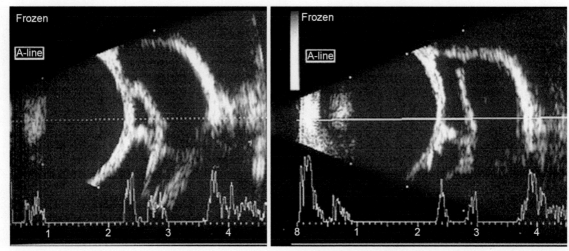

Fig. 18: Transocular B scan of lymphangioma which is a diffuse mass having multiple lymph filled large interspaces and more compressible in comparison to cavernous hemangioma.

of the increased venous pressure in the prone position for the direct coronal scan. Occasionally, a Valsalva maneuver during the scan may be necessary to visualize the lesion. Contrast enhancement is seen, and the lesion may be identified after contrast only.

They present as intermittent proptosis, exacerbated with bending of the head or performance of a Valsalva maneuver (Figs. 20 and 21).

Arteriovenous malformations and carotid cavernous fistulas are characterized by ipsilateral enlargement of the cavernous sinus, superior ophthalmic vein, and extraocular muscles, causing proptosis. Arteriovenous malformations also show irregular tortuosities with marked contrast enhancement, and intracranial component may also be evident on brain CT.

Neural Tumors

Optic Nerve Lesions

On B scan, the optic nerve is best displayed with the probe placed on the globe temporally and to compare the two eyes a similar probe orientation is used.

Retrobulbar optic nerve disorders can cause widening of optic nerve pattern due to the thickening of optic nerve parenchyma (e.g. tumor or inflammation) and thickening of perineural sheaths (e.g. tumor or inflammation), and increased subarachnoid fluid (e.g. pseudotumor cerebri). The differentiation is based on the degree of thickening, internal reflectivity, structure of the nerve, and thirty degree test shown in Table 6.[22]

Thirty Degree Test[23]

Ossoinig et al. described the test to differentiate increased subarachnoid fluid from thickening of optic nerve

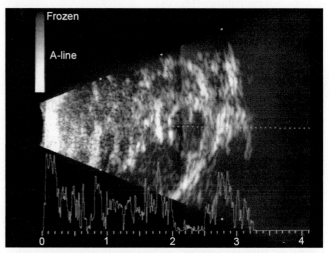

Fig. 19: Paraocular scan of lymphangioma.

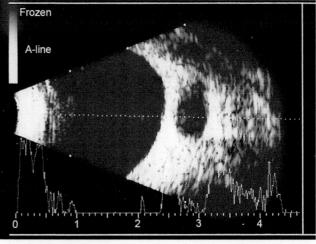

Fig. 20: Orbital varix before Valsalva maneuver.

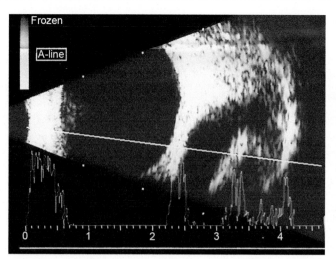

Fig. 21: Orbital varix showing dilatation of superior ophthalmic vein after Valsalva maneuver.

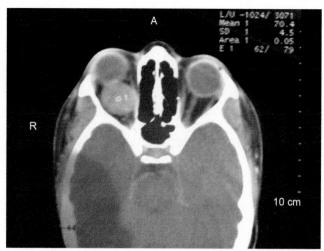

Fig. 22: Axial CT scan showing optic nerve glioma.

TABLE 6: Difference on the basis of degree of thickening, internal reflectivity, structure of the nerve and thirty degree test.

Disorder	Reflectivity	Internal structure	Thirty degree test
Increased subarachnoid fluid	Variable	Irregular	Positive
Glioma	Low-medium	Regular	Negative
Meningioma	Medium-high	Irregular	Negative

parenchyma or perineural sheaths using A scan technique. The maximum thickness of the optic nerve is measured in primary gaze and with the patient fixating 30° or more toward the probe. The test is considered positive if the nerve pattern decreases by at least 10% at 30° gaze as compared to the primary gaze as in increased subarachnoid fluid.

Optic nerve glioma is usually a tumor of childhood that is benign, well differentiated, and slow growing. Neuroimaging is crucial to determine the posterior extent of the lesion and whether intracanalicular, chiasmal, or deep intracranial involvement is present. CT shows a well-defined, fusiform enlargement of the optic nerve with smooth margins (Fig. 22). A sinusoidal appearance with a kinking, tortuous enlargement is characteristic of the childhood form.[21,24] Calcification is very rare. These tumors usually show uniform and moderate enhancement with contrast, but the enhancement may be nonhomogenous from areas of tumor infarction. With intracanalicular extension, bone molding and canal dilation may be seen.[4]

The lesions are generally isointense or slightly hypotense on T1-weighted images and hyperintense on T2-weighted images.[25]

Primary optic nerve meningiomas are usually benign, slow-growing, and unilateral tumors. They have three radiographic patterns. The most common is tubular enlargement with irregular margins, but a fusiform swelling or globular enlargement may also be seen.[4] CT demonstrates calcification in up to 25% of lesion. The "railroad" or "tram-track" appearance of the optic nerve on axial sections occurs because the optic nerve has a relatively lower density than the surrounding tumor.[4] Contrast enhancement occurs and is useful in determining intracranial extension. Intracranial sphenoid wing meningiomas show hyperostosis and calcification on CT. On MRI studies, meningioma is isointense to brain on T1-weighted and T2-weighted images with uniform and often very intense contrast enhancement (Fig. 23).[26]

Neurilemoma (schwannoma) are peripheral nerve sheath tumors that can occur anywhere along the course of a peripheral, cranial, or sympathetic nerve (Fig. 24). CT demonstrates a well-circumscribed round or ovoid mass. The tumor has a heterogenous density depending on lipid deposition, cysts, degenerated tumor, and (rarely) calcification.[27] Mild enhancement occurs with contrast. Bony remodeling may be seen.

On B scan, schwannoma (neurilemmoma) appears as oval, encapsulated with low-medium reflectivity, regular internal reflectivity, moderate sound attenuation, and with some degree of vascularity (Fig. 25).

Plexiform neurofibroma is irregularly shaped with irregular internal structure, high internal reflectivity, and minimal sound attenuation (Figs. 26 and 27).

Rhabdomyosarcoma (Fig. 28)

Rhabdomyosarcoma is the most common orbital malignancy of childhood. The superonasal quadrant is the most common site. On CT, they are irregular, moderately well-

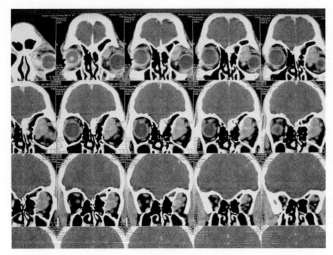

Fig. 23: Coronal CT scan showing supero-nasal orbital meningioma.

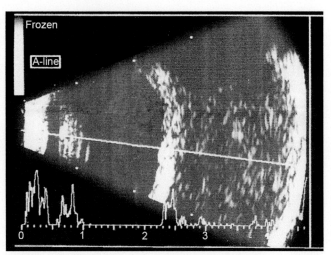

Fig. 25: Schwannoma of the orbit is a solid mass with regular, homogenous structure showing low to medium internal reflectivity with indentation of the globe.

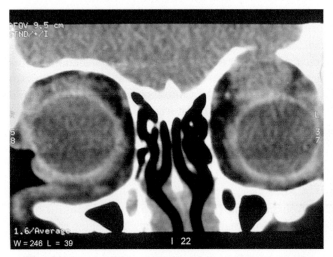

Fig. 24: Coronal CT scan showing schwannoma in the left superior orbit.

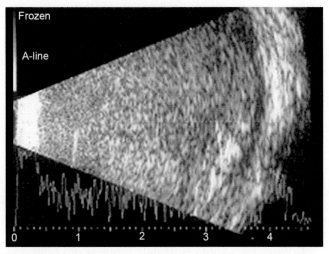

Fig. 26: Paraocular scan of plexiform neurofibroma showing an ill-defined heterogenous solid mass in the lid region with multiple interfaces.

circumscribed masses, and often quite large because of their rapid growth. They invade bone, and may invade the brain or sinuses. There is uniform enhancement with contrast.[28]

On B scan a well circumscribed, variable shape, low-medium internal reflectivity, moderate sound attenuation, and internal blood flow is seen.

Lacrimal Fossa Lesions

Inflammatory and lymphoid lesions of the lacrimal gland show diffuse enlargement conforming to the shape of the globe. In addition, there is marked contrast enhancement, but the adjacent bone is normal. In general, such lesions involve the entire lacrimal gland including the palpebral

lobe, and thus often extend anteriorly. There may be a ring of uveo-scleral enhancement of the adjacent ocular coats in such cases.

Pleomorphic adenoma on CT scans reveals a globular, circumscribed mass, often oval or round in shape (Fig. 29). The shape and contour of these lesions help to differentiate them from inflammatory or lymphoid lesions. Inflammatory and lymphoid lesions tend to elongate, mold to the globe, and do not appear encapsulated. For small lesions, it is helpful to compare with the contralateral side because these tumors are rarely bilateral and have the same density of normal lacrimal gland. Larger lesions that have been present for some time show pressure expansion of the

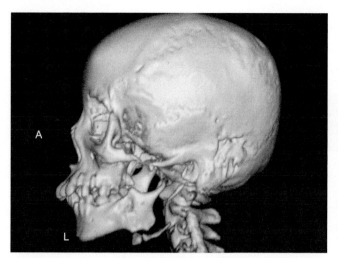

Fig. 27: 3 D-reconstruction showing sphenoid wing dysplasia in plexiform neurofibromatosis.

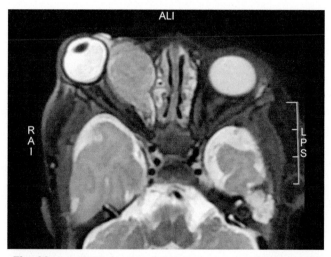

Fig. 28: Axial MRI showing rhabdomyosarcoma of right medial rectus muscle

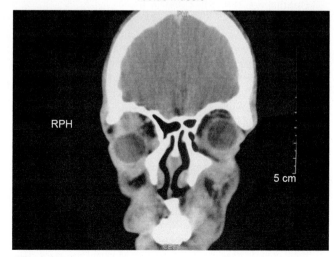

Fig. 29: Coronal CT scan showing right pleomorphic adenoma.

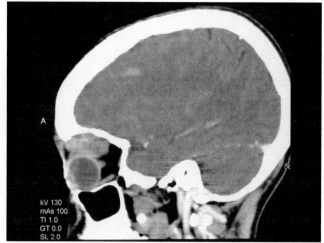

Fig. 30: Sagittal CT scan showing left adenocarcinoma of lacrimal gland. There is infiltration of adjacent structures, calcification and irregular erosion and destruction of bone.

lacrimal fossa but no bone destruction. Calcification may be seen.

Adenoid cystic carcinoma on CT scans reveals a globular or rounded mass, with irregular borders, that invades bone and soft tissue (Fig. 30). Bony changes occur in 80% of cases.[4,29] Calcification is common. Because of the bone changes and calcification, CT is the modality of choice in evaluating these lesions.[4]

Secondary Tumors

Secondary orbital tumors refer to those lesions that extend from an adjacent area into the orbit. Nasopharyngeal angiofibromas are the most common benign neoplasms of the nasopharynx, with the propensity for aggressive local growth. This highly vascular tumor predominantly occurs in adolescent males (Figs. 31A to C).

Basal cell, squamous cell, sebaceous cell carcinomas, and malignant melanomas may extend posteriorly from the eyelids. CT scans are preferred over MR imaging because they image the details of the bone better. Mucoceles are benign, cystic, and slowly expanding lesions originating from the sinuses, most commonly from the ethmoid or frontal sinus. On CT, they appear as a mass expanding into the orbit from an opacified sinus.

Metastatic Tumors

The most common primary tumors that are metastatic to the orbits in adults are breast in women and lung in men. Neuroblastoma and Ewing's sarcoma are the most common tumors with orbital metastases in children. CT and MR imaging demonstrate metastatic tumors as either a focal mass or an infiltrative lesion. Metastasis can occur in any

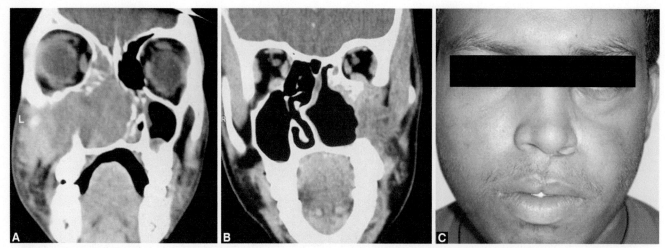

Figs. 31A to C: Nasopharyngeal angiofibroma. (A) Coronal CT showing the left sided mass; (B) Coronal CT after the surgery; (C) Postoperative clinical photograph showing the lateral rhinotomy incision.

location in the orbit. Bone destruction is commonly seen with metastatic breast carcinoma.

CONCLUSION

Computed tomography and MRI complement each other in evaluation of orbital lesions and may need to be combined with ultrasonography in some cases. Doppler ultrasonography provides specific information regarding blood flow. Larger venous abnormalities and orbitocranial vascular malformations and fistulas can be visualized on MR venography. Arteriography is the gold standard for diagnosis of arterial lesions like aneurysm or arteriovenous malformation. MR angiography on the other hand, though less sensitive than direct arteriography in identification of carotid and dural cavernous sinus fistulas, is frequently used because of lesser invasiveness.

The best approach is a combination of clinical judgment supplemented with appropriate orbital imaging.

REFERENCES

1. Fergenson JM, Mandell N, Abrahams JJ. The orbit. In: Haaga JR, Lanzieri CF, Gilkeson RC (Eds). CT and MR Imaging of the Whole Body, 4th edition. Missouri: Mosby; 2003. pp. 474-94.
2. Dutton JJ. Atlas of clinical and surgical orbital anatomy. Philadelphia: WB Saunders; 1994. pp. 201-32.
3. Hesselink JR, Karampekios S. Normal computed tomography and magnetic resonance imaging anatomy of the globe, orbit, and visual pathways. Neuroimaging Clin N Am. 1996;6(1):15-27.
4. Purdy EP, Bullock JD. Magnetic resonance imaging and computed tomography in orbital diagnosis. Ophthalmol Clin North Am. 1991;4:89-111.
5. Yousem DM. Orbit: Embryology, anatomy, and pathology. In: Som PM, Curtin HD (Eds). Head and Neck Imaging, 4th edition. St Louis, MO: Mosby–Elsevier Science; 2003. pp. 1-544.
6. Mafee MF. Imaging of the orbit. In: Valvassori GE, Mafee MF, Carter B (Eds). Imaging of the Head and Neck. Stuttgart: Georg Thieme; 1995. pp. 248-327.
7. Miraldi F, Sims MS, Wiesen EJ. Imaging principles in computerized tomography. In: Haaga JR, Lanzieri CF, Gilkeson RC (Eds). CT and MR Imaging of the Whole Body. Vol 1, 4th edition. USA: Mosby; 2003. pp. 2-36.
8. Lee AG, Brazis PW, Garrity JA, et al. Imaging for neuro-ophthalmic and orbital disease. Am J Ophthalmol. 2004;138(5):852-62.
9. Muller-Forell W, Pitz S. Orbital pathology. Eur J Radiol. 2004;49(2):105-42.
10. Lagouros PA, Langer BG, Peyman GA, et al. Magnetic resonance imaging and intraocular foreign bodies. Arch Ophthalmol. 1987;105(4):551-3.
11. Gilbard SM, Mafee MF, Lagouros PA, et al. Orbital blowout fractures. The prognostic significance of computed tomography. Ophthalmology. 1985;92(11):1523-8.
12. Polito E, Leccisotti A. Diagnosis and treatment of orbital hemorrhagic lesions. Ann Ophthalmol. 1994;26(3):85-93.
13. Chandler JR, Langenbrunner DJ, Stevens ER. The pathogenesis of orbital complications in acute sinusitis. Laryngoscope. 1970;80(9):1414-28.
14. Mafee MF, Inoue Y, Mafee RF. Ocular and orbital imaging. Neuroimaging Clin N Am. 1996;6(2):291-318.
15. Weiss RA. Orbital disease. In: McCord CD, Tanenbaum M, Nunery WR (Eds). Oculoplastic Surgery, 3rd edition. New York: Raven Press; 1995. pp. 417-76.
16. Kahaly GJ. Imaging in thyroid-associated orbitopathy. Eur J Endocrinol. 2001;145(2): 107-18.
17. Byrne SF, Green RL. Extraocular muscles. In: Ultrasound of the Eye and Orbit, 2nd edition. USA: Mosby; 1992. pp. 1-576.

18. Byrne SF, Gendron EK, Glaser JS, et al. Diameter of normal extraocular recti muscles with echography. Am J Ophthalmol. 1991;112(6):706-13.

19. Yuen SJ, Rubin PA. Idiopathic orbital inflammation: Ocular mechanisms and clinicopathology. Ophthalmol Clin North Am. 2002;15(1):121-6.

20. Weber AL, Romo LV, Sabates NR. Pseudotumor of the orbit: Clinical, pathologic, and radiologic evaluation. Radiol Clin North Am. 1999;37(1):151-68, xi.

21. Leib ML. The continuing utility of computed tomography in ophthalmology. Ophthalmol Clin North Am. 1994;7271-6.

22. Byrne SF, Green RL. Optic Nerve in Ultrasound of the Eye and Orbit. USA: Mosby Year Book; 1992. pp. 1-403.

23. Ossoinig KC, Cennamo G, Byrne SF. Echographic differential diagnosis of optic nerve lesions. In: Ultrasonography in Ophthalmology, Doc Ophthalmol Proceed Series, Vol 29. Dordrecht, NL: Dr W Junk Publishers; 1981. pp. 327-35.

24. Jakobiec FA, Depot MJ, Kennerdell JS, et al. Combined clinical and computed tomographic diagnosis of orbital glioma and meningioma. Ophthalmology. 1984;91:137-55.

25. Haik BG, Saint Louis L, Bierly J, et al. Magnetic resonance imaging in the evaluation of optic nerve gliomas. Ophthalmology. 1987;94(6):709-17.

26. Zimmerman RD, Fleming CA, Saint Louis LA, et al. Magnetic resonance imaging of meningiomas. AJNR Am J Neuroradiol. 1985;6(2):149-57.

27. Rootman JA, Goldberg C, Robertson W. Primary orbital schwannomas. Br J Ophthalmol. 1982;66(3):194-204.

28. Geoffray A, Vanel D, Masselot J, et al. Contribution of computed tomography (CT) in the study of 24 head and neck embryonic rhabdomyosarcomas in children. Eur J Radiol. 1984;4(3):177-80.

29. Jakobiec FA, Yeo JH, Trokel SL, et al. Combined clinical and computed tomographic diagnosis of primary lacrimal fossa lesions. Am J Ophthalmol. 1982;94(6):785-807.

Congenital Orbital Anomalies

Sumit Kumar, Ruchi Goel

INTRODUCTION

The orbits are formed by seven different bones namely frontal, zygomatic, sphenoid, ethmoidal, maxillary, lacrimal, and palatine.

NORMAL GROWTH OF INTERORBITAL REGION

Development of the interorbital region:
- The superior portion of the interorbital region is influenced by the enlargement of the neurocranium to about three times from birth to maturity
- *Growth of sutures*: The frontal-ethmoid suture is the critical suture for interorbital growth
- The medial orbital margin smoothens and there is decrease in the width of the interorbital region
- Pneumatization of bone and development of paranasal air sinuses
- The eye ball increases 3.25 times between birth and adulthood. Removal of eyeball prior to completion of orbital growth results in development of contracted orbit
- Initially, the fetal face, orbit, and globe have a linear growth curve
- There occurs rapid change in the size and shape of the orbit between 6 months of gestational age and 18 months after birth.

MORPHOLOGICAL LANDMARKS OF THE ORBITS

The interorbital distance is the shortest distance between the inner walls of the orbits.

The interorbital measurements are measured on CT scan, Waters (half axial projection), or from posteroanterior cephalograms.

Clinically, the following landmarks help in evaluation of the interocular distances:
- Interpupillary distance
- Inter inner canthal distance
- Outer inter canthal distance
- Horizontal palpebral length
- *Farkas canthal index*: Inner to outer intercanthal ratio × 10. Canthal index is higher than 42 in hypertelorism and lower than 38 in hypotelorism.

CONGENITAL ABNORMALITIES AND SYNDROMES OF THE ORBIT

The developmental defects may occur at any time after conception. A profound abnormality indicates that the disturbance occurred in early part of development.

Abnormalities of Distance between the Eyes and Orbits (Fig. 1)

Hypotelorism

Hypotelorism is defined as a decreased distance between the medial orbital walls (interorbital distance), with abnormally short inner and outer canthal distances. It may develop due to skull malformation or a failure in brain development is associated with numerous syndromes like:
- *Trigonocephaly*: A rare craniosynostosis with premature closure of the metopic sutures. *Features*—hypotelorism, a triangular skull, and a prominent frontal protuberance

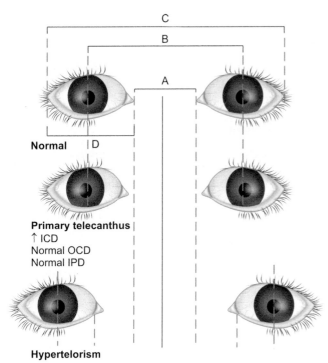

Fig. 1: Abnormal distances between the eyes: A—Inter canthal distance (ICD); B—Inter pupillary distance (IPD); C—Outer inter canthal distance (OCD); D—Horizontal palpebral fissure length (HPL).

- *Holoprosencephaly*: A rare major brain malformation with abnormal cleavage and morphogenesis during the third week of fetal development.

Hypertelorism

Hypertelorism is defined as an increased distance between the medial orbital walls (interorbital distance), with abnormally increased inner and outer canthal distances (not of the inner canthi only).

Three potential mechanisms of hypertelorism include:
1. The orbits change from being widely divergent 180° during early development to 70° at birth. Early ossification of the lesser wings of the sphenoid may result in fixing the orbits in the fetal position.
2. The failure of development of nasal capsule causes protrusion of primitive brain vesicle into this space like in frontal encephalocele.
3. There may occur disturbance in the development of skull base as seen in craniosynostosis syndromes like Apert and Crouzon syndromes; midfacial malformations such as frontonasal dysplasia or craniofacial dysplasia.

Hypertelorism may be associated with more than 550 disorders.

Telecanthus

Telecanthus is defined as increased distance between the two medial canthi compared with the interorbital distance. It can be objectively calculated as Mustardé ratio [intercanthal distance/interpupillary distance (ICD/IPD)] greater than 0.55.

Primary telecanthus: ↑ distance between the inner canthi with normally spaced outer canthi and normal interpupillary measurement.

Secondary telecanthus: ↑inner canthi distance associated with ocular hypertelorism.

Dystopia Canthorum

The lateral displacement of the inner canthi (telecanthus) is associated with lateral displacement of the lacrimal puncta. The puncta are displaced to such an extent that if an imaginary vertical line is drawn through the puncta it cuts the cornea.

Waardenburg syndrome type 1 is an autosomal dominant syndrome with variable expressivity. It is associated with the following:
- Dystopia canthorum (characteristic feature)
- A broad nasal root
- Poliosis (often a white forelock)
- Heterochromia irides
- Various degree of sensorineural hearing loss.

Waardenburg type 2 is differentiated from Waardenburg type 1 by the absence of dystopia canthorum. The *type 3* is a variant of type 1 with limb anomalies and *type 4* is associated with Hirschsprung disease.

Abnormalities of the Eyes in Relation to their Respective Orbits

Prominent Eyes

Prominent eyes occur due to protrusion of normal globes beyond the normal orbital margin denoted as proptosis or with a normal globe in the setting of reduced orbital depth (shallow orbit).

Prominent eyes occur in:
- *Craniosynostosis syndromes* due to underdevelopment of the orbital ridges and midfacial bones that reduces the orbital volume, e.g. Apert and Crouzon syndrome
- *Midfacial retrusion or hypoplasia* seen in conditions such as:
    - Maternal consumption of drugs (warfarin, retinoic acid, etc.)
    - *Stickler syndrome*, autosomal dominant condition characterized by variable presentation that can include:
        - Midfacial hypoplasia
        - Prominent eyes
        - Cleft palate

- Micrognathia
- Sensorineural deafness with high tone loss
- Spondyloepiphyseal dysplasia.

The prominence of eyes is heightened by high-degree myopia and abnormalities of vitreous gel architecture.

– *Schinzel-Giedion syndrome* is characterized by:
- Prominent eyes
- Central nervous system degeneration
- Skeletal, cardiac, and renal anomalies
- Bitemporal narrowing
- A deep groove under the eyes causes figure-eight appearance of the midface.

Sunken Eyes

Overtly prominent orbital ridges and walls, insufficient development of the globes, or loss of fatty tissue within the orbit can result in sunken eyes. Sunken eyes can be associated with Cockayne syndrome.

Cockayne syndrome is an autosomal recessive premature aging disorder of DNA repair with the following features:
- Sunken eyes secondary to melting of orbital fat
- Sensorineural hearing loss
- Cataracts
- Pigmentary retinopathy
- Cutaneous photosensitivity
- Dental caries.

Abnormalities of the Size

An abnormal shape or size of one or both orbits may result from:
- Primary developmental defect of bone, e.g. craniosynostosis
- Secondary changes in bony orbit occurring in utero or postnatally due to primary intraorbital process.

Increased Size of the Orbit

Increased size of the orbit typically unilateral occurs in presence of a mass present in the orbit (encephalocele, cystic eye, and tumor).

Small Orbit

The small size of the orbit may occur unilaterally or bilaterally and often coexists with microphthalmia or anophthalmia.

Anophthalmia

True anophthalmia is defined as a total absence of tissues of the eye. Three types of anophthalmia have been described as:
1. *Primary anophthalmia* is rare and often bilateral. Failure of the primary optic vesicle to grow out from the cerebral vesicle at the 2 mm stage of embryonic development may result in primary anophthalmia.
2. *Secondary anophthalmia* is rare and lethal and is a result of gross abnormality in the anterior neural tube.
3. *Consecutive anophthalmia* probably occurs due to secondary degeneration of the optic vesicle.

The adnexal structures may also fail to develop and remain hypoplastic in anophthalmia.

Microphthalmia

Microphthalmia is commoner than anophthalmia and is defined by the presence of a small eye with axial length that is at least two standard deviations below the mean axial length for age. It may occur as an isolated defect or as part of a syndrome.

Asymmetric Orbits

Congenital craniofacial tumors such as in sphenoid wing dysplasia in neurofibromatosis type 1 or orbital hamartomas in Proteus syndrome may result in asymmetric orbits.

Other causes of asymmetric orbits include craniofacial clefting anomalies.

Congenital Craniofacial Clefting Anomalies Affecting Orbit

Clefting syndromes that involve the orbit and eyelids are the oculoauriculovertebral spectrum that includes:
- Hemifacial microsomia
- Oculoauriculovertebral dysplasia (Goldenhar syndrome)
- Mandibulofacial dysostosis (Treacher Collins–Franceschetti syndrome)
- Midline clefts with hypertelorism.

The bones of the skull or orbit may also have congenital clefts through which the intracranial contents can herniate, e.g. meninges *(meningocele)*, brain tissue *(encephalocele)*, or both meninges and brain tissue *(meningoencephalocele)*.
- A subcutaneous protrusion may occur near the medial canthus or over the bridge of the nose.
- The mass may increase in size on straining or crying and the globe may be displaced inferolaterally
- Pulsation of the globe may be seen.

FURTHER READING

1. Dollfus H, Verloes A. Dysmorphology and the orbital region: A practical clinical approach. Surv Ophthalmol. 2004;49(6):547-61.
2. Farkas LG, Ross RB, Posnick JC, et al. Orbital measurements in 63 hyperteloric patients. Differences between the anthropometric and cephalometric findings. J Craniomaxillofac Surg. 1989;17(6):249-54.
3. Morin JD, Hill JC, Anderson JE, et al. A study of growth in the interorbital region. Am J Ophthalmol. 1963;56:895-901.

Orbital Infection and Inflammation

Smriti Bansal, Sima Das

INTRODUCTION

Orbital infections and inflammations include a broad spectrum of disorders which can affect any age group. Orbital infection is also a form of orbital inflammation caused by specific pathogens and therefore these disorders can have similar presentations. The characteristic signs of orbital inflammation are proptosis, extraocular muscle movement limitation, pain, red eye, and ophthalmoplegia. In severe forms, signs of optic nerve involvement can also be elicited. In both the groups detailed history and complete physical examination form the backbone for narrowing the list of differential diagnosis and further laboratory and radiological investigation can supplement the way to reach proper diagnosis.

RELEVANT SURGICAL ANATOMY

Orbit is a pyramidal shaped structure and due to its anatomical correlations it is commonly affected by infection and inflammatory processes:

Orbit lies in close vicinity to paranasal sinuses. There is a papery thin plate of bone between medial wall of orbit and ethmoid sinus. Superiorly roof of the orbit is directly related to floor of frontal sinus and floor of orbit shares a common wall with roof of maxillary sinus. In children frontal sinus is not developed till 8 years of age so ethmoid sinus is the main cause of infection.[1] This thin bone can also get disrupted in cases of trauma, tumors or through some surgical intervention (Fig. 1A).

- The venous system surrounding orbit also has a unique feature of being valveless in nature and therefore it leads to a two way communication between face, nasal cavity, sinuses, pterygoid region, and orbit itself. Superior ophthalmic vein continues as nasofrontal vein which in turn anastomose with angular vein.[1] Any infection affecting the mid face can spread to orbit and can also lead to cavernous sinus thrombosis (Fig. 1B).

ORBITAL INFECTIONS

Infections affecting orbit is not an uncommon entity. Orbital infections should be kept as first differential diagnosis whenever a patient presents with signs of orbital inflammation. Orbital cellulitis is potentially a sight-threatening condition especially in young children and therefore prompt identification and appropriate treatment is the key to success. Orbit can get inoculated by infections through various routes:

- *Direct inoculation of infection:* This occurs when the pathogen directly infects the orbital structures leading to infection. This happens in cases of external hordeolum, acute dacryocystitis, internal hordeolum and trauma or penetrating injury, etc.
- *Hematogenous spread:* The infection travels through the blood vessels most commonly through veins and affects the orbital structures like in cases of dental infection, subacute bacterial endocarditis, etc.
- *Extension of infection from the surrounding sinuses:* This commonly spreads through paranasal sinuses most common being ethmoid sinus since there is only a papery thin bone separating ethmoid sinus and orbit. Infection of lacrimal sac can also lead to development of orbital infection

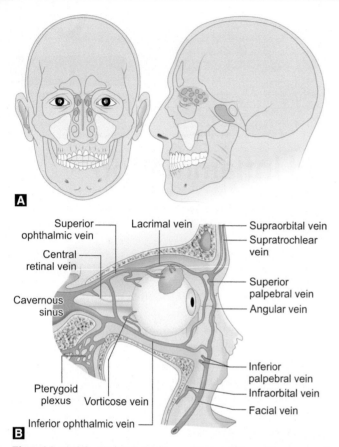

A

Superior ophthalmic vein
Lacrimal vein
Supraorbital vein
Supratrochlear vein
Central retinal vein
Superior palpebral vein
Cavernous sinus
Angular vein
Pterygoid plexus
Vorticose vein
Inferior palpebral vein
Infraorbital vein
Facial vein
Inferior ophthalmic vein

B

Figs. 1A and B: (A) Orbital walls and their relation with paranasal sinuses—Maxillary sinus (blue), frontal sinus (green), ethmoid sinus (purple), sphenoid sinus (red); (B) Orbital venous drainage system.

Orbital Cellulitis

Etiology

Orbital infections are most commonly caused by bacteria worldwide. Around two decades back haemophilus influenzae B (HiB) was the most common cause but with the advent of the vaccine against HiB its incidence has reduced drastically.[2] Most common group of pathogens leading to orbital infections nowadays includes *Staphylococcus aureus* and *Streptococcus* species. In pediatric population *Streptococcus aeruginosa* is the emerging pathogen.[3] Incidence of methicillin resistant *Staphylococcus aureus* (MRSA) is increasing dramatically due to irrational use of antibiotics. In a retrospective study conducted in United States population has shown 75% of infectious cases were affected by MRSA and in orbital cellulitis also major pathogen was the same.[4]

Clinical Staging

Orbital infection is further divided into five stages by Chandler for the ease of diagnosis and treatment (Table 1).[1]

- *Stage 1—Preseptal cellulitis:* Infection limited to orbital septum is classified as preseptal cellulitis. Orbital septum (palpebral fascia) is a membranous sheet or a fibrous band which forms the anterior boundary of orbit. It extends from orbital rim to eyelids. In upper eyelid it fuses with levator palpebrae aponeurosis and in lower lid with the tarsal plate. It is commonly seen after direct inoculation of the infection to the orbit and if not treated on time, infection can break the barrier and affects the orbital cavity. Clinically patients presents with lid edema and lid erythema, pain, periorbital swelling and erythema of the surrounding skin. Vision remains unaffected in this stage (Fig. 2)

- *Stage 2—Orbital cellulitis:* This happens when inflammation crosses the eyelid septum and goes into the orbit. Soft tissue is involved without any abscess formation. This condition commonly is seen due to extension of infection from the surrounding sinuses. In this condition patient presents with proptosis, chemosis, restriction of extraocular motility, and compromised visual functions. At this stage patient needs aggressive treatment as optic nerve is at risk (Fig. 3)

- *Stage 3—Subperiosteal abscess:* Periosteum covering the orbital bony walls also referred to as periorbita is a soft tissue membrane which forms the only barrier between sinuses and orbital cavity. There is collection of inflammatory products between periorbita and bony walls of the orbit. It usually presents with proptosis and dystopia where globe is displaced to the opposite direction of the abscess. This condition usually requires drainage of the abscess if accessible. Garcia and Harris have described several indication of drainage (Table 2).[5] These indications are—if there is failure of response to parenteral antibiotic; if there is suspicion or presence of foreign body; if the pressure effect of abscess is causing visual compromise or there are chances of its spread to the cranial cavity

- *Stage 4—Orbital abscess:* This is collection of pus and inflammatory products within orbital soft tissues. Patient presents with proptosis, complete ophthalmoplegia, visual compromise, and papilledema on fundus examination

- *Stage 5—Cavernous sinus thrombosis:* Only 1% of the orbital infection cases actually progresses to this condition. In this condition patients present with neurological deficits because of involvement of 3rd, 4th, 5th, and 6th cranial nerves along with proptosis, severe pain, visual compromise, and complete internal and external ophthalmoplegia. Despite giving parenteral therapy mortality rate is as high as 30% in these cases.[6]

TABLE 1: Chandler's clinical staging with their clinical features and treatment.

Stages	Clinical features	Treatment
Stage 1: Preseptal cellulitis	• Inflammatory eyelid edema, pain, and tenderness • Absence of orbital signs like proptosis, limitation of extraocular movement, and chemosis • Vision remains unaffected	Broad-spectrum oral antibiotic + nonsteroidal anti-inflammatory drugs
Stage 2: Orbital cellulitis	• Inflammatory eyelid edema with chemosis • Restriction of extraocular movement • Displacement of globe • Vision can be affected • May have relative afferent pupillary defect	Intravenous broad-spectrum antibiotic + nonsteroidal anti-inflammatory drugs + topical antibiotic
Stage 3: Subperiosteal abscess	• Displacement of globe in opposite direction of collection of pus • Vision can be affected • Pain, limitation of extraocular motility • May have relative afferent pupillary defect	Intravenous broad-spectrum antibiotic + nonsteroidal anti-inflammatory drugs +/– drainage
Stage 4: Orbital abscess	• Vision decreases, color vision is affected • Axial or nonaxial proptosis depending upon site of abscess • Ophthalmoplegia • Relative afferent pupillary defect	Intravenous broad-spectrum antibiotic + nonsteroidal anti-inflammatory drugs +/– drainage
Stage 5: Cavernous sinus thrombosis	• Bilateral proptosis • Severe pain • Meningeal signs may present • Vision decreases • Ophthalmoplegia • Relative afferent pupillary defect	Intravenous broad spectrum antibiotic + nonsteroidal anti-inflammatory drugs +/– drainage

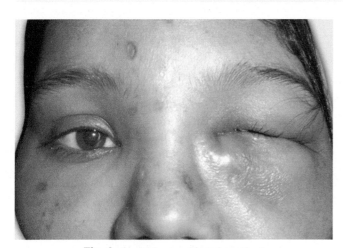

Fig. 2: A middle-aged female patient with left preseptal cellulitis.

Clinical Features

There is a generalized preponderance of males getting affected by orbital infections as compared to females with no explainable cause. The mean age of involvement is 7 years. Acute rhinosinusitis is the most common cause leading to development of orbital infections in children with ethmoid sinus being the most common. This explains the medial orbit to be most common site of involvement.

A detailed history and examination is the key to success to reach a particular diagnosis and for proper management as delay in management can lead to poor visual outcome.[7]

History: It includes onset and duration of symptoms. Any history of fever, associated upper respiratory tract infection, lacrimal outflow obstruction or any tumor should be asked. In children tumors like rhabdomyosarcoma or retinoblastoma can also present like orbital cellulitis. Systemic history should be thoroughly asked to rule out diabetes or any other immunocompromised condition.

Examination: Complete ophthalmological examination is to be done.
- *Vision:* Visual acuity with appropriate refractive error, color vision, and diplopia to be documented
- *Pupillary reaction:* Both direct and consensual reflex to be taken. A note of relative afferent papillary defect to be made
- *Extraocular motility:* Movement of extraocular movements with proper grading should be taken into account everyday as it can be used as an indicator of response to treatment
- *Fundus:* Detailed fundus findings should be documented. Any signs of disk edema need prompt and aggressive treatment to prevent permanent visual loss

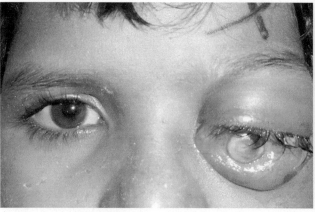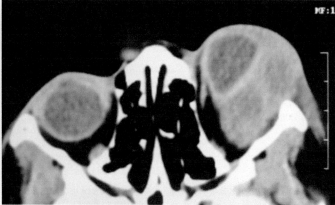

Fig. 3: A child presenting with typical features of orbital cellulitis with corresponding axial scan of CT scan showing soft tissue swelling compressing optic nerve.

TABLE 2: Indications for surgical drainage in case of subperiosteal abscess.

1	Large subperiosteal abscess
2	Patients age >9 years
3	Frontal sinusitis
4	Nonmedial SPA
5	Suspicion of anaerobic infection
6	Recurrence of SPA once drained
7	Any signs of optic nerve compromise
8	Infection of dental origin

- *Ocular adnexal examination*: Eyelids in cases of preseptal cellulitis should be properly examined to rule out any localized stye which has led to periorbital swelling. Acute dacryocystitis should also be kept as one of important differential diagnoses if swelling is localized to inferomedial part of orbit particularly presenting below medial canthus.

Investigations: Ancillary investigations including complete blood counts with blood sugar, blood culture, and pus culture should be sent. A computed tomography scan is essential to look for sinus involvement. MRI plays an important role if clinician suspects any intracranial extension or cavernous sinus involvement. Investigations like lumbar puncture are to be preserved specifically for cases showing signs of meningitis.

Treatment

Conservative management: The therapy depends upon the age of patient, stage of presentation, site of origin, and suspected organism. The patient does not require an inpatient care if he presents in the phase of preseptal cellulitis.

- *Antibiotic:*
  - *Oral antibiotic*: Empirically a broad-spectrum antibiotic is started. A combination of amoxicillin and clavulanic acid is given in the dose of 20–40 mg/kg body weight in 2–3 divided doses in children and 625 mg three times a day in adults for 10–14 days. This mainly provides protection against *Staphylococcus* and *Streptococcus* species. This also provides coverage for haemophilus influenzae which once was the most common cause of orbital cellulitis in children but after vaccination the cases have substantially decreased
  - *Intravenous antibiotic*: This is needed in cases of orbital cellulitis when there are signs of visual compromise. Broad-spectrum antibiotics are started. The preferred regimen nowadays is to start on third generation cephalosporins (100 mg/kg/day in two divided doses) and vancomycin (40–60 mg/kg/day in four divided doses)
- *Nonsteroidal anti-inflammatory drugs:* A combination of a nonsteroidal anti-inflammatory and serratiopeptidase is given three times a day. For children a combination of oral ibugesic (0.5 mg/kg/dose) and paracetamol (15 mg/kg/dose) is preferred three times a day
- *Nasal decongestants:* Oxymetazoline nasal drops are prescribed four times a day
- *Hot fomentation.*

Surgical management: Surgical debridement or drainage is mainly indicated in cases of abscess formation and if patient does not respond to the conservative management (Figs. 4A to C).

Orbital Tuberculosis

Orbital and adnexal tuberculosis (TB) is a rare form of extrapulmonary tuberculosis. Its incidence has increased

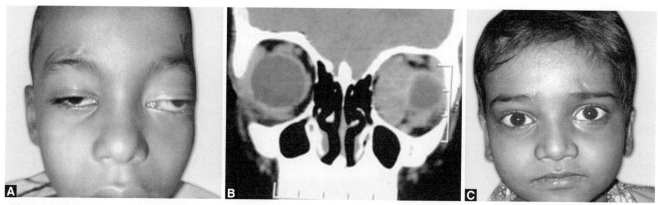

Figs. 4A to C: (A) A child presented with complete ocular motility limitation with laterally displaced globe; (B) Coronal section of CT orbit showing a subperiosteal abscess in the medial orbit; (C) Complete recovery after 1 week of drainage.

in present day because of increasing HIV infections and increasing cases of drug resistance in tuberculosis. Orbit can get involved either by hematogenous spread to orbital periosteum or soft tissue or by direct spread from paranasal sinuses. The disease process can involve bony orbits, lacrimal apparatus or soft tissue. Clinically, orbital TB can be classified into five categories:[8]

1. *Classical periostitis:* This type of orbital TB presents as chronic ulceration or discharging fistula in the periorbital area. The surrounding skin can get thickened and edematous which can lead to cicatricial ectropion. On imaging bony erosions and irregular thickening of bone are frequently seen (Fig. 5).

2. *Orbital soft tissue tuberculoma or cold abscess with no bony destruction:* In this subtype patients present with proptosis, palpebral orbital mass, diplopia, and pain. It can be associated with visual loss depending upon the site of tuberculoma. Radiologically, a well-defined isodense soft tissue mass is seen affecting a particular area of orbit.

3. *Orbital TB with evidence of bony involvement:* In this form soft tissue mass is associated with massive bony destruction (Fig. 6).

4. *Orbital spread from the paranasal sinuses:* Proptosis is the most common presentation with globe displacement to the opposite side of the mass. Maxillary antrum is the most common cause which spreads to the orbit.

5. *Dacryoadenitis:* It presents as a soft tissue palpable mass in the superotemporal quadrant of orbit.

Management

Complete hemogram with chest X-ray and Mantoux test can help in diagnosing systemic TB but for orbital TB biopsy is recommended in all cases for confirmation. Antitubercular (ATT) drugs according to the standard regimens are started once the histopathological diagnosis confirms the presence of mycobacterium.

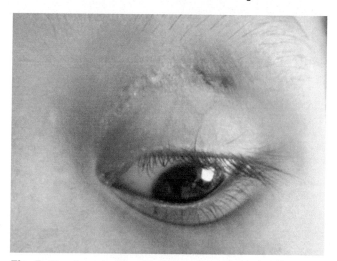

Fig. 5: Classic periostitis with discharging sinus and surrounding skin is tethered to the orbital rim.

Fungal Orbital Cellulitis

Fungal orbital cellulitis is most commonly seen among immunocompromised individuals and is associated with high mortality. The risk factors include uncontrolled diabetes, HIV positive patients, malnutrition, kidney transplant, and some chronic disorder. Orbit is most commonly affected by mucormycosis and aspergillosis. Table 3 describes specific clinical features of each of the groups with their specific treatment.

Parasitic Cyst

Parasites invading eye is not uncommonly seen especially in tropical and subtropical parts of world where environmental conditions and poor sanitation favor parasitism between man and animal. Nowadays they are popularly known as zoonotic helminthes affecting eyes. According to WHO more than 1.5 billion people (24% of world's population) is affected by these helminthes which are transmitted through

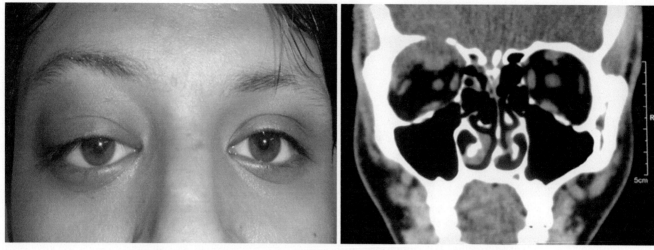

Fig. 6: A young male presented with globe dystopia and superior orbital fullness.
Coronal section of CT scan showing isodense lesion with superior orbital rim destruction.

TABLE 3: Features of different organisms causing fungal orbital cellulitis.[9]

Species of fungi	Mucormycosis (rhino-orbital-cerebral-mucormycosis	Aspergillosis
Type of fungus	Nonseptate filamentous fungi	Septate filamentous fungi
Pathogenesis	These are angioinvasive fungi which cause endothelial damage, ischemia, and finally leading to tissue necrosis	This group includes aerobic fungi which leads to bony destruction and invades orbit through surrounding paranasal sinuses This is commonly associated with allergic sinusitis
Mode of spread to orbit	Invasion from adjacent paranasal sinus or direct inoculation	Invasion from adjacent paranasal sinuses
Risk factors	• Uncontrolled diabetes • Patients with iron overload (desferrioxamine therapy, hemochromatosis, hemodialysis) • Intravenous drug abuse • Bone marrow or kidney transplant • Neutropenia	• Neutrophil count less than $1,000/mm^3$ • T-cell defects (AIDS) • Hematological malignances • Elderly aged people or endemic areas • Steroids therapy or any prosthetic device in body
Clinical features	• Features of orbital cellulitis including proptosis, decrease in visual acuity, and ophthalmoplegia • In later stages they may develop black eschar over nasal mucosa and soft palate	• Painful gradual progressing proptosis • Restriction of ocular movements • Visual loss is rare
Investigations	• KOH mount shows nonseptate-branched fungal hyphae at right angle • Culture on Sabouraud's agar without cycloheximide • Histopathology shows thrombosed artery with fungi invading the vessel wall • PCR • Blood sugars	• KOH mount shows septate hyphae with dichotomous branching at 45° • Culture on SDA to show type of *Aspergillus* species. (*A. fumigatus* has gray green colonies and *A. flavus* has yellow-green colonies). • PCR
Imaging	CT scan can show thrombosed superior ophthalmic vein with an orbital mass.	CT scan shows a heterogenous soft tissue mass with calcification and bony erosion.
Management	• *Intravenous amphotericin B:* 0.7–1 mg/kg body weight. Kidney function test should be monitored. • *Liposomal amphotericin B:* More effective against ROCZ complex. • *Topical amphotericin B:* Irrigation and packing of orbit with 1 mg/ml can be done • *Posaconazole:* Oral antifungal can be used in combination with amphotericin B in refractory cases. • Surgical debridement helps in decreasing the surgical load.	• *Intravenous liposomal amphotericin B:* Dose of 0.7–1 mg/kg body weight. Kidney function test should be monitored. • Oral voriconazole 6 mg/kg twice on day 1 followed by 4 mg/kg for 1 week and then 200 mg twice a day for 12 weeks • Surgical debridement may help in reducing fungal load but its role is not proven.

(PCR: polymerase chain reaction; SDA: Sabouraud dextrose agar)

soil. They are mainly transmitted through eggs present in human feces of the affected person where sanitation is poor. There have been case reports of eye getting affected by almost each and every species of helminthic group but we will be restricting ourselves to helminthes involved with orbital infection. Man always remains an accidental host in all these infections.

Orbital Hydatid Cyst (Echinococcosis)

Orbit is affected in less than 1% of all cases of hydatid cyst affecting humans.[10] The most common organs are liver (60%) and lungs (20%). This is caused by echinococcus genus in helminthic group. There are mainly four species involved in affecting humans:

- Cystic echinococcosis, also known as hydatid disease or hydatidosis, caused by infection with *Echinococcus granulosus*
- Alveolar echinococcosis, caused by infection with *E. multilocularis*
- Polycystic echinococcosis, caused by infection with *E. Vogeli*
- Unicystic echinococcosis, caused by infection with *E. oligarthrus.*

Life cycle: Cystic echinococcosis is the most common form of hydatid cyst affecting humans followed by alveolar echinococcosis.

Definite host of echinococcus: Dogs and canine group of species

Intermediate host: Sheep, goat, swine, etc.

Accidental host: Humans
Humans ingest eggs and they enter into the blood stream after penetrating the intestinal lumen. From blood these eggs travel to different organs and get lodged in various tissues where they are transformed into larvae. This larva develops into fluid-filled cavity leading to formation of hydatid cyst in different organs. This cyst is made of three layers namely, pericyst, ectocyst (outer germinal layer), and endocyst (inner germinal layer) and the fluid is clear pale yellow in color which contains scolices, hooklets, and hydatid sand and is antigenic in nature.

Clinical features: Orbital hydatid cyst is commonly seen in countries like Africa, eastern Europe, Mediterranean countries, middle east, and Iran. It generally presents in people who are involved in rearing sheeps and cattles. It mainly affects children and young adults with mean age of 16 though there have been case reports in which hydatidosis was seen in elderly patients of 74 years.[11] It is uncommon to see hydatid cyst in any other part of the body along with orbital involvement.

- Orbital hydatid cyst commonly presents as unilateral slowly progressive, nonpulsatile, nonreducing orbital mass in a young adult. Vision is affected in most of the cases. Other features may include chemosis, extraocular motility, papilledema, and optic atrophy
- *Location:* Orbital hydatid cyst most commonly presents in retrobulbar area either in intraconal space (60%) or extraconal space. Common location is in the superior part of the orbit which can either be superomedially or superolaterally.[10] The cyst can erode orbital roof and can go intracranially. Cases affecting extraocular muscles are rare though cases reporting hydatid cyst in inferior and medial rectus are present. Orbital hydatid cyst presenting as subconjunctival mass is also rare[12]
- *Investigations:* Casoni's intradermal serological test for detecting antibodies used to be gold standard test but it is only 50–60% specific. Eosinophilia can also be seen in 20–25% of cases
- *Ultrasound features:* Orbital mode ultrasound will show an anechoic cystic lesion. Betharia et al. has characteristically described a double-walled sign in orbital cyst corresponding to the layers of the cyst wall[13]
- On computed tomography, it appears as a hypodense well-defined fluid-filled cystic lesion which is commonly thin walled and unilocular in the orbit. We can also see peripherally a ring enhancing lesion from the fibrous cyst wall. CT scan forms an important tool of investigation as it provides exact location of the cyst and hence aids in planning the treatment (Figs. 7A to C)
- On MRI, hypointense cystic lesion is seen on T1 images whereas a high intensity lesion is present on T2 images
- Color Doppler is the new imaging modality which can detect the alteration in blood flow through central retinal artery, posterior and short ciliary artery, and help us in knowing the compression effects caused due to cyst.

Treatment: The primary treatment for orbital hydatid cyst is complete surgical excision. Depending upon the location of the cyst approach to orbit should be decided. The cyst should be removed in toto without rupture as spillage of contents can lead to anaphylaxis and also increases risk of recurrence. During surgery if cyst ruptures then proper irrigation with 0.9% saline should be thorough. Following surgery, adjuvant therapy with antihelminthes is given. Albendazole in the dose of 30 mg/kg is preferred over mebendazole and given for 28 days with 2 weeks of break and continued like this for 3 months to prevent recurrences.

Orbital Cysticercosis

The other parasitic infection commonly seen in Indian subcontinent is cysticercosis which is caused by cysticercosis cellulosae. This is a larval form which can get inoculated in

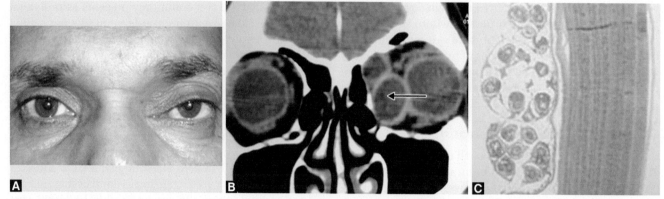

Figs. 7A to C: (A) A middle-aged patient presented lateral displacement of globe; (B) Coronal section of the CT scan showing a well-defined encapsulated isodense lesion in the medial orbit; (C) On H and E stain 20x shows numerous scolices and cyst of hydatid along with the fibrous wall.

various tissues of the body and inciting an inflammatory reaction which leads to various symptoms depending upon the site of infection. The most common systemic form is neurocysticercosis following ocular cysticercosis and then in subcutaneous tissue.

Pathogenesis: Cysticercosis cellulosae is the larval form of *taenia solium* belonging to class cestode of platyhelminthic group. This condition is also endemic in countries with poor sanitation and humans become intermediate host on consuming uncooked pork meat or beef.

Prevalence: Human cysticercosis is also seen in tropical and subtropical counties as seen in hydatidosis though it is much more common than orbital hydatidosis. In India 78% of the ocular cysticercosis is seen in Andhra Pradesh and Pondicherry though commonly seen in other parts of the country as suggested by different case reports.[14] Orbital and adnexal cysticercosis constitute around 13–46% of the systemic disease.[15] In western countries intraocular cysticercosis is common but it is just opposite for Indian subcontinent where extraocular cysticercosis is seen. It is again rare to find cysticercosis associated with any other part of the body when patient presents with ocular symptoms (as seen with hydatid cyst too) but there are case reports of neurocysticercosis coexisting with ocular infection.

Clinical features: Cysticercosis commonly affects children and young adults of age group from 10 years to 30 years and it is rare to find it after 40 years of age group. No gender predilection is seen. We will be discussing only the orbital and adnexal symptoms of cysticercosis and will not go into details of intraocular cysticercosis.

- The most common symptom is periocular swelling and pain depending upon the location of the cyst
- Patients present with limitation of extraocular motility (most common presentation), proptosis, diplopia, ptosis (mechanical), displacement of globe, subconjunctival cyst, and may be squint

- *Site of cyst:* It most commonly occupies anterior orbit followed by subconjunctival space and then posterior orbit in that order. In anterior orbit extraocular muscles are the most common site where superior rectus is most frequently involved followed by inferior rectus, medial rectus, and lateral rectus.[15] In subconjunctival space also it usually presents at the insertion of the muscle. Cases of cysticercosis involving optic nerve are also reported[16]
- Vision remains unaltered in extraocular cases though one can loose vision if cyst is present in vitreous cavity due to the inflammatory reaction
- On examination, following things should be done on every visit:
  - Vision
  - Exophthalmometry
  - Diplopia charting
  - Complete ptosis measurements
  - Thorough fundus examination via indirect ophthalmoscope
  - Motility of extraocular muscles
  - Squint measurements
  - Amount of globe displacement.

Investigation:
- *Lab investigations:* Serum enzyme-linked immuno-sorbent assay (ELISA) for anticysticercal antibodies can be done but it is only 50% specific in ocular cysticercosis. A complete blood count is also insignificant and might show eosinophilia[17]
- *Ultrasound:* It forms a relatively specific and cheaper modality of investigation. On B scan it shows a well-defined cystic lesion with clear contents and hyper reflective echodense shadow in between representing scolex and on A scan there is high reflective spike from cyst wall and scolex. It also forms an important tool in follow up of patient

- *CT scan*: CT scan characteristically shows a well delineated cystic hypodense lesion with a hyperdense shadow in between the lesion suggestive of scolex. Inflammation of the surrounding soft tissues can be seen if cyst is ruptured. Corresponding brain scan should be done to rule out neurocysticercosis[18]
- *MRI*: MRI shows a hypointense cystic lesion with a hyperintense shadow in between the lesions.

Treatment: Medical treatment with antihelminthic and oral corticosteroids remains the main stay of treatment for orbital and adnexal cysticercosis. Oral albendazole 15 mg/kg is prescribed along with oral corticosteroids (1.5 mg/kg/day in tapering doses) for a month.[19] Involuting cyst produces inflammation; therefore corticosteroids are added along with antihelminthics. If any residual cyst persists then oral albendazole can be given till 6 weeks though it is being said that complete resolution can take around 12 weeks.

Surgical excision: It can be done for cysts present in subconjunctival space though excision is difficult as cyst is adherent to the extraocular muscle and care should be taken during excision though required rarely (Figs. 8 to 11).

ORBITAL INFLAMMATION

Orbital inflammatory disorders represent a broad spectrum of disorders and one of the common noninfective presentations to an ophthalmologist. They have various cardinal signs including pain, redness, swelling, proptosis, and ophthalmoplegia. Vision may or may not be affected. There are many causes for orbital inflammation and can be divided into vascular, infective, inflammatory, and neoplastic but a major group is represented by idiopathic variant. Different orbital infections have already been discussed. So in this section we will concentrate on noninfective causes.

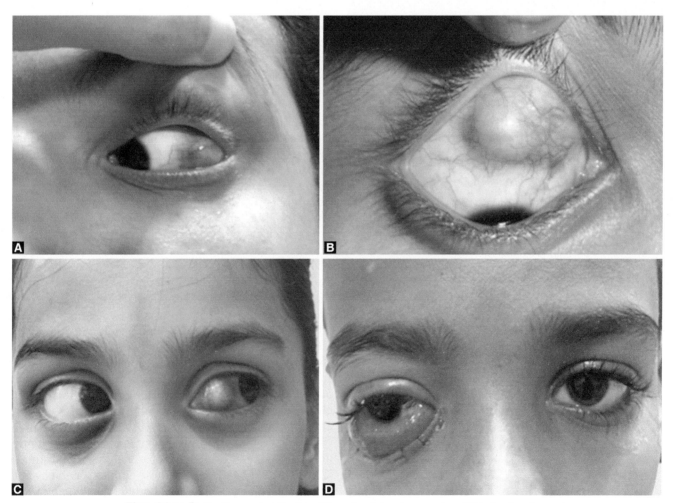

Figs. 8A to D: Cysticercosis affecting different extraocular muscles: (A) Lateral rectus; (B) Superior rectus; (C) Medial rectus; (D) Inferior rectus.

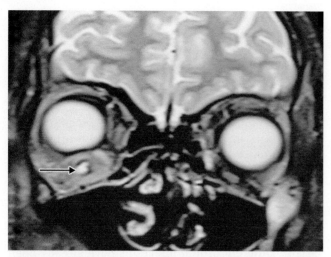

Fig. 9: A well-defined isointense lesion in the inferior rectus with a hyperintense shadow in center of the lesion depicting scolex.

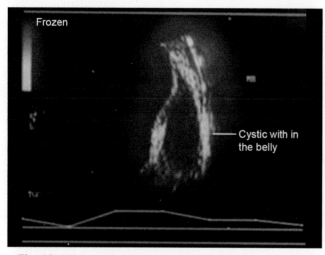

Fig. 10: Ultrasound of the orbit showing a cystic lesion in the belly of extraocular muscle.

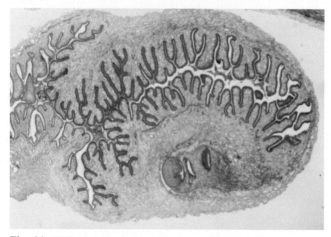

Fig. 11: H&E 10x showing an intact cyst with internal invaginations of cysticercosis cellulosae along with fibrous tissue.

Idiopathic Orbital Inflammation Syndrome

Idiopathic orbital inflammation or orbital pseudotumor is an idiopathic, nonspecific, and benign inflammatory condition. The term orbital pseudotumor was first described by Gleason in 1903 but was more popularized when Birch and Hirschfeld published a case series analyzing 30 similar cases in 1930.[20,21] This is the third most common orbital disease after thyroid orbitopathy and lymphoproliferative disorders and accounts for 5% of all orbital disorders.[22,23]

Pathology

The etiology of orbital pseudotumor is not clear but it is said that it could either be infectious or immune mediated. Idiopathic orbital inflammation syndrome (IOIS) has been observed in association with upper respiratory tract infection and flulike viral illness but the exact pathogenesis is unknown.[24] Similarly, there are evidences showing the role of immune-mediated processes leading to orbital inflammation.[25] There have been cases where orbital inflammation is reported in association with a number of systemic diseases like Crohn's disease, systemic lupus erythematosus, diabetes mellitus, rheumatoid arthritis, myasthenia gravis and ankylosing arthritis.[26-32] An underlying autoimmune mechanism has also been proposed in which they say that there are either circulating antibodies against eye muscles or there is production of fibrogenic cytokines leading to aberrant wound healing causing fibrosis leading to sclerosing variant of IOIS.[33] Histologically, in acute form the disease consists of polymorphous infiltrates mainly mature lymphocytes, plasma cells, macrophages, and neutrophils whereas in chronic phase there is increased amount of fibrovascular stroma and rarely inflammatory cells are seen.

Clinical Features

The presenting feature of the patient mainly depends upon the ocular part which has been affected by the inflammatory process. The disease can affect at any age and is seen in all ethnic groups. IOIS typically presents unilaterally in adults whereas bilateral presentation is more common in children. For the ease of making clinical diagnosis we can subdivide them anatomically into anterior and posterior orbit involvement. Anterior orbit constitutes lacrimal gland (dacryoadenitis), extraocular muscles (myositis), and anterior scleritis whereas in posterior orbit structures which can be affected are posterior sclera, optic nerve (optic perineuritis), and orbital apex (orbital apex syndrome). We will further be discussing these entities separately but in general, patients with anterior orbital inflammation will present as pain with redness, eyelid and periorbital swelling, and limitation of ocular motility. Vision remains unaffected in anterior orbital inflammatory process whereas posterior orbital inflammation presents as proptosis, compromised visual acuity, and ophthalmoplegia.

Anterior Orbit

Dacryoadenitis: In dacryoadenitis the focus of inflammation is lacrimal gland. The lacrimal gland is located in superotemporal part of orbit and is divided into orbital and palpebral part. This gland is mainly responsible for formation of aqueous layer of tear film. Approximately 50% cases of IOIS present as dacryoadenitis and idiopathic dacryoadenitis is the diagnosis in 30% of the total lacrimal gland biopsies.[34]

Clinical features:
- Acute dacryoadenitis can be unilateral or bilateral (Fig. 12). Bilateral presentation should raise suspicion of some underlying systemic condition
- *History*: Patient presents with pain and swelling in upper eyelid and specifically gives history of increase of swelling in the morning
- *Examination*: On examination there will be a mass palpable in superotemporal orbit giving a characteristic S-shaped deformity of the upper eyelid associated with redness and pain. There can be limitation of extraocular motility with chemosis and discharge. Patients can have proptosis or displacement of globe in inferomedial direction. On everting the lid enlarged palpebral lobe of the gland can be visualized
- *Imaging*: On CT scan there is a homogenously enlarged lacrimal gland in superotemporal part of the orbit. The gland generally molds itself according to the surrounding structures, and infiltration can be seen in lateral rectus muscle and Tenon's capsule. Compression over globe and bone erosion is rare.

Myositis: Orbital myositis is an inflammatory process localized to extraocular muscles. It is the most common cause after thyroid orbitopathy involving orbital muscles.[35] It can have varied presentation which may be unilateral or bilateral, acute or chronic, mild or severe, and involving one muscle or multiple muscles.

Clinical features:
- It is more common in third decade with a female predominance
- Clinically, patients present with complaints of pain, diplopia, proptosis, eyelid swelling and conjunctival congestion. Pain typically increases on ocular movement and is observed in 85–100% of patients whereas diplopia is the most frequent sign seen secondary to the muscle affected
- The horizontal recti muscles (29-37%) are more commonly affected (medial rectus > lateral rectus)

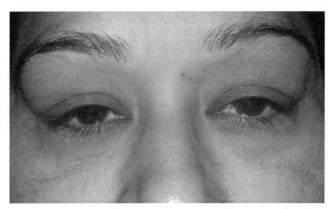

Fig. 12: Bilateral palpebral lacrimal gland.

than vertical recti muscles (0–23%).[24] Oblique muscle involvement is rare whereas isolated levator palpebrae superioris presenting as ptosis is commonly seen[5]
- *Imaging*: On CT and MRI there is diffuse enlargement of the affected muscle involving the muscle belly and tendon which forms an important differentiating feature from thyroid orbital myopathy
- *Biopsy*: Patients with atypical presentation or not showing any response to conventional treatment may require biopsy for a more definitive diagnosis.

Posterior Orbit

The posterior orbital involvement presents mainly with signs of optic neuropathy and orbital apex syndrome.

Clinical features:
- Patients present with proptosis, pain, vision loss, and limitation of ocular movements
- Signs of optic nerve can be seen like decreased visual acuity, optic disk edema, relative afferent pupillary defect, visual field, and color vision defects. Isolated optic nerve involvement is rarely seen
- *Imaging*: On CT scan the most common feature is infiltration of retro-orbital fat with proptosis, orbital apex inflammation, enlargement of extraocular muscles, and edematous optic nerve sheath.[36]

Tolosa Hunt Syndrome

Tolosa hunt syndrome is characterized by painful ophthalmoplegia due to nonspecific inflammation involving cavernous sinus or superior orbital fissure.

Features:
- This syndrome is rarely seen in first two decades of life and commonly involves adults over 20 years of age[37]
- Clinically patients present with retrobulbar pain and painful limitation of extraocular motility which is acute in onset. This can be associated with diplopia and vision loss

- Paresthesias over the forehead area can also be noticed by patients because of involvement of first division of trigeminal nerve
- *Imaging*: MRI (with or without contrast) is the investigation of choice for diagnosing soft tissue swelling around cavernous sinus.[38] Inflammatory changes are seen around cavernous sinus, superior orbital fissure, and apex of the orbit.

Extraorbital Extension

Extraorbital extension is seen in 8.6% of the cases.[39] Inflammation can spread to the cranial cavity via orbital apex or to the adjacent paranasal sinuses through the small communicating blood vessels or through erosion of the adjacent bone. There have been case reports of patients presenting with hypopituitarism, cranial nerve palsies, and transient ischemic attacks as complication associated with intracranial extension. Maxillary and ethmoid sinus are the most commonly affected paranasal sinuses though cases with spread to sphenoid sinus and pterygopalatine fossa have also been there in literature.

Sclerosing Idiopathic Orbital Inflammation

There is a rare variant of IOIS called sclerosing form of idiopathic inflammation which has very few cases reported in literature with incidence of around 5–7.8% of inflammatory orbital lesions.[40] It is characterized by insidious onset of inflammation resulting in synthesis of fibers and collagen, with injury of orbital structures. There is no gender predominance and it commonly presents in middle aged people with 44 years as mean age of presentation.[41] Its clinical features are similar to idiopathic inflammation but are more aggressive in nature. The most common presentation is proptosis, palpebral edema, and orbital pain (Figs. 13A to D).

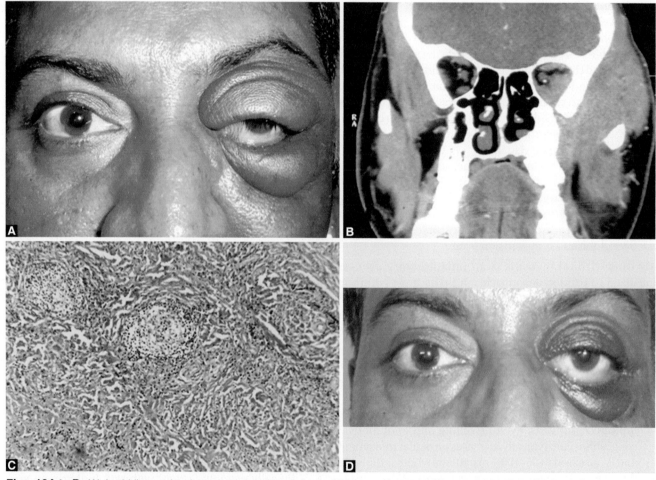

Figs. 13A to D: (A) A middle-aged patient presented with proptosis of left eye with surrounding eyelid swelling; (B) On CT scan there was an ill-defined lesion in the orbital cavity and extending till the temporal fossa; (C) On biopsy, section 10x shows abundant fibromuscular tissue with interspersed chronic inflammatory cells comprising of lymphocytes and plasma cells, also seen are collections of histiocytes surrounded lymphoplasmocytic cells; (D) Clinical picture showing improvement after a course of intravenous methylprednisolone and oral steroids for 4 weeks.

Pediatric Orbital Inflammatory Disorder

Idiopathic orbital inflammatory syndrome in pediatric age group is an uncommon entity with around 100 cases reported in literature. The clinical presentation varies in this age group. The mean age of presentation is 11 years ranging from 5 years to 17 years with no sex predominance.[42] Bilateral involvement is more common in pediatric patients than in adults and is unlikely to be associated with the underlying systemic disease as seen in adult group. The most frequent ophthalmic findings are palpable mass and decreased extraocular motility. Pain is more common in older children. Other signs commonly seen are proptosis, eyelid swelling, iritis, optic disk edema, and eosinophilia. Children most often present with dacryoadenitis and myositis form of IOIS and constitutional symptoms like fever, headache, malaise, vomiting, abdominal pain, and anorexia are often associated. Chances of having recurrence are as high as 76% as reported in literature probably due to common bilateral presentation.[43] In pediatric population infectious and neoplastic causes like rhabdomyosarcoma, leukemia, Langerhans cell histiocytosis (LCH), lymphangioma, and ruptured orbital dermoid should be kept in mind as differential diagnosis and thorough investigations should rule out all the causes before labeling it as idiopathic.

Diagnosis of IOIS

Idiopathic is a Greek work which means arising spontaneously without any cause, and therefore idiopathic diseases are diagnosis of exclusion when all other causes are negated. A meticulous history and proper examination play a very important role in ruling out other diseases and subsequent laboratory and radiological investigation help in supplementing the findings (Table 4).

Treatment of IOIS

In IOIS, the basic pathology is the underlying inflammation which affects different target tissues. This inflammation leads to localized cellular damage which leads to release of mediators like arachidonic acid and the treatment of IOIS is mainly focused on controlling the inflammation

Corticosteroids: Corticosteroids form the mainstay for treatment of such an idiopathic form of inflammatory process where they inhibit the cascade of inflammation and immune response at every level and suppress the proinflammatory cytokines.[43,44] There are various routes for steroid administration though oral route is the most preferred one.

Dose of steroids: Steroids are started at dose of 1–1.5 mg/kg of body weight/day and continued for 2–3 weeks till the inflammation subsides. After that, the dose is tapered over

TABLE 4: Investigation and differential diagnosis of orbital inflammatory disorder.

S. no.	Disease	Laboratory investigation
1.	Infectious disorders: Bacterial and fungal orbital cellulitis, orbital tuberculosis.	Complete blood count with erythrocyte sedimentation rate (ESR), Montoux test, blood and urine culture
2.	Endocrine disorders: Thyroid ophthalmopathy	Thyroid profile (TSH, T3, T4)
3.	Inflammatory causes: Sarcoidosis, Wegeners granulomatosis, xanthogranulomatosis, orbital foreign body granuloma, rheumatologic disorder	Antinuclear antibodies (ANA), antineutrophil cytoplasmic antibody (cANCA and pANCA), C-reactive protein (CRP), serum angiotensin-converting enzyme (ACE) levels, serum calcium, serum lysozyme
4.		Radiological investigation (CT/MRI)
5.		Orbital biopsy

weeks to months and reduction by 5–10 mg per week is generally advocated.

Side effects: Oral steroids lead to various side effects most common being gastritis, weight gain, cushingoid features, and mood swings. Its use can also exacerbate or induce diabetes, hypertension, glaucoma, or cataract. Prolonged use of steroids can also cause osteoporosis. Therefore, oral steroids should always be prescribed along with antacids like ranitidine and calcium or vitamin D supplements.

Nonsteroidal anti-inflammatory drugs: Patients with anterior orbital inflammation like dacryoadenitis and anterior myositis can also respond to NSAIDs like indomethacin. However, studies have reported high chance of recurrence with this group of drugs and corticosteroids still form the drug of choice. NSAIDs can be given for persistent pain later on when inflammation has subsided.[45]

Radiotherapy: Radiation in low doses can be used in patients in whom corticosteroids are contraindicated medically or in refractory cases that do not respond to steroids.

Dose: The recommended dose for orbital inflammation is around 1,000–3,000 cGy. Many lesions respond to 1,500–2,000 cGy of radiation, however, a higher dose of 2,500–3,000 cGy is needed for IOIS extending to intracranial cavity.[46-48] This dose should be administered in fractionated form over 10–14 days to avoid complications.

Side effects: Potential side effects associated with radiotherapy are cataract formation, retinopathy, and dry eye. To avoid complication, globe should be properly shielded and fractionated dose is recommended.

Immunosuppressive drugs: This category of drugs is becoming popular in cases where steroids does not work or are contraindicated. These are classified as (Table 5):

- *Antimetabolites*—methotrexate and azathioprine
- *Alkylating agents*—cyclophosphamide and chlorambucil
- *T-cell inhibitors*—cyclosporine and tacrolimus
- *Biological immunomodulators*—infliximab and etanercept.

Specific Orbital Inflammations

Wegener's Granulomatosis

Wegener's granulomatosis is a necrotizing granulomatous inflammation. This disease falls in the category of focal small vessel disease affecting multiple organs. A classical triad has been described for diagnosing disseminated Wegener's which includes necrotizing granulomatous inflammation affecting upper and lower respiratory tract with glomerulonephritis.[49]

Features:

- Ocular involvement is commonly seen in around 50% of the patients in the form of conjunctivitis, keratitis, uveitis, scleritis, and retinal vasculitis[49]
- Orbital signs are also seen in 40–50% patients with ocular signs. Patients commonly present with proptosis, pain, erythematous eyelid edema, and limitation of extraocular motility
- Orbit can get primarily affected by the disease or it could be contiguous spread from the paranasal sinuses
- Extraconal compartment is more commonly involved than intraconal
- On CT scan there is an orbital mass which is homogenous and isodense with the extraocular muscles[50]
- *Diagnosis:* For specific diagnosis ANCA levels are useful which are found to be positive in 60–96% of the patients in disseminated form but only 60–70% in focal or localized form of disease.[51,52] Histopathological confirmation is always recommended. Classically on histopathology necrotizing granulomatous vasculitis with giant cells is seen

TABLE 5: Mechanism and doses of immunosuppressive drugs in IOIS.

Drug category	Mechanism of action	Dose	Side effects
Antimetabolites:			
Methotrexate[53]	Interferes with folic acid mechanism during RNA and DNA synthesis	7.5–15 mg/kg weekly dose	Gastrointestinal disturbances, fatigue, and headache Liver enzymes should be monitored Folic acid at 1 mg per day should be added as supplement
Azathioprine	Inhibits purine synthesis	2–3 mg/kg body weight/day orally	Fever and chills, unusual bleeding and bruising including bleeding from gums and blood in urine and stools
Alkylating agents:			
Cyclophosphamide[54]	Stops cell growth by forming cross links between DNA strands and induce apoptosis	100 mg/day	Gastrointestinal disturbances, temporary hair loss
T-cell inhibitors:			
Cyclosporin[55]	Prevents transcription of interleukin-2 and inhibits lymphokine production	4 mg/kg/day	Nephropathy and hypertension. Kidney function test should be monitored
Mycophenolate mofetil[56]	Inhibits de novo purine synthesis and prevents B and T lymphocyte replication	1–2 g/day	
Biologic immunomodulators:			
Infliximab[57]	Blocks tumor necrosis factor-alpha which is a cytokine involved in pathophysiology of inflammation	3–5 mg/kg/day at, 2 and 6 weeks and to be continued 4–8 weeks thereafter till inflammation subsides	Rash, headache, respiratory congestion, and hypotension

- It is important to diagnose the disease as it is related to high mortality rate specially if disseminated form is present. It can be fatal within 2 years of diagnosis. Wegener's respond very well to systemic corticosteroids. In case of refractory cases cyclophosphamide is the drug of choice.

Sarcoidosis

Sarcoidosis is a multisystemic granulomatous disorder which is characterized by presence of noncaseating granulomas affecting different organs. Ocular involvement is seen in around 25% of patients with systemic sarcoidosis.[58] Anterior ocular involvement in the form of anterior uveitis is the most common presentation. Orbital and adnexal sarcoidosis are not uncommon entity.

Clinical features:
- The mean age of involvement is around 50–70 years of age group with female predominance
- Lacrimal gland is the most common site of presentation. Besides that, infiltration can be seen in extraocular muscles, orbital fat, and optic nerve
- Clinically, patients present with orbital mass, proptosis, diplopia, pain, and restriction of ocular motility.

Investigation: For diagnosing orbital sarcoidosis histopathology remains the main stay. However, systemic investigations are necessary to rule out systemic involvement. Elevated levels of serum ACE, serum lysozyme, and serum calcium with chest X-ray showing hilar lymphadenopathy are diagnostic for systemic sarcoidosis.

Histopathology: Biopsy shows noncaseating granulomatous inflammation with epithelioid cells, giant cells, and lymphocytes.

IgG4-related Orbital Disease

Immunoglobulin G4-related orbital disease represents a spectrum of disorders where serum IgG4 levels are elevated which causes IgG4-related lymphoplasmacyte infiltration in different parts of the body. It was first described in relation to autoimmune pancreatitis but was later found to involve almost all organs of the body including thyroid, lungs, kidney, and liver. Orbit is commonly affected with IgG4-related diseases.[59]

Features:
- It commonly affects middle aged men with median age of 59 year (30–60 years)
- Patient commonly presents with chronic eyelid selling and proptosis. Lacrimal gland (69%) is the most commonly affected part of the orbit. It can also involve extraocular muscles leading to ocular motility restriction

- Pathogenesis is poorly understood but probable hypothesis is supporting it to be either an autoimmune-mediated disease or could be related to some kind of allergies
- On histopathology typically three characteristic features are described:
  1. Dense lymphoplasmacytic infiltrate
  2. Storiform fibrosis
  3. Obliterative fibrosis with phlebitis or increased eosinophilia.
- *Treatment:* Oral corticosteroids are the main stay for treatment. In these patients relapses are often seen; therefore a combination of steroids and immunosuppressants is given.

Adult Orbital Xanthogranulomatous Disorder

Adult orbital xanthogranulomatous disease (AOXGD) is a rare group of syndromes with a poorly understood pathophysiology. It affects patients from 17 years to 85 years of age with no specific gender predisposition.[60] Clinically, AOXGD is divided into four subtypes:

1. *Adult onset granuloma (isolated lesion without any systemic lesion):* This is the least common form of AOXGDs and is limited to middle aged patients (40–80 years). This is a self-limiting disorder and does not require any kind of aggressive form of therapy.
2. *Adult onset Asthma and periocular xanthogranuloma:* This is a rare form of AOXGDs which is often associated with bilateral yellow-orange nonulcerated orbital masses. It can lead to involvement of extraocular muscles and lacrimal gland. This condition is commonly associated with adult onset asthma and is more likely to affect males than females. The underlying pathophysiology is not known but hypothesis of deranged immune mechanism is proposed. Vision remains unaffected in these patients.
3. *Necrobiotic xanthogranuloma:* This group is characterized by specific skin lesions which ulcerate leading to fibrotic changes. It affects adults from 20 years to 80 years of age and is commonly seen in association with paraproteinemia and multiple myeloma.
4. *Erdheim-Chester disease:* An idiopathic condition characterized by lymphohistiocytic infiltration of orbital tissues and various internal organs like heart, retroperitoneum, lungs, and bones. Patient should be appropriately investigated as this is a fatal condition leading to death due to cardiomyopathies, renal failure, or severe lung problems.

Histopathology: Orbital xanthogranulomatous disorders are characterized by common histopathological features which is constituted by sheets of mononucleated foamy histiocytes (xanthoma cells) infiltrating the orbicularis muscles and the orbital tissue. Touton giant cells are seen scattered amongst these sheets of histiocytes. These cells are positively stained by Oil Red O. Immunohistochemically these foamy cells are positive for CD68, CD163, and Factor XIIIa and negative for CD21, CD35, S100, and CD1a.[60]

Treatment: Intralesional corticosteroids remain the mainstay of treatment. Other modalities include chemotherapy with cyclophosphamide, vincristine, and doxorubicin. Recent treatment also includes management with interferon alpha and methotrexate too.

Drug-related Orbital Inflammation

Orbital inflammation has been reported after taking bisphosphonate group of drugs (zoledronic acid and pamidronate) and allergic response to hyaluronidase.[24,61] Patients typically present from day 1 to day 6 after getting exposed to the drug. They present with complaints of eyelid swelling, orbital pain, and diplopia. The mechanism is unknown. Apart from these drugs there have been case reports of orbital involvement after taking etanercept, intraorbital injection of alcohol, and periocular fillers which can migrate and cause inflammatory reaction (Figs. 14A and B).

Langerhans Cell Histiocytosis

Langerhans cell histiocytosis represents an uncommon form of orbital mass which is characterized by accumulation of histiocytes in various tissues. It mainly involves children with age range from 1 year to 4 years but can affect any age group with worse prognosis if present in infancy.[62]

Features:
- Three clinical forms of LCH has been described namely:
    1. Eosinophilic granuloma
    2. Hand-Schuller-Christian disease
    3. Letterer–Siwe disease.

- Orbit can be a unifocal site or can be a part of multisystem disorder. In orbit mainly bones are affected with frontal bone being the most common site followed by zygomatic, sphenoid, and maxillary in that order
- Ophthalmologist should be well versed with this condition specially if a young child presents with proptosis as thorough systemic evaluation is the mainstay for timely diagnosis
- Clinically they present with proptosis, eyelid edema, ptosis, and globe dystopia with pain
- Complete surgical excision is not required as they respond very well to chemotherapy once the diagnosis is established
- For diagnosis, biopsy is helpful which characteristically shows birbeck granules on electron microscopy and shows typical Langerhans cells on histopathology.

Secondary Orbital Inflammations

Inflammatory processes can affect orbit primarily or due to any secondary cause which can present in the form of orbital inflammation. Several lymphoproliferative disorders can involve orbit as a part of systemic illness or can just be a primary presentation. There can be other conditions like ruptured orbital dermoid, orbital foreign body, orbital tumors, etc. which can initially present as orbital inflammation and later on after proper investigations diagnosis is made.

Orbital Lymphoproliferative Disorder

Orbital lymphomas are most common tumor affecting orbit. It has been said in around 30–35% of cases orbit and adnexal lymphomas are associated with systemic lymphomas.[63] These lesions present with clinical features of orbital inflammation, so steroids should not be started without performing biopsy in such patients. In general B

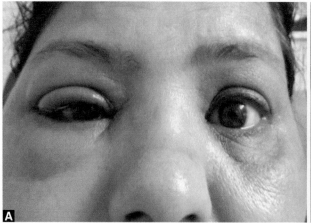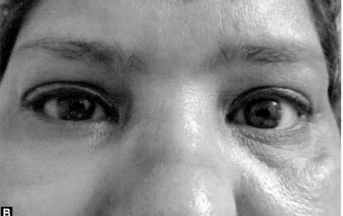

Figs. 14A and B: (A) Right lid swelling following lignocaine hypersenstivity; (B) Subsidence of inflammation following antihistaminic administration.

cell type of lymphoma is more common than T-cell in orbit with low-grade marginal zone B cell subtype being the most common. Clinically, patient presents with painless

proptosis, insidious in onset, diplopia, and limitation of ocular motility. Vision is usually preserved till late stages. These lesions commonly involve anterior superior orbit. Treatment in such cases is based on the type of lymphoma (Fig. 15).

Orbital Foreign Body

Orbital foreign bodies can present with orbital inflammations as a delayed presentation specially in children who do not give history of any past injury. A CT or MRI can rule out any foreign body. Treatment is foreign body removal (Figs. 16A to C).

Orbital hemorrhage: Acute onset orbital hemorrhage with proptosis and motility limitation can be caused by varices and lymphangioma.

Summary

Orbital infections and inflammations can present with same features but can have variety of underlying etiologies. One should be aware of all the conditions and treatment should

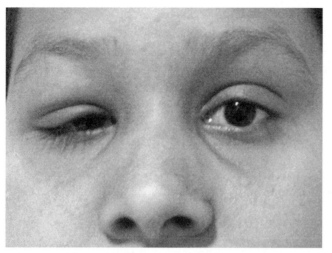

Fig. 15: A young female presented with orbital inflammation localized to superior orbit, that was later diagnosed as B cell lymphoma on biopsy.

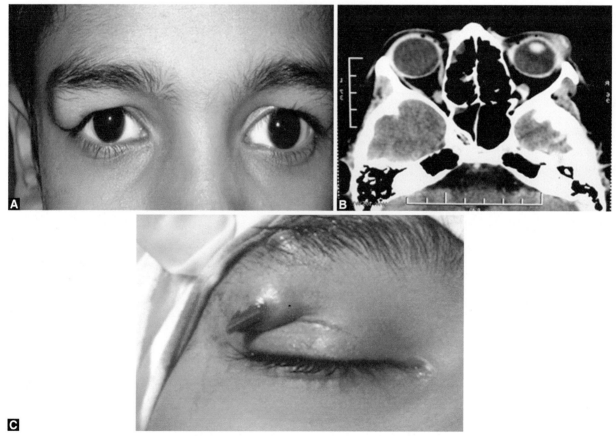

Figs. 16A to C: (A) A 12-year-old child presented with nonresolving superotemporal orbital inflammation for 2 months; (B) Axial section of CT scan showed a hyperdense shadow in a well-defined isodense lesion in superotemporal quadrant; (C) On exploration a wooden foreign body was found.

only be started after confirming the diagnosis either through laboratory investigations or biopsy. Corticosteroids are the mainstay of treatment in cases of orbital inflammatory lesions but one should be cautious before starting and should always rule out infectious etiologies (Flowcharts 1 and 2).

Flowchart 1: Treatment protocol for patient presenting with typical signs and symptoms of idiopathic orbital inflammatory syndrome.

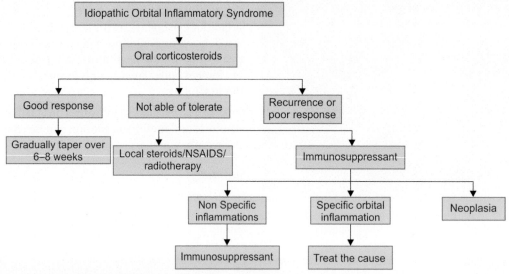

(NSAIDs: nonsteroidal anti-inflammatory drugs)

Flowchart 2: Treatment protocol for patients with orbital cellulitis.

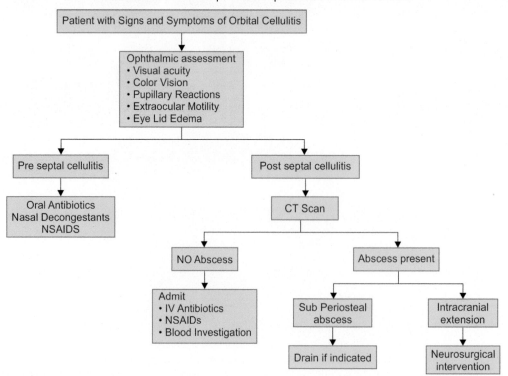

(NSAIDs: nonsteroidal anti-inflammatory drugs)

REFERENCES

1. Chandler JR, Langenbrunner DJ, Stevens ER. The pathogenesis of orbital complications in acute sinusitis. Laryngoscope. 1970;80(9):1414-28.

2. Ambati BK, Ambati J, Azar N, et al. Periorbital and orbital cellulitis before and after the advent of *Haemophilus influenza* type B vaccination. Ophthalmology. 2000;107(8):1450-3.

3. Seltz LB, Smith J, Durairaj VD, et al. Microbiology and antibiotic management of orbital cellulitis. Pediatrics. 2011;127(3):e566-72.

4. McKinley SH, Yen MT, Miller AM, et al. Microbiology of pediatric orbital cellulitis. Am J Ophthalmol. 2007;144(4):497-501.

5. Garcia GH, Harris GJ. Criteria for nonsurgical management of subperiosteal abscess of the orbit: Analysis of outcomes 1988-98. Ophthalmology. 2000;107(8):1454-8.

6. Ahmad R, Salman R, Islam S, et al. Cavernous sinus thrombosis as a complication of sphenoid sinusitis: A case report and review of literature. Internet J Otorhinolaryngol. 2009;12(1):11770.

7. Tabarino F, Elmaleh-Bergès M, Quesnel S, et al. Subperiosteal orbital abscess: Volumetric criteria for surgical drainage. Int J Pediatr Otorhinolaryngol. 2015;79(2):131-5.

8. Madge SN, Prabhakaran VC, Shome D, et al. Orbital tuberculosis: A review of the literature. Orbit. 2008;27(4):267-77.

9. Mukherjee B, Raichura ND, Alam MS. Fungal infections of the orbit. Indian J Ophthalmol. 2016;64(5):337-45.

10. Nimir AR, Saliem A, Ibrahim IA, et al. Ophthalmic parasitosis: A review article. Interdiscip Perspect Infect Dis. 2012;2012:587402.

11. Limaiem F, Bellil S, Bellil K, et al. Primary orbital hydatid cyst in an elderly patient. Surg Infect (Larchmt). 2010;11(4):393-5.

12. Mehta M, Sen S, Sethi S, et al. Large orbital hydatid cyst presenting as subconjunctival mass. Ann Trop Med Parasitol. 2010;104(7):601-4.

13. Betharia SM, Sharma V, Pushkar N. Ultrasound Findings in Orbital Hydatid Cysts. American journal of ophthalmology. Am J Ophthalmol. 2003;135(4):568-70.

14. Bodh SA, Kamal S, Kumar S, et al. Orbital cysticercosis. Del J Ophthalmol. 2012;23(2):99-103.

15. Rath S, Honavar SG, Naik M, et al. Orbital cysticercosis: Clinical manifestation, diagnosis, management, and outcome. Ophthalmology. 2010;117(3):600-5.

16. Sudan R, Muralidhar R, Sharma P. Optic nerve cysticercosis: Case report and review of current management. Orbit. 2005;24(2):159-62.

17. Foster S, Vitale A. Cysticercosis. In: Diagnosis and Treatment of Uveitis, 2nd edition. New Delhi, India: Jaypee-Brothers Medical Publishers; 2013. pp. 1-1290.

18. Sekhar GC, Honavar SG. Myocysticercosis: Experience with imaging and therapy. Ophthalmology. 1999;106(12):2336-40.

19. Sotelo J, Escobedo F, Penagos P. Albendazole vs praziquantel for therapy for neurocysticercosis. A controlled trial. Arch Neurol. 1988;45(5):532-4.

20. Gleason J. Idiopathic myositis involving the intraocular muscles. Ophthalmol Rec. 1903;12:471-8.

21. Birch-Hirschfeld A. Handbuch der Gesamten Augenheikunde. Berlin, Germany: Julius Springer; 1930. p. 9.

22. Henderson JW. Orbital tumors. In: Decker BC (Ed). New York, NY: Thieme-Stratton; 1980. pp. 68-70.

23. Weber AL, Romo LV, Sabates NR. Pseudotumor of the orbit. Clinical, pathological, and radiologic evaluation. Radiol Clin North Am.1999;37(1):151-68, xi.

24. Yuen SJ, Rubin PA. Idiopathic orbital inflammation: Distribution, clinical features, and treatment outcome. Arch Ophthalmol. 2003;121(4):491-9.

25. Mombaerts I, Koorneef L. Current status in the treatment of orbital myositis. Ophthalmology. 1997;104(3):402-8.

26. Reese AB. Tumors of the eye. New York, NY: Harper & Row; 1951. pp. 68-143.

27. Easton JA, Smith WT. Non-specific granuloma of orbit ("orbital pseudotumor"). J Pathol Bacteriol. 1961;82:345-54.

28. Serop S, Vianna RN, Claeys M, et al. Orbital myositis secondary to systemic lupus erythematosus. Acta Ophthalmol (Copenh). 1994;72(4):520-3.

29. Squires RH Jr. Zweiner RJ, Kennedy RH. Orbital myositis and Crohn's disease. J Pediatr Gastroenterol Nutr.1992;15(4):448-51.

30. Van de Mossetaer G, Van Deuren H, Dewolf-Peeters C, et al. Pseudotumor orbitae and myasthenia gravis. A case report. Arch Ophthalmol.1980;98(9):1621-2.

31. Weinstein JM, Koch K, Lane S. Orbital pseudotumor in Crohn's colitis. Ann Ophthalmol. 1984;16(3):275-8.

32. Young RS, Hodes BL, Cruse RP, et al. Orbital pseudotumor and Crohn's disease. J Pediatr.1981;99(2):250-2.

33. Atabay C, Tyutyunikov A, Scalise D, et al. Serum antibodies reactive with eye muscle membrane antigens are detected in patients with nonspecific orbital inflammation. Ophthalmology. 1995;102(1):145-53.

34. Andrew NH, Kearney D, Sladden N, et al. Idiopathic dacryoadenitis: Clinical features, histopathology, and treatment outcomes. Am J Ophthalmol. 2016;163:148-153.e1.

35. Costa RM, Dumitrascu OM, Gordon LK. Orbital myositis: Diagnosis and management. Curr Allergy Asthma Rep. 2009;9(4):316-23.

36. Patankar T, Prasad S, Krishnan A, et al. Isolated optic nerve pseudotumor. Australas Radiol. 2000;44(1):101-3.

37. Zanus C, Furlan C, Costa P, et al. The Tolosa-Hunt syndrome in children: A case report. Cephalalgia. 2009;29(11):1232-7.

38. Mormont E, Laloux P, Vauthier J, et al. Radiotherapy in a case of Tolosa Hunt syndrome. Cephalalgia. 2000;20(10):931-3.

39. Tay E, Gibson A, Chaudhary N, et al. Idiopathic orbital inflammation with extensive intra- and extracranial extension presenting as 6th nerve palsy—a case report and literature review. Orbit. 2008;27(6):458-61.

40. Hsuan JD, Selva D, McNab AA, et al. Idiopathic sclerosing orbital inflammation. Arch Ophthalmol. 2006;124(9):1244-50.

41. Corrêa CM, Cunha AD Junior, Machado R, et al. Sclerosing orbital pseudotumor: Pseudotumor esclerosante de órbita. Rev Bras Oftalmol. 2016;75(5):398-400.

42. Spindle J, Tang SX, Davies B, et al. Pediatric idiopathic orbital inflammation: Clinical features of 30 cases. Ophthalmic Plast Reconstr Surg. 2016;32(4):270-4.

43. Harris GJ. Idiopathic orbital inflammation: A pathogenetic construct and treatment strategy: The 2005 ASOPRS Foundation Lecture. Ophthalmic Plast Reconstr Surg. 2006;22(2):79-86.

44. Mombaerts I, Schlingemann RO, Goldschmeding R, et al. Are systemic corticosteroids useful in the management of orbital pseudotumors? Ophthalmology. 1996;103(3):521-8.

45. Nobel AG, Tripathi RC, Levine RA. Indomethacin for the treatment of idiopathic orbital myositis. Am J Ophthalmol. 1989;108(3):336-8.

46. Sergott RC, Glaser JS, Charyulu K. Radiotherapy for idiopathic inflammatory orbital pseudotumor. Indications and results. Arch Ophthalmol. 1981;99(5):853-6.

47. Orcutt JC, Garner A, Henk JM, et al. Treatment of idiopathic inflammatory orbital pseudotumours by radiotherapy. Br J Ophthalmol. 1983;67(9):570-4.

48. Lanciano R, Fowble B, Sergott RC, et al. The results of radiotherapy for orbital pseudotumor. Int J Radiat Oncol Biol Phys. 1990;18(2):407-11.

49. Ostri C, Heegaard S, Prause JU. Sclerosing Wegener's granulomatosis in the orbit. Acta Ophthalmol. 2008;86(8):917-20.

50. Provenzale JM, Mukherji S, Allen NB, et al. Orbital involvement by Wegener's granulomatosis: Imaging findings. AJR Am J Roentgenol. 1996;166(4):929-34.

51. Nolle B, Specks U, Ludemann J, et al. Anticytoplasmic autoantibodies: Their immunodiagnostic value in Wegener's granulomatosis. Ann Intern Med. 1989;111:28-40.

52. Pulido JS, Goeken JA, Nerad JA, et al. Ocular manifestation of patients with circulating antineutrophil cytoplasmic antibodies. Arch Ophthalmol. 1990;108(6):845-50.

53. Smith JR, Rosenbaum JT. A role for methotrexate in the management of non-infectious orbital inflammatory disease. Br J Ophthalmol. 2001;85(10):1220-4.

54. Garrity JA, Kennerdell JS, Johnson BL, et al. Cyclophosphamide in the treatment of orbital vasculitis. Am J Ophthalmol. 1986;102(1):97-103.

55. Zacharopoulos IP, Papadaki T, Manor RS, et al. Treatment of idiopathic orbital inflammatory disease with cyclosporine-A: A case presentation. Semin Ophthalmol. 2009;24(6):260-1.

56. Hatton MP, Rubin PA, Foster CS. Successful treatment of idiopathic orbital inflammation with mycophenolate mofetil. Am J Ophthalmol. 2005;140(5):916-8.

57. Miquel T, Abad B, Badelon I, et al. Successful treatment of idiopathic orbital inflammation with infliximab: An alternative to conventional steroid-sparing agents. Ophthalmic Plast Reconstr Surg. 2008;24(5):415-7.

58. Vagn. Sarcoidosis of the orbit. Acta Ophthalmol. 1957:416-9.

59. Kubota T, Moritani S. Orbital IgG4-related disease: Clinical features and diagnosis. ISRN Rheumatol. 2012;2012:412896.

60. Guo J, Wang J. Adult orbital xanthogranulamatous disease: Review of the literature. Arch Pathol Lab Med. 2009;133(12):1994-7.

61. Pirbhai A, Rajak SN, Goold LA, et al. Bisphosphonate-induced orbital inflammation: A case series and review. Orbit. 2015;34(6):331-5.

62. Herwig MC, Wojno T, Zhang Q, et al. Langerhans cell histiocytosis of the orbit: Five clinicopathologic cases and review of the literature. Surv Ophthalmol. 2013;58(4):330-40.

63. Lam Choi VB, Yuen HK, Biswas J, et al. Update in pathological diagnosis of orbital infections and inflammations. Middle East Afr J Ophthalmol. 2011;18(4):268-76.

Thyroid-associated Orbitopathy

Ruchi Goel, Amit Goel

INTRODUCTION

Thyroid-associated orbitopathy (TAO) or thyroid eye disease (TED), an autoimmune inflammatory disorder, is the most common disease affecting the orbit. TAO may be associated with Graves' hyperthyroidism (90%), primary hypothyroidism (1%), Hashimoto thyroiditis (3%), or the patient may be euthyroid (6%). Though most patients with TED have hyperthyroidism at presentation, eventually, only 30% of patients with hyperthyroidism will develop TAO. It is six times more common in women. The peak incidence in females is observed in 40–44 years and 60–64 years age group whereas in males it occurs in 45–49 years and 65-69 years. It is seven times more common in smokers. Although TAO is more common in women, the severity is more in men. It accounts for ~85% of cases of bilateral exophthalmos. A genetic predisposition is indicated with positive family history in 20–60% patients.

Graves' disease (GD) is a syndrome consisting of hyperthyroid goiter, thyroid-associated orbitopathy, and dermopathy. Factors associated with increased risk and severity of ophthalmopathy in GD are tobacco use, genetics, type of treatment for hyperthyroidism, thyrotropin/thyroid-stimulating hormone (TSH) receptor (TSH-R) antibody levels, advanced age, and stress; *cigarette smoking being the strongest modifiable risk factor for developing TAO.* Other related autoimmune diseases like myasthenia gravis are 50 times more common in patients with TAO. Presence of myasthenia gravis is associated with worse prognosis. Patients with concurrent diabetes mellitus have a higher predisposition to dysthyroid optic neuropathy (DON).

PATHOGENESIS[1]

The normal thyroid hormone function starts at the hypothalamus. Thyroid-releasing hormone (TRH) is released through the hypothalamic-hypophyseal portal system to the anterior pituitary gland resulting in release of TSH.

Thyroid-stimulating hormone on release into the blood, travels to the thyroid gland, and directly binds to the *TSH-R on the basolateral aspect of the thyroid follicular cell.* TSH-R is a G-protein coupled receptor, and its activation results in activation of adenylyl cyclase and intracellular levels of cyclic adenosine monophosphate (cAMP) which in turn activates the follicular cells of the thyroid gland, the enzyme thyroid peroxidase (TPO), synthesis of thyroglobulin, and uptake of iodide from the bloodstream and formation of T3 and T4 (Flowchart 1).

The normal reference range of thyroid hormones is as follows:

Serum T4	4.6–12 µg/dL
Serum T3	80–180 ng/dL
Serum TSH	0.5–6 mIU/L

Graves' disease is an autoimmune thyroid disease caused by the production of IgG autoantibodies directed against the thyrotropin receptor (TSHR). These antibodies bind to the thyrotropin receptor and cause its activation leading to autonomous production of thyroid hormones.

It is postulated that thyroid and orbital tissue may share a common antigen. These antigens could be thyroglobulin, the TSH receptor, insulin-like growth factor (IGF-1) receptor, or extraocular muscle antigens. TED is triggered by binding and activation of orbital fibroblasts by autoantibodies.

Types of orbital fibroblasts:
- *Thy-1+ orbital fibroblasts:* These generate higher levels of PGE_2 and show exaggerated expression of

Flowchart 1: Steps involved in regulation of thyroid hormone release.

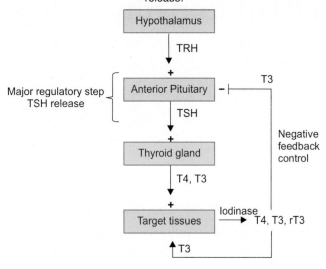

prostaglandin-endoperoxide H synthase (PGHS)-2, and are responsible for robust fibrosis
- Thy-1- orbital fibroblasts express high levels of IL-8 and have adipogenic potential.

Activated orbital fibroblasts release chemokines (Fig. 1).

Chemokines recruit T-lymphocytes into the orbit. These lymphocytes then interact with fibroblasts, the mutual activation results in promotion of cytokine production and secretion of T-cell activating factors. The synthesis of hyaluronan and glycosaminoglycan (GAG) is increased. This results in the deposition of extracellular matrix molecules, fibroblast proliferation, and adipogenesis.

On exposure of orbital fibroblasts to cigarette extract, there is increased production of GAGs and adipogenesis. Cessation of smoking prevents worsening of orbitopathy.

CLINICAL FEATURES

The natural course of TAO is self-limited. There is an active phase of inflammation and progression that stabilizes spontaneously within 3–5 years of onset. Reactivation of inflammation occurs in 5–10% patients over their lifetime.

Rundle described the orbital changes in three phases:[2]

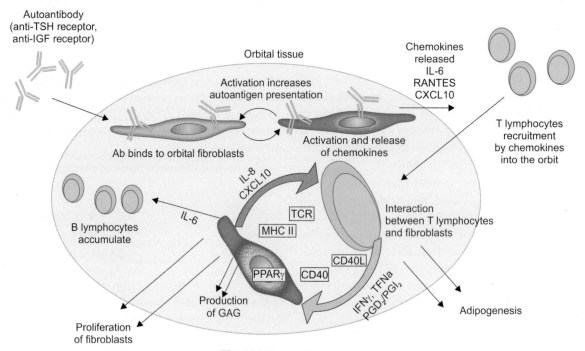

Fig. 1: Pathogenesis of TAO.

1. *Initial phase:* Orbital and periorbital signs including proptosis and eyelid retraction are present.
2. *Static phase:* There is little clinical improvement despite reduced inflammation.
3. *Quiescent phase:* Gradual improvement in ocular motility and lid retraction. Improvement of upper lid retraction occurs in majority of cases but course of recovery of ocular motility is variable. Proptosis mostly shows slight improvement.

Initial symptoms are complaints of foreign-body sensation, tearing, or photophobia. Periorbital inflammation occurs early in the disease course. The most characteristic signs (Table 1) are eyelid erythema and swelling, caruncular and conjunctival injection, and edema. In active disease the upper or lower eyelid swelling may fluctuate. In congestive ophthalmopathy there is chronic swelling in the absence of erythema. Proptosis and lid retraction with lateral eyelid flare (pathognomonic of TAO) can present during any phase of Graves' orbitopathy (GO) that results in the characteristic staring appearance. Lid retraction (Dalrymple's sign is

the most frequent sign in TAO which affects 90–98% of patients). Lid retraction is known to occur due to increased sympathetic stimulation of Muller's muscle, contraction of the levator muscle, and scarring between the lacrimal gland fascia and levator, which specifically gives rise to the lateral flare (Fig. 2 and Table 1).

Other common findings include lid lag in which the excursion of the upper eyelid lags behind eyeball movement

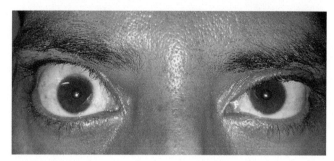

Fig. 2: Right upper lid retraction with lateral flare.

TABLE 1: Common signs of thyroid eye disease.

Facial and general signs	Joffroy's sign	Absent crease on forehead on upgaze
	Kocher's sign	Staring appearance (Fig. 3)
	Vigouroux sign	Eyelid fullness of puffiness (Fig. 4)
	Rosenbach's sign	Tremors of eyelids when closed
	Riesman's sign	Bruit over the lids
Upper eye lid signs	Von Graefe's sign	Upper lid lag on down gaze (Fig. 5)
	Dalrymple's sign	Upper eye lid retraction (Fig. 6)
	Stellwag's sign	Incomplete or infrequent blinking
	Grove sign	Resistance to pulling the retracted upper lid
	Boston sign	Uneven jerky movements of upper lid on inferior gaze
	Jellinek's sign	Abnormal pigmentation of the upper lid
	Gifford's sign	Difficulty in everting the upperlid
	Means sign	Increase superior scleral show on upgaze
Lower eyelid signs	Enroth's sign	Edema of the lower lid
	Griffith's sign	Lower lid lag on upgaze
Extraocular muscle movement signs	Moebius's sign	Inability to converge the eyes
	Ballet's sign	Restriction of one or more extraocular muscle
	Suker's sign	Poor fixation on abduction
	Jendrassik's sign	Paralysis of all extraocular muscles
Conjunctival signs	Goldzeiher's sign	Conjunctival injection (Fig. 7)
Pupillary signs	Knies sign	Uneven pupillary dilatation in dim light
	Cowen's sign	Jerky contraction of pupil to light
	Lowi's sign	Dilatation of pupil with weak epinephrine solution

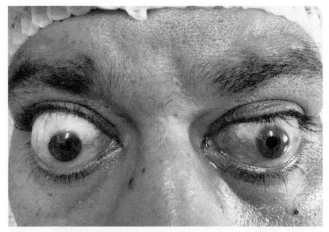

Fig. 3: Staring appearance: Kocher's sign.

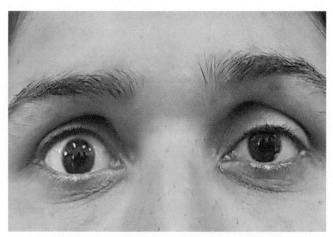

Fig. 6: Right upper lid retraction: Dalrymple's sign.

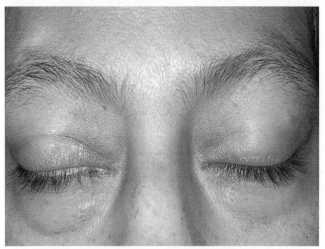

Fig. 4: Eyelid fullness of puffiness: Vigouroux sign.

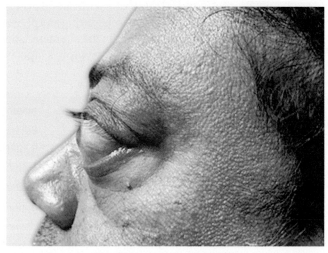

Fig. 7: Conjunctival injection.

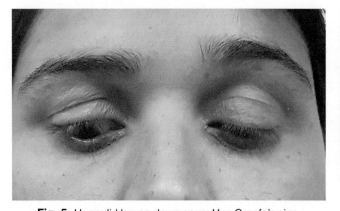

Fig. 5: Upper lid lag on down gaze: Von Graefe's sign.

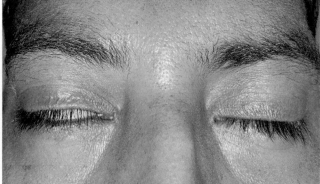

Fig. 8: Lagophthalmos.

on vertical downward pursuit and remains high; incomplete eyelid closure (lagophthalmos) (Fig. 8); and exposure symptoms (foreign body sensation, grittiness, photophobia, and lacrimation) secondary to the wide palpebral aperture combined with poor blinking, leading to increased tear evaporation.

Conjunctival and caruncle signs usually suggest active disease. Conjunctival signs include deep temporal injection, enlarged vessels over the insertion of the medial and lateral rectus muscles, and chemosis.

Exophthalmos occurs following increase in soft tissue mass within the bony orbit in the form of enlargement of the extraocular muscles or increased orbital fat volume. It is almost always bilateral and usually relatively symmetrical. Retropulsion, that is, attempts to push the globe back into the orbit are met with firm resistance because of the inflammatory orbital changes that preclude displacement of the fat.

Limitation of ocular motility results due to involvement of extraocular muscles. The inferior rectus muscle is involved most commonly, followed by the medial rectus and the superior rectus. Radiological evidence of muscle involvement may precede clinical presentation.

Intraocular pressure may increase on gaze in the opposite direction of the restricted muscle. In particular, this is seen on up gaze with inferior rectus restriction.

Diminished tear production resulting from lacrimal gland infiltration and lagophthalmos from proptosis or loss of Bells phenomenon from inferior rectus infiltration can also complicate management.

Orbital swelling at the apex can cause pressure on the optic nerve leading to DON. DON is only seen in severe disease with crowding of the orbit apex by enlarged extraocular muscles and it affects only 5% of clinical TAO patients. Risk factors for optic neuropathy include older age, smoking, male gender, and significant strabismus with mild proptosis.

DIAGNOSIS OF THYROID EYE DISEASE

Diagnosis of TED is made on presence of two of the following three signs:
1. Concurrent or recently treated immune-related thyroid dysfunction (one or more of the following):
   i. Graves' hyperthyroidism
   ii. Hashimoto thyroiditis
   iii. Circulating thyroid antibodies without a coexisting dysthyroid state, TSH-R antibodies, thyroid-binding inhibitory immunoglobulins (TBII), thyroid-stimulating immunoglobulins (TSI), and antimicrosomal antibody.
2. Typical orbital signs (one or more of the following):
   i. Unilateral (U/L) or bilateral (B/L) eyelid retraction with typical temporal flare
   ii. U/L or B/L proptosis (on comparison with old photographs)
   iii. Restrictive strabismus in a typical pattern
   iv. Compressive optic neuropathy

   v. Fluctuating eyelid edema/erythema
   vi. Chemosis/caruncular edema.
3. Radiological evidence: U/L or B/L fusiform enlargement of one or more of the following:
   i. Inferior rectus muscle
   ii. Medial rectus muscle
   iii. Superior rectus muscle
   iv. Lateral rectus muscle.

Computed tomography (CT) is the preferred imaging technique for evaluating Graves' orbitopathy (Fig. 9). CT is more sensitive than magnetic resonance imaging (MRI) in identifying enlarged extraocular muscles. Typically there is enlargement of the muscle belly with sparing of the tendinous insertions, an apparent increase in orbital fat volume, and crowding of the optic nerve at the orbital apex. Imaging helps in assessment of the degree of extraocular muscle and orbital fat involvement and delineation of sinus and skull base anatomy prior to radiation therapy or decompressive surgery.

TED is often confused with pseudotumor (idiopathic orbital inflammatory disorder). The features shown in Table 2 help in differentiation.

CLASSIFICATION OF THYROID-ASSOCIATED ORBITOPATHY

Various classifications have evolved over the time.
• Based on types (Table 3):[3]
• NO SPECS was classification given by Werner in 1969[4] (Table 4).
Weaknesses of NO SPECS classification limiting its prognostic value:

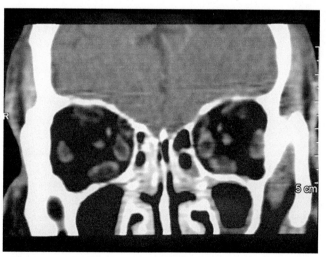

Fig. 9: Coronal view CT scan showing bilateral enlargement of all the recti.

TABLE 2: Differences between pseudotumor and Graves orbitopathy.

Variable	Pseudotumor	Graves orbitopathy
Sex predilection	None	More common in females
Mode of onset	Typically, acute but can be subacute or chronic	Subacute to chronic
Pain	Usually present	Painless unless there is keratitis or marked orbital congestion
Laterality	Usually unilateral	Usually bilateral
Lid signs	Edema, erythema, ptosis	Edema, retraction, lagophthalmos
Systemic symptoms	Possible malaise	Those of thyroid disease
Response to steroids	Often immediate	Less dramatic
Radiographic signs	Infiltrative or mass lesion, uveoscleral enhancement, Extraocular muscle is involved at the tendon	Extraocular muscle is involved at the belly sparing the tendon, expanded orbital fat compartment, bulging orbital septum
Ultrasonography	Uveoscleral thickening with tenon's edema (T sign)	Enlarged extraocular muscle

TABLE 3: Classification based on types.

Types	
I	Minimal inflammation and restrictive myopathy
II	Significant orbital inflammation and restrictive myopathy

TABLE 4: Werner's NOSPECS classification.

Class	Grade	
0		No signs or symptoms
1		Only signs
2	0	Soft tissue involvement, with symptoms and sign
	A	Absent
	B	Minimal
	C	Moderate
		Marked
3	0	Proptosis
	A	<23
	B	23–24 mm
	C	25–27 mm
		≥28 mm
4	0	Extraocular muscle involvement
	A	Absent
	B	Limitation of motion in extremes of gaze
	C	Evident restriction of movement
		Fixed eyeball
5	0	Corneal involvement
	A	Absent
	B	Stippling of cornea
	C	Ulceration
		Clouding
6	0	Sight loss
	A	Absent
	B	20/20–20/60
	C	20/70–20/200
		<20/200

Box 1: Van Dyke's RELIEF classification.

Resistance to retropulsion

Edema of conjunctiva and caruncle

Lacrimal gland enlargement

Injection over the horizontal rectus muscle insertions

Edema of the eyelids

Fullness of the eyelids

- Patients may fall into more than one class and may not follow a systematic progression from class 1 to class 6
- Absence of marked proptosis or other signs of severe disease even in patients with visual loss from compressive optic neuropathy.

- Van Dyke refined the class 2 of NO SPECS soft tissue findings with the mnemonic RELIEF[5] (Box 1)
- Clinical activity score (CAS) described by Mourits and colleagues is widely utilized[6,7] (Table 5). It attempts to identify patients with active disease who are likely to respond to medical therapy. Each symptom or sign is assigned equal weight; the score is a simple summation. A score of 3 or less is considered as inactive and 4 or more is active eye disease and thus is supposedly more likely to respond to immunosuppression.

Limitation of CAS:
- Depends on subjectivity of both patient and clinician
- Fails to account for active improvement or worsening of the disease.

Advantage of CAS: Inexpensive and can be done instantly in a clinic.

- VISA classification by Dolman and Rootman is based on the international working group's suggestion to follow four disease endpoints that can be used in the

TABLE 5: Clinical activity score described by Mourits.

Clinical activity score is the sum of all items present	
Pain	• Painful, oppressive feeling on or behind the globe during the last 2 weeks • Pain on attempted up, side or down gaze during the last 4 weeks
Redness	• Redness of the eyelids • Diffuse redness of the conjunctiva covering at least one quadrant
Swelling	• Swelling of the eyelids • Chemosis • Swollen caruncle • Increase of proptosis ≥2 mm during a period of 1–3 months
Impaired function	• Decrease of eye movements in any direction ≥5° during a period of 1–3 months • Decrease of visual acuity of ≥1 line on the snellen chart during a period of 1–3 months

office setting to record changes and to guide and assess therapy (Table 6)

These clinical points include vision, inflammation, strabismus, and appearance (VISA).[8]

Advantages:
- Each section records subjective and measurable objective inputs that aid in planning ancillary testing and treatment
- It helps direct appropriate management for patients with GO in a logical sequence.
• European Group on Graves' orbitopathy (EUGOGO) classification (Table 7).

MANAGEMENT

Treatment of Thyroid Gland Dysfunction

Restoration and maintenance of euthyroidism should be done promptly. Thyroid profile is repeated every 4–6 weeks. Antithyroid drugs are used for treating hyperthyroidism. Intolerance or ineffectiveness of antithyroid drugs is an indication for radioactive iodine (RAI). Worsening of TED with RAI may occur due to release of TSH-R antigens which incite immune response. Also, irreversible hypothyroidism may occur after RAI treatment.

A prophylactic steroid cover should be given to patients with active GO on administration of radioiodine.

Supportive Measures

• Lubricant eye drops during the day and/or lubricant ointments at night-time, cool compresses, and head elevation when sleeping
• Prisms for symptomatic diplopia

• 5% guanethidine sulfate drops transiently improve mild eyelid retraction (side effect—worsened ocular redness and pain)
• Botulinum toxin injection for upper lid retraction.

Medical Management

Glucocorticoids

Used for their anti-inflammatory and immunosuppressive actions with response rate from 63% to 77%. IV steroids have higher effectiveness and fewer side effects and are now the mainstay of treatment. Pulse therapy with intravenous methylprednisolone 500 mg weekly for 6 weeks followed by 250 mg weekly for next 6 weeks is used widely.

As the response to intravenous steroids is usually seen within 1–2 weeks of commencement of treatment, absence of response justifies rapid withdrawal of medication, avoiding longer term side effects. The cumulative dose of IV steroids should be no more than 6–8 g. Routine liver assessment is performed to rule out liver toxicity during and after treatment. Recurrences are not infrequent, thus repeated dosing is often required.

Radiotherapy

This has a nonspecific anti-inflammatory effect. It destroys the radiosensitive lymphocytes and reduces GAGs production. A cumulative dose of 20 Gy per eye fractioned in 10 daily doses over 2 weeks is usually used. The transient exacerbation of inflammation can be avoided by simultaneous steroid administration.

Antioxidants

Nicotinamide and allopurinol have been successfully used in mild and moderately severe, newly diagnosed active disease.

Somatostatin Analogs

Somatostatin analogs such as octreotide and lanreotide bind to certain somatostatin receptors on surface of various orbital cells like lymphocytes, fibroblasts, and muscle cells, thereby altering their immunologic and metabolic activities.

Targeted Antibody-based Therapies

Targeted antibody-based therapies are recently gaining lot of attention due to lesser side effects and promising results (Table 8).

Steroid-sparing Immunosuppressive Drugs

Cyclosporine affects both cell-mediated and humoral immune reactions. But the effect of cyclosporine given as

TABLE 6: VISA classification by Dolman and Rootman.

Visa Classification Date	Visit #			Patient Label:
ORBITOPATHY Time since onset: Progress: Tempo: Symptoms: Therapy:	THYROID Time since onset: Progress: Status: Symptoms: Anti-thyroid meds: Radioactive iodine:			GENERAL Smoking: Family Hx: Medical Hx: Allergies: Meds:

Subjective	Objective	OD	OS	
VISION Vision: n/abn Color vis: n/abn Fundus Progress: s/b/w	Central vision: sc/cc/ph with manifest Color vision errors (AO) Pupils (afferent defect) Optic nerve: Edema pallor	20/___ 20/___ y/n y/n y/n	20/___ 20/___ y/n y/n y/n	Refractions Wearing ___+___×___ ___+___×___ Manifest ___+___×___ ___+___×___ Normal <4
INFLAMMATORY Retrobulbar ache At rest (0–1) with gaze (0–1) Lid swelling AM: y/n Progress: s/b/w	Chemosis (0–2) Conjunctival injection (0–1) Lid injection (0–1) Lid edema upper (0–2) Lower (0–2)			Inflammatory index (worst eye/eyelid) Chemosis (0–2): Conjunctival injection (0–1): Lid injection (0–1:) Lid edema (0–2): Retrobulbar ache (0–2) Total (8):
Strabismus/Motility Diplopia: None (0) With gaze (1) Intermittent (2) Constant (3) Head turn: y/n Progress: s/b/n	Ductions (degrees): Restriction > 45° 30–45° 15–30° < 15°	+ 0 1 2 3	+ 0 1 2 3	Prism Measure: ↑ ← ↓ →
Appearance/Exposure Lid retraction y/n Proptosis y/n Tearing y/n FB Sensation y/n	Lid retraction (upper): MRD- 4 (lower scleral show): Levator function Lagophthalmos Exophthalmometry (Hertel) Corneal ulcers IOP – straight –Up	mm mm mm mm mm y/n y/n mmHg mmHg	mm mm mm mm mm y/n y/n mmHg mmHg	Fat prolapse and eyelid position: Base:
Disease Grading V (optic neuropathy) I (inflammation) 0-8 S (strabismus) 0-3 (restriction) 0-3 A (appearance/exposure)		Grade y/n /8 /3 /3 mid/mod/ severe	Progress/Response s/b/w s/b/w s/b/w s/b/w s/b/w	
MANAGEMENT			FOLLOW-UP INTERVAL:	

TABLE 7: European group on Graves' orbitopathy (EUGOGO) classification.

Sight-threatening GO	Patients with dysthyroid optic neuropathy (DON) and/ or corneal breakdown. This category warrants immediate intervention.
Moderate-to-severe GO	These patients usually have any one or more ot the following: lid retraction >2 mm, moderate or severe soft tissue involvement, exophthalmos >3 mm above normal for race and gender, inconstant, or constant diplopia.
Mild GO	These patients usually have only one or more of the following: Minor lid retraction (<2 mm), mild soft tissue involvement, exophthalmos < 3 mm above normal for race and gender, transient or no diplopia, and corneal exposure responsive to lubricants.

TABLE 8: Targeted antibody-based therapies for thyroid associated ophthalmopathy.

Immunotherapeutic agent	Target receptor against which antibody acts
Rituximab	CD-20
Adalimumab	Tumor necrosis factor alpha
Infliximab	Tumor necrosis factor alpha
Tocilizumab	Interleukin- 6
Teprotumumab	Insulin like growth factor 1

TABLE 9: Management of TAO depending on disease severity.[9]

Disease severity	Intervention
Mild	Observation Lifestyle changes Smoking cessation Elevation of head end of the bed Wearing sunglasses Ocular surface lubrication
Moderate	Topical cyclosporine Eyelid taping at night Moisture goggles Prisms/selective ocular patching Moderate dose oral steroid therapy
Severe	High dose oral steroid therapy or intravenous steroid therapy Surgical orbital decompression followed by strabismus surgery and eyelid surgery Periocular radiotherapy
Refractory	Steroid sparing immunomodulators

monotherapy has been found to be inferior to prednisone. Methotrexate is given in doses of 5–25 mg once per week.

Surgical Management

Surgical treatment of Graves' ophthalmopathy includes decompression of the orbit, strabismus surgery, and eyelid retraction repair.

Orbital Decompression

Surgical decompression creates more space for the swollen tissues by expanding the walls of the orbit (bony decompression) or by removing excess orbital fat (fat decompression). (for details refer to chapter 9)

Strabismus Surgery

Due to incomitant nature of strabismus, surgery is aimed at resolution of diplopia in primary position and downgaze. Surgery is performed once the disease has been inactive for at least 6 months. The restricted muscle is released by recession rather than resection. The use of adjustable sutures is recommended due to unpredictable results.

Eyelid Surgery

The upper lid retraction is treated by graded Muller's and levator aponeurosis weakening. Lower lid lengthening is indicated in lower lid retraction and is treated by recession of lower lid retractors alone or interposition of graft or spacer.

Blepharoplasty

Blepharoplasty is the final surgical procedure in the rehabilitation.

Summarization of Management of TAO

The management of TAO has been described in Table 9 and Flowchart 2.

SUMMARY

Thyroid-associated orbitopathy is a self-limiting autoimmune disease that is usually associated with hyperthyroidism, but also with hypothyroid and euthyroid states. It is more common in females and smoking is the strongest modifiable risk factor. Orbital fibroblasts play an active role in modulating the inflammatory process. The upregulation of GAG synthesis is the essential pathology. Current therapeutic modalities include local supportive measures, corticosteroids, external beam radiation, and steroid-sparing immunosuppressive agents for reducing the inflammation during active disease. Surgical rehabilitation

Flowchart 2: Management synopsis of TAO.[10]

Management synopsis for patient with Thyroid Association Orbitopathy

1. Restore euthyroidism
2. Urge to stop smoking

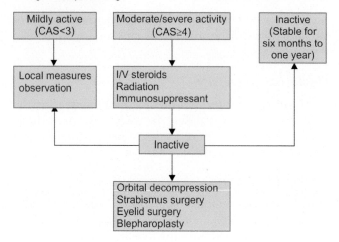

consists of orbital decompression, squint surgery, correction of lid retraction, and blepharoplasty.

REFERENCES

1. Lehmann GM, Garcia-Bates TM, Smith TJ, et al. Regulation of lymphocyte function by PPARgamma: Relevance to thyroid eye disease-related inflammation. PPAR Res. 2008;2008:895901.

2. Rundle FF, Wilson CW. Development and course of exophthalmos and ophthalmoplegia in Graves' disease with special reference to the effect of thyroidectomy. Clin Sci. 1945;5(3-4):177-94.

3. Ing E, Abuhaleeqa K. Graves' ophthalmopathy (thyroid-associated orbitopathy). Clinical and Surgical Ophthalmology. 2007;25:386-92.

4. Werner SC. Classification of the eye changes of Graves' disease. Am J Ophthalmol. 1969;68(4):646-8.

5. Van Dyk HJ. Orbital Graves' disease. A modification of the "NO SPECS" classification. Ophthalmology. 1981;88(6):479-83.

6. Mourits MP, Koornneef L, Wiersinga WM, et al. Clinical criteria for the assessment of disease activity in Graves' ophthalmopathy: A novel approach. Br J Ophthalmol. 1989; 73(8):639-44.

7. Mourits MP, Prummel MF, Wiersinga WM, et al. Clinical activity score as a guide in the management of patients with Graves' ophthalmopathy. Clin Endocrinol (Oxf). 1997;47(1):9-14.

8. Dolman PJ, Rootman J. VISA Classification for Graves orbitopathy. Ophthalmic Plast Reconstr Surg. 2006;22(5):319-24.

9. American Academy of Ophthalmology. Orbital inflammatory and infectious disorders. In: Cantor LB, Rapuano CJ, Cioffi GA (Eds). Orbit, Eyelids, and Lacrimal System, BCSC, Section 7. San Francisco, CA: AAO; 2012-2013. pp. 43-66.

10. Maheshwari R, Weis E. Thyroid associated orbitopathy. Indian J Ophthalmol. 2012;60(2):87-93.

Orbital Fractures: A Conceptual Approach

Gangadhara Sundar

INTRODUCTION

Orbital fractures are commonly seen following midfacial injuries and account for about 3% of all emergency room visits globally. They are frequently encountered following road traffic accidents, assaults, industrial accidents, sports injuries, and domestic accidents, both in adults and children. The spectrum of orbital fractures includes simple small fractures which only warrant conservative management to complex orbitofacial fractures which require multidisciplinary management. Occasionally high velocity induced orbital fractures, especially involving the orbital roof and medial wall, may be vision and even life-threatening and thus of great medical and medicolegal significance. All ophthalmologists should thus have a conceptual approach to the diagnosis and management of orbital fractures, identify and treat related ophthalmic emergencies, and become an integral part of the cranio-maxillo-facial team managing complex cranio-orbito-facial fractures. Likewise they should also be comfortable managing simple orbital blow-out and blow-in fractures along with other common midfacial fractures like zygomatico-maxillary complex and naso-orbito-ethmoidal fractures.

DEFINITION

Any cortical bone disruption of the rim and/or the walls of the orbit which may be associated with intraorbital soft tissue injuries including the globe and the optic nerve and not infrequently adjacent periorbital soft tissue and bones of the midface, cranial or even the entire facial skeleton. Although clinically suspected and diagnosed,

they are confirmed and best characterized by computerized tomography (CT scan) of the face and orbits.

APPLIED ANATOMY

The human orbits, paired and symmetrical, are comprised of an anterior frame (rims) and the walls. While there are four walls anteriorly, the medial wall and floor form a common wall posteriorly, with the orbital shape being described as a "Quadrilateral Triangle". The junction of the medial wall and floor, the internal orbital buttress, is termed inferomedial orbital strut. The angle between the two walls is variable between individuals and has been described as the angle of inferomedial orbital strut (AIOS) which is crucial for preoperative assessment and guides reconstruction to restore symmetry. The orbital cavity may also be divided into the anterior third (rim—inferior orbital fissure), middle (length of inferior orbital fissure), and the apex (posterior extent of inferior orbital fissure to the optic foramen), each with its implications for volume expansion and risks of reconstruction. The floor and often times the medial wall has a variable convexity posteriorly (S-contour) also described as the postbulbar construction or as the psotero-medial bulge, which should be accurately reconstructed to minimize postoperative enophthalmos. Finally, the posterior ledge, often present even in large fractures, representing the vertical process of the palatine bone, is a landmark that should be identified in all floor and medial wall fractures prior to placement of implant. Of course the various soft tissue structures including the globe, extraocular muscles, and the neurovascular bundles along the floor (infraorbital) and medial wall (anterior and posterior ethmoidal) should also be kept in mind, during clinical and radiological assessment and intraoperatively as well.

MECHANISM OF ORBITAL FRACTURES

Multiple mechanisms may predispose to the variety and spectrum of orbital fractures (Table 1), which may be unilateral or bilateral and may be present in isolation or in combination with other fractures of the craniofacial skeleton. While penetrating injuries may predispose to isolated and more localized orbital wall injuries, most orbital fractures are caused by either low impact or high impact blunt injuries. Blow-out fractures of the orbital walls are caused by low to medium impact blunt injuries with varying combinations of both a "hydraulic" and a "buckling" mechanism. Most complex fractures are caused by medium to high velocity injuries such as high speed motor vehicle accidents, fall from heights or projectile, and blast injuries. Blow-out fractures are commonly caused by objects larger than the size of the orbital aperture (e.g. closed fist, tennis/cricket balls, etc.). While the floor and/or the medial wall of the orbit are most frequently involved the lateral wall and less frequently the roof of the orbit may all be involved. Children, less than 7 years of age, owing to the relatively prominent forehead (well-developed brain) are more prone to sustain orbital roof fractures compared to older children and adults. Isolated orbital roof fractures are rare in adults and may be present either in combination with cranioorbital injuries or with other midfacial injuries.

DIAGNOSIS AND IMAGING

Although frequently diagnosed based on the history and clinical signs on examination, they are confirmed by radiological investigations. Plain X-rays although used as in the past, have a very limited role in modern practice given its various limitations. These include variable quality, high false negatives and of limited use for surgical planning and execution. Thus its role is limited to emergency rooms as a screening tool, especially when intraorbital foreign bodies are to be ruled out.

Computerized tomography (CT) scans, noncontrast enhanced, remain the mainstay and the modality of choice for diagnosing and characterizing orbital and orbito-facial fractures. Modern scanners are spiral CT scans with images acquired in the axial format and subsequently formatted into coronal, sagittal, and when necessary 3D reconstructions as well. When acquired in less than 1 mm cuts with the gantry at 0°, this Image Guidance Surgery (IGS) protocol is useful for a complete diagnosis, treatment planning and when necessary, stereolithographic (STL) model printing and even for postoperative image fusion for quality control.

Magnetic resonance imaging (MRI) has limited role in acute trauma and only performed when additional soft tissue imaging is required, e.g. suspect optic nerve sheath hematoma. Ferromagnetic foreign bodies, MRI incompatible cardiac pacemakers, and claustrophobia are contraindications for this modality of imaging.

CLASSIFICATION

Broadly, orbital fractures may be classified into "simple" orbital fractures and "complex" orbital fractures.

Simple (pure, internal) orbital fractures are fractures that may involve one or more walls without involvement of the orbital frame/rim(s). They may be classified into the following:

- *Linear fractures:* These are crack fractures without displacement, entrapment or herniation of orbital contents. They are often missed on plain X-rays, sometimes even on CT scans, usually clinically insignificant and do not require surgical intervention
- *Blow-out fractures:* These are orbital fractures where one, two or rarely three walls of the orbit are disrupted without involvement of the orbital rims. The bone fragments are typically displaced towards the adjacent region (maxillary sinus for floor fractures, ethmoidal sinus for medial wall fractures, and frontal sinus/anterior cranial fossa for roof fractures), often with herniation/prolapse of orbital contents. While small fractures without entrapment (<1/3 of one orbital wall—"small") may be clinically insignificant, larger fractures (1/3–1/2 of one wall—"medium" and >1/2 of one wall—"large") often result in enophthalmos, double vision, or other structural deformities and thus often justifying intervention. Isolated blow-out fractures most commonly involve the orbital floor (Fig. 1) or the medial wall (Fig. 2), although not infrequently involve both of them with disruption of the inferomedial orbital strut (Fig. 3)
- Trapdoor fractures are a subtype of blow-out orbital fractures which result in herniation and entrapment of the orbital soft tissue contents along with either the adjacent rectus muscle (inferior rectus—floor

TABLE 1: Mechanisms of orbital fractures.

Blunt injury a. Hydraulic mechanism b. Buckling mechanism c. Combination	Low (to intermediate) velocity injury (blow-out fractures) (Intermediate to) High velocity injury (complex orbital fractures)
Penetrating injury	Isolated localized orbital wall fractures with contiguous involvement (foreign bodies, intracranial injuries, etc.)

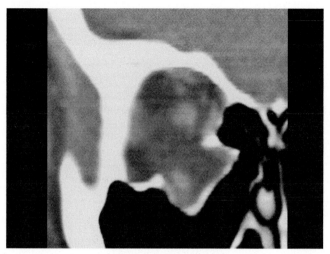

Fig. 1: Blow-out orbital floor fracture.

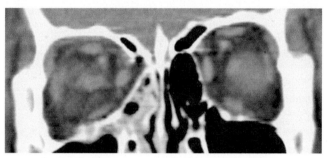

Fig. 2: Blow-out orbital medial wall fracture.

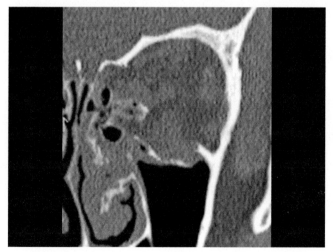

Fig. 3: Combined medial wall and orbital floor fracture.

fractures, medial rectus—medial wall fractures) and / or the adjacent intermuscular septum. These fractures radiologically are typically small as the bony fragment springs back to the original position after trapping the contents. When this occurs in children and young

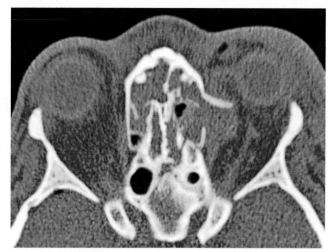

Fig. 4: Medial wall blow in fracture.

adults with minimal ocular or periorbital injection or ecchymosis, it is termed a "White eyed blow-out fracture", which requires urgent surgical intervention
• Blow-in fractures are those where there is disruption of one or more walls, typically only one, without orbital rim involvement. The bone fragments are displaced intraorbitally (Fig. 4) and often impinge against an orbital soft tissue structure. These may include the inferior rectus, the medial rectus, the superior rectus, the superior oblique or even the globe and thus often require surgical intervention.

Complex orbital fractures are fractures that involve one or more of the orbital walls with involvement and displacement of the orbital rims. They are often associated with other midfacial, cranial or panfacial fractures. These fractures often require the evaluation and comanagement with the cranio-maxillo-facial surgeon and surgery optimally performed by a multidisciplinary team.

An overview of the classification and types of orbital fractures is shown in Table 2.

While the ophthalmologist is often involved in the management of pure/internal orbital fractures, they are far less common than complex orbital fractures underlying the need for close collaboration with cranio-maxillo-facial surgeons.

Some orbital and ocular adnexal soft tissue considerations with complex fractures are shown in Table 3.

PRESENTATION

Most patients present with a reliable history, either witnessed or unwitnessed. Incomplete and inaccurate history may be encountered with unconscious patients or in young children. A summary of common symptoms and signs with their clinical correlation is shown in Tables 4 and 5.

TABLE 2: Classification of Orbitofacial fractures.

Simple	Complex
Linear fractures	Zygomatico-maxillary complex (ZMC) fracture
Blow-out fractures a. Orbital floor blow-out fractures b. Medial wall blow-out fractures c. Combined floor-medial wall blow-out fractures	Naso-orbito-ethmoidal (NOE) fracture a. Type I b. Type II c. Type III
Blow-in fractures a. Orbital floor blow-in fracture b. Medial wall blow-in fracture c. Orbital roof blow-in fracture	Cranio-orbital fracture (skull base and orbital fracture)
	Orbito-facial fracture (orbit and midface)
	Panfacial fracture (upper, mid and lower facial fractures)

TABLE 3: Complex midfacial fractures and their associations.

Zygomatico-maxillary complex fractures (Fig. 5)	Malar depression, lateral canthal dystopia, pseudoenopthhalmos, pseudoproptosis
Naso-orbito-ethmoidal fractures (Fig. 6)	Telecanthus, medial canthal webbing, nasolacrimal disruption, CSF leak
Cranio-orbital fracture (Fig. 7)	Growing fracture (children), supraorbital paresthesia, CSF leak, late frontal mucoceles

Some common emergencies that may be associated with orbital fractures are shown in Box 1. They should be recognized and appropriately managed.

WORK UP

All patients should have a detailed history elicited along with the details of circumstances of trauma including witness reports, and a detailed personal medical history for comorbidities. Substance abuse should be suspected and documented as appropriate. A police report may be justified in road traffic accidents, suspected assaults at home or elsewhere or when in doubt. Life-threatening and neurosurgical injuries should be addressed and managed when present.

A complete ophthalmological examination including best elicited visual acuity, globe assessment with alignment, and pupillary evaluation and when possible a dilated fundus examination should be performed with photographic documentation. In more extensive injuries or when patient is unconscious a complete neurological and facial examination should also be performed. With suspected orbitofacial trauma a craniomaxillofacial surgeon should also be consulted.

TABLE 4: Common symptoms in orbital fractures.

Symptoms	Cause
Pain	
Bleeding	Laceration
Blurred vision	Closed globe injury Open globe injury Optic neuropathy
Double vision	EOM contusion Cranial neuropathy EOM/intermuscular septum entrapment
Nausea and vomiting	Hyphema with secondary glaucoma Entrapment of inferior rectus/medial rectus (Trapdoor fracture) Oculocardiac reflex
Epistaxis	Medial wall/floor fracture

TABLE 5: Common signs in orbital fractures.

Signs	Cause
Periorbital ecchymosis	
Infraorbital step off/point tenderness	Rim involvement (complex fractures)
Crepitus	Orbital emphysema
Infraorbital hypoesthesia	Floor fracture
Supraorbital hypoesthesia	Roof fracture
Proptosis	Orbital hemorrhage
Enophthalmos	Large orbital fracture with globe displacement
Hypoglobus	Large orbital floor fracture with globe prolapse
Limitation of ocular motility	Pain Entrapment Contusion of extraocular muscle(s)
Anisocoria	Sphincter rupture, traumatic iritis, etc.
Relative afferent pupillary defect	Traumatic optic neuropathy, open globe injury, retinal detachment, etc.
Clear nasal discharge	Suspect CSF leak

Following a complete clinical assessment, a CT scan of the face and orbits, ideally by an image guidance surgery (Sub mm) protocol with gantry at 0° should be performed. MRI is contraindicated in most traumas unless embedded ferromagnetic foreign bodies have been ruled out and detailed soft tissue assessment (globe, optic nerve sheath, and intracranial injuries) is necessary.

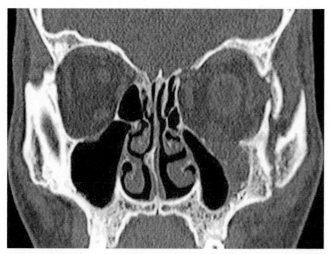

Fig. 5: Comminuted displaced left zygomatico-maxillary complex (ZMC) fracture.

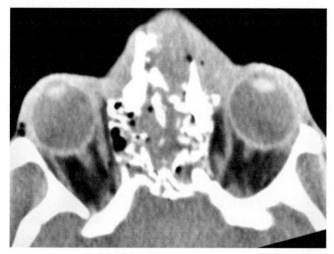

Fig. 6: Comminuted displaced (Type III) bilateral naso-orbito-ethmoid (NOE) fracture.

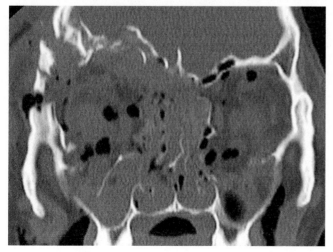

Fig. 7: Cranio-orbito-facial fracture.

Box 1: Ophthalmic/Oculoplastic emergencies.

1. Closed globe injury with hyphema, vitreous hemorrhage, retinal detachment, optic nerve avulsion, etc.
2. Open globe injuries (soft globe, excessive chemosis, poor vision, etc.).
3. Traumatic optic neuropathy (RAPD with intact globe).
4. Orbital compartment syndrome (Retrobulbar hemorrhage) from laceration of the infraorbital, supraorbital or anterior/ posterior ethmoidal arteries (Tense orbit with intact globe, poor vision and RAPD).
5. White-eyed blow-out fractures with entrapment myopathy (children and young adults).

In patients presenting to the clinic in a subacute setting a dilated fundus examination along with detailed assessment of the visual fields, documentation of ocular motility with Hess charting and field of binocular single vision (BSV) should be performed.

Finally, when a patient is determined to be a good candidate for surgery, a general assessment for fitness for general anesthesia with optimization of any underlying medical condition is warranted.

MANAGEMENT

As a general rule, life-threatening systemic, cervical or neurological injuries should be managed first. Vision threatening injuries (severe closed globe injury, open globe injuries, and traumatic optic neuropathy) should be managed next. Orbital fractures which are minimally displaced or small, without herniation or entrapment of contents may be managed conservatively. All significantly displaced orbital walls, with or without rim involvement, with prolapse of orbital soft tissue generally require surgical intervention. Complex orbital fractures (comminuted displaced multiple wall fractures, displaced ZMC fractures, unilateral or bilateral NOE fractures with displacement, cranio-orbital or panfacial fractures with displacement) will benefit from surgical intervention by a multidisciplinary approach. The primary goal of surgery is anatomical correction which in turn helps functional restoration. These, in turn, aid esthetic and psychological rehabilitation of the patient.

Medical Management

Patients should be advised against nose blowing and prescribed nasal decongestants. Although routine systemic antibiotics may not be indicated, they may be prescribed, especially when overlying lacerations are present, frank contamination is present in the presence of intraorbital or facial foreign bodies. Analgesics and antiemetics should be prescribed as appropriate.

Surgical Management

Indications for surgical management are mentioned above. General timings of intervention for common orbital fractures are shown below:

- Trapdoor white-eyed   As soon as possible blow-out fracture
- Zygomatico-maxillary   Within 5–7 days complex fractures
- Naso-orbito-ethmoidal   Within 5–7 days, as soon fracture as patient is stable
- 1 or 2 wall blow-out   Within 2 weeks fractures

The requisites for proper surgical management include making an accurate radiological and clinical diagnosis, detailed discussion with the patient and family regarding the nature of injury with various treatment options, an informed consent regarding potential risks, benefits, alternatives and complications, and photographic documentation. Under general anesthesia, the most direct and minimally invasive approach to the respective orbital rim(s)/wall(s) should be employed with good visualization of the fracture fragments and prolapsed content which should be completely reduced, with intraoperative verification. Bony rim and wall reconstruction are then performed with a permanent or bioresorbable implant as indicated. Intraoperatively, preincision and postwound closure forced duction testing should be performed to ensure adequate release and absence of tissue incarceration.

APPROACHES TO THE ORBIT

Incisions and approaches to the various walls of the orbit are widely varied. Factors determining them include specialty of practice, training, and experience. A brief overview of various approaches to the walls and rims of the orbit is shown in Table 6.

IMPLANTS IN ORBITAL FRACTURES

A wide variety of implants and biomaterials are available for orbital reconstruction. Some common implants, their advantages and disadvantages, are mentioned in Table 7. While other permanent implants including silicone, nylon

TABLE 6: Incisions and exposure in orbital fractues.

Fracture	Incision
Orbital floor	Direct transconjunctival approach (with or without a lateral canthotomy and inferior cantholysis). Subciliary approach (less ideal).
Medial wall	Retrocaruncular approach. Lynch incision (not recommended). Inferior transconjunctival approach. Coronal approach (for NOE, cranio-orbital fractures).
Combined orbital floor and medial wall	Swinging eyelid approach (with or without a retrocaruncular incision, with or without disinsertion of the inferior oblique tendon). Subciliary approach (less ideal).
ZMC fracture	Swinging eyelid approach with upper blepharoplasty incision. Swinging eyelid approach with trans/sub brow incision. Coronal, transbuccal approach with swinging eyelid approach (extensive comminuted fractures).
Orbital roof fracture	Coronal approach (cranio-orbital fractures)—subfrontal approach. Upper eyelid crease incision (blow in fractures).
Panfacial fractures with orbital involvement	Coronal approach, swinging eyelid approach, transoral approach.

TABLE 7: Implants and biomaterials used for orbital reconstruction.

Permanent implants	Advantages	Disadvantages
Titanium (Fig. 8)	Permanent, osseointegration Inert, biologically compatible Strength Time tested Anatomical, 3-dimensional implant, can be customized Porous (low risk of compartment syndrome) 1 or 2 wall fractures	Permanent: late exposures, late infections (with chronic sinusitis) Palpability (rim implants with thin overlying soft tissue) Adhesion syndrome (Titanium mesh, not anatomical plates) Difficult to remove Expensive

Contd...

Contd...

Permanent implants	Advantages	Disadvantages
	Orbital rim reconstruction Radiologically visible Various sizes	
Porous polypropylene (Medpor) (Fig. 9)	Time tested Inert Tissue integration	Permanent (late hematoma, exposure, etc.) Memory (not suitable for 3 dimensional 1 wall or 2 wall reconstruction) Radiologically invisible Compartment syndrome (risk) Expensive
Composite (hybrid) implants (Fig. 10) (porous polypropylene with titanium) Titan®, Synpor®	Advantages of both biomaterials Anatomical 3-dimensional configuration Radiologically visible	Permanent Memory (less than ideal 3-dimensional contouring) Compartment syndrome Expensive
Bioresorbable implants		
Poly L/DL Lactide 85:15 (Rapidsorb) (Fig. 11)	Thermolabile, can be anatomically customized and contoured 1 wall, 2 wall reconstruction (small to medium sized fractures) Absorbed in 15–18 months Bony healing	Expensive Unproven benefit with large fracture defects
Poly L/DL Lactide 70:30 (Polymax)	Thermolabile, can be anatomically customized and contoured 1 wall, 2 wall reconstruction (small to medium sized fractures) Absorbed in 24 months Bony healing	Delayed absorption Expensive Unproven in large orbital fracture defects
Polycaprolactone (PCL, Osteomesh®) (Fig. 12)	Porous implant (reduced compartment syndrome) Ideal for small defects	Non-thermolabile Not ideal for 3-dimensional 1 wall or 2 wall reconstruction, medium—large defects Supple implant
Polydioxanone (PDS)	Readily available Inexpensive Small—medium fractures	Pseudocapsule formation Inadequate support for large fractures
Bone graft	Autologous Inert "Bioresorbable"	Donor site morbidity Increased operating time Inability for 3-dimensional contouring

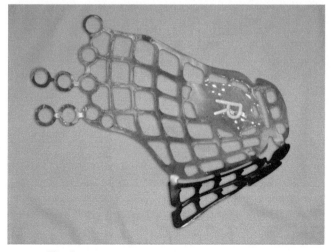

Fig. 8: Anatomical prefabricated titanium implant.

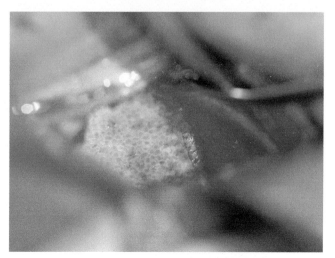

Fig. 9: Porous polypropylene implant.

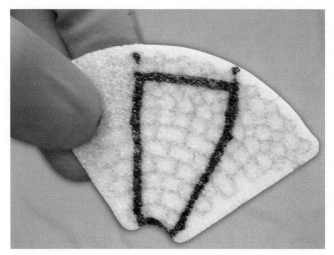

Fig. 10: Composite (porous polypropylene-titanium) implant.

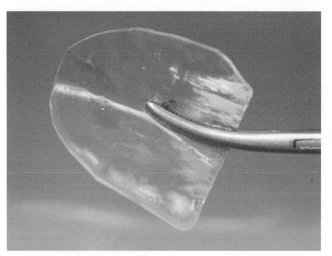

Fig. 11: Polylactide bioresorbable implant.

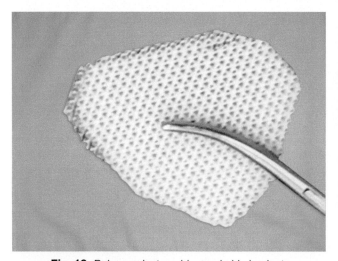

Fig. 12: Polycaprolactone bioresorbable implant.

(Suprafoil®), and other materials have been used, they are no longer recommended owing to their various limitations. Figures 13 and 14 demonstrate ideal placement of orbital implants following orbital reconstruction.

COMPLICATIONS OF ORBITAL FRACTURE REPAIR

Several complications are associated with orbital trauma and also with repair and reconstruction of orbital and orbitofacial fractures. It is thus imperative that the patients are counseled regarding both the common and the serious complications. These are highlighted in Table 8.

Most orbital fractures when appropriately managed surgically, yield gratifying results both for the patient and the surgeon. Despite numerous advances, there are potential limitations which have been overcome by the advent of newer techniques and technology. Some of these are highlighted in Table 9.

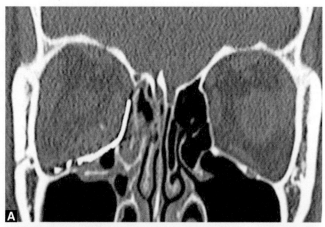

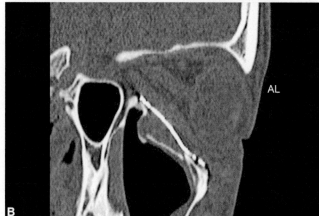

Figs. 13A and B: (A) Prebent anatomical titanium implant coronal view; (B) Prebent anatomical titanium implant sagittal view, showing implant placement on the posterior ledge.

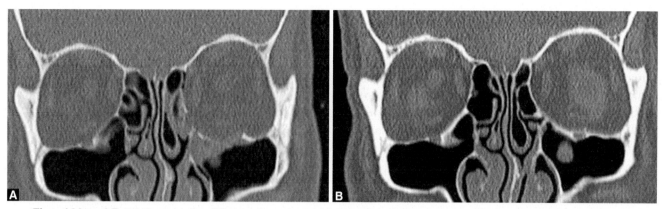

Figs. 14A and B: (A) Preoperative CT scan shown in a right orbital floor fracture. (B) Postoperative CT scan demonstrated well healed fracture with absorption of the implant.

TABLE 8: Pitfalls/complications of orbital fracture repair/reconstruction.

Preoperative	Intraoperative	Postoperative
Missed diagnosis	Anesthetic considerations	Early
Timing of intervention	Incision	Hemorrhage–Compartment syndrome
a. Blow-out fractures (too early)	a. Visible skin incisions	Infection
b. Pediatric white eyed blow-out fracture (too late)	b. Too large an incision	Visual loss
	Bleeding	Diplopia (transient vs. permanent
Poor primary management	a. Infraorbital artery	Wound complications (dehiscence,
a. Systemic/neurotrauma	b. Anterior/posterior ethmoidal artery	infection)
b. Incomplete ophthalmic exam	Incomplete release of entrapped/herniated	Implant malposition
c. Wound management	tissue	Late
Incomplete imaging study (only orbital	Not identifying the posterior ledge	Scarring (cutaneous incisions)
CT when facial CT should have been	Poor implant choice	Enophthalmos (incomplete reduction,
performed)	a. Material	incomplete fracture repair, malpositioned
Poor informed consent	b. Size	implant)
	c. Shape	Implant complications
	Poor implant placement	Diplopia
	Globe, extraocular muscle, optic nerve injury	

TABLE 9: Recent advances in orbital fractures.

Minimally invasive orbital surgery	Small, direct approaches (direct forniceal, retrocaruncular incisions) Faster surgeries with access to orbital defect Faster wound healing Increased patient acceptance Well executed with expertise
Intraoperative navigation	Real-time intraoperative guidance Optical or electromagnetic tracking systems Identify and confirm anatomical landmarks, e.g. posterior ledge, orbital apex, skull base, etc. Increased accuracy of reduction, delivery of outcomes
3-dimensional anatomic implants	3-dimensional floor, medial wall reconstruction Reduced postoperative enophthalmos Ideal for combined medial wall and floor fractures with disruption of the orbital strut
Patient specific (customized) implants	For complex and late reconstruction during secondary reconstruction
Intraoperative imaging	Ensure adequacy and completeness of reconstruction prior to closure and recovery from GA to avoid postoperative surprises and minimize postoperative implant related complications

SUMMARY

Orbital fractures are common, yet often poorly managed in inexperienced hands. The role of an ophthalmologist and an orbital surgeon is crucial in managing these patients individually as a part of a craniomaxillofacial surgeon. A methodical, comprehensive, and systematic approach to clinical assessment, appropriate imaging, treatment planning, patient counseling, and management is essential for the best outcome possible. When managed well complete structural, functional, esthetic, and psychological rehabilitation can be achieved.

Disclosures: The author has no financial conflicts of interests in any of the impants, devices and technology mentioned in the chapter. The author receives royalties from the book 'Orbital Fractures: Principles, concepts and management', Ed Sundar G. Imaging Science Today, USA ISBN 978-0997781922.

8
CHAPTER

Orbitotomy

Ruchi Goel

INTRODUCTION

Improvements in imaging and instrumentation have greatly reduced the risks of orbital surgery and the focus has now shifted toward cosmetically better approaches.

The orbit can be divided into three surgical zones—anterior, middle, and deep or apical.

SURGICAL ZONES OF THE ORBIT (FIG. 1)

Anterior: Approached by anterior orbitotomy.

Middle: Often requires removal of lateral orbital wall. Lateral orbitotomy may be combined with superior or inferior anterior orbital lesions to affect greater exposure.

Apical: Transcranial approach.

Deeply placed medial lesions can be accessed by medial orbitotomy and external ethmoidectomy.

PREOPERATIVE EVALUATION AND INFORMED CONSENT

A detailed examination and imaging help in:
- Detection of mass
- Differentiation between thyroid orbitopathy, metastatic tumor, and orbital inflammation
- Whether encapsulated
- Assessment of relationship of the mass to the surrounding bony structures, paranasal sinuses, and brain
- Planing incision biopsy or complete removal
- Finding the proximity to the optic nerve
- Planning the surgical approach
    - To allow most direct access to the lesion
    - To allow optimal scar camouflage.

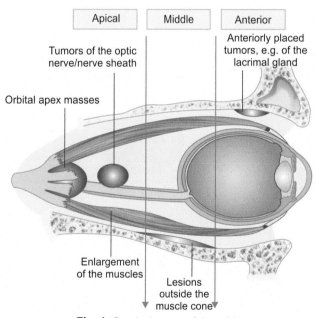

Fig. 1: Surgical zones of the orbit.

The initial choice for evaluation is CT scan which may be complemented with MRI and ultrasonography.

A detailed informed consent including risk of losing vision, diplopia, ptosis, and hypoesthesia should be explained to the patient. Orbitotomies are performed under general anesthesia; so risk of anesthesia should also be discussed.

SURGICAL APPROACHES

- Anterior orbitotomy
    - Transcutaneous

- Transconjunctival
- Eyelid split
- Medial orbitotomy
  - Transcutaneous
  - Transconjunctival
  - Transcaruncular
  - Endoscopic
- Lateral
- Combined
- Transcranial
- Endoscopic.

Anterior Orbitotomy

Transcutaneous

A skin crease or sub-brow incision in the upper lid allows access to the superior extraconal or subperiosteal space (Fig. 2). Subciliary or skin crease incision in the lower lid allows access to the anterior inferior orbit (Figs. 3A to C).

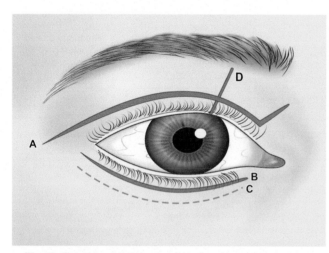

Fig. 2: Anterior orbital approaches: A—skin crease incision; B—subciliary; C—lower lid crease; D—eyelid split.

Transconjunctival

Conjunctival incision is made in the inferior fornix. The swinging eyelid approach is a variation of the trans-conjunctival approach combined with a lateral canthotomy (Figs. 4A to D). It provides excellent exposure of inferior and lateral orbital wall and is especially useful in orbital floor repair and lateral wall decompression. Inferior fornicial incision may be extended to transcaruncular incision.

Eyelid Split Technique

For intraconal or superomedial extraconal access a vertically oriented incision of the upper eyelid only divides the muscles and allows appropriate function postoperatively. The vertical incision should be perpendicular to the tarsus at the junction of medial third and lateral two-thirds (Fig. 2). Meticulous closure ensures appropriate realignment of the tarsus and lid border to provide cosmesis. A transverse upper eyelid approach provides access to this area, but at the expense of transecting the levator apparatus leading to postoperative ptosis.

Medial Orbitotomy (Fig. 5)

Transcutaneous

Used for medial extraconal or subperiosteal lesions. It is especially useful for drainage of a subperiosteal abscess or repair of the medial wall fracture.

Lynch incision: A curvilinear skin incision is placed midway between the line joining medial canthal angle to the bridge of the nose.

Gull wing incision: A dacryocystorhinostomy incision may be combined with a Lynch incision meeting at the medial canthus in a gull wing fashion to provide access to medial orbit, ethmoid sinus, and orbital apex.

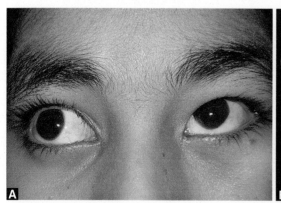
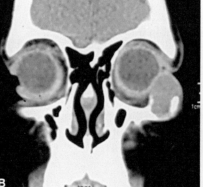
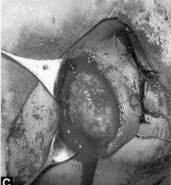

Figs. 3A to C: (A) Clinical photograph showing displacement of globe upward and medially; (B) Coronal view CT scan showing an intraosseous mass; (C) Transcutaneous anterior orbitomy.

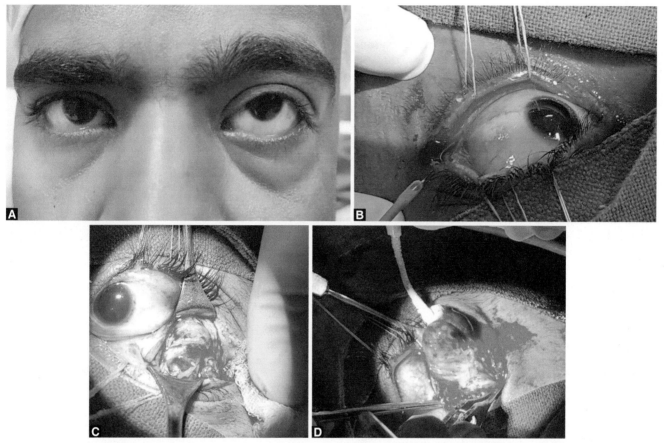

Figs. 4A to D: (A) Clinical photograph with displacement of left globe upwards; (B) Swinging eye lid incision—lateral canthotomy being performed with radiofrequency knife; (C) Swinging eye lid incision—incision extended to inferior fornix with exposure of mass; (D) The lesion being lifted with a cryoprobe.

The periosteum is incised and elevated with medial canthal tendon and lacrimal sac. Medial orbital wall is fractured posterior to lacrimal fossa and the opening is enlarged posteriorly. The anterior ethmoidal vessels are visualized at the superior border of the operative field and above this lies the anterior cranial fossa. Any injury to the underlying dura may result in cerebrospinal leak.

Transconjunctival

It is used for gaining access to Tenon's or extraconal space or for performing optic nerve decompression. A medial 180° peritomy is performed and radial relaxing incisions are given. Medial rectus may be disinserted if required and reattached later (Fig. 6).

Transcaruncular (Baylis) Incision

This is used for repair of medial wall fracture, to perform ethmoidectomy, as part of orbital decompression or optic nerve sheath decompression. The incision is made between the caruncle and the plica. The medial orbital wall posterior to the posterior lacrimal crest is exposed.

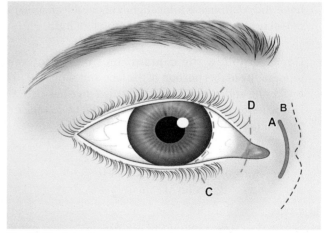

Fig. 5: Medial orbitotomy approaches: A—Lynch incision; B—gull using incision; C—transconjunctival incision; D—transcaruncular incision.

Lateral Orbitotomy

It provides an excellent access to intraconal and extraconal space lateral to the optic nerve. It is used for removal of lacrimal gland tumors, intraconal tumors, and as part of orbital decompression.

The crux of the surgery is manipulation of a hinged bone flap, "wedge shaped" to provide access to the middle and anterior part of apical surgical zone. The margin of the orbital rim is the base of the bony wedge. The superior extent is just above the zygomaticofrontal suture in the zygomatic process of frontal bone and inferior extent is at base of frontal process of zygomatic bone just above its arch. The bone is hinged to the skin-fascia-muscle flap of the temporal area that provides nutrition to the bone when the flap is replaced and sutured. The upper lid crease incision is the most popular approach nowadays. However, lateral orbitotomy has been described using the following approaches:

- Standard Krönlein incision
- Modified Krönlein incision
- T–shaped incision
- Berke-Reese incision
- Guyton incision
- Kocher incision
- Stallard-Wright incision.

Standard Krönlein Incision (Fig. 7)

- Crescentic with convexity directed anteriorly
- Superior and inferior ends of the incision are 3 cm anterior to the ear
- Curved inferior arm corresponds to superior border of the zygomatic arch
- Superior arm commences in the temporal fossa along the semi-circular ridge of the lateral face of the frontal bone and continues as a line slightly above the imaginary dorsal projection of the superior orbital margin.

Criticism:
- Does not follow the contour lines of skin or the topography of this portion of the face and skull
- Puckering and furrowing of the healed incision
- Due to its location, the ugly scar could not be concealed by clothing or change in hair style.

Modified Krönlein Incision (Fig. 8)

- Lengthening of the radius of curvature
- Reversing the direction of convexity dorsal ward.

Advantage:
- Blended with the contours of the skin
- Less noticeable when healed.

Criticism: Less exposure.

T–Shaped Incision (Fig. 9)

- Addition of a horizontal arm to the modified Krönlein incision.

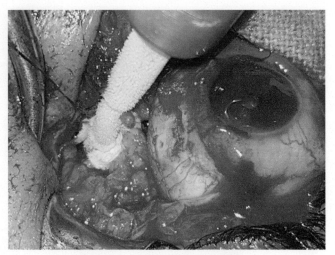

Fig. 6: Transconjunctival approach.

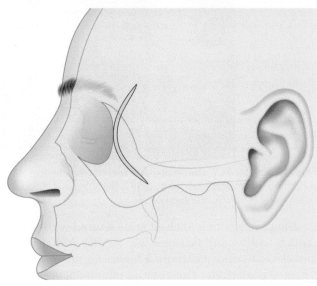

Fig. 7: Standard Krönlein incision.

Criticism: Difficult to obtain a good cosmetic closure of the skin at the junction of the vertical and horizontal cuts.

Berke Incision (Fig. 10)

- Straight horizontal cut 30–40 mm in length extending from lateral canthus toward the ear and passing over the mid-point of the lateral orbital rim at the level of insertion of lateral palpebral raphae
- A lateral canthotomy is included at the ocular end of the incision.

Criticism: Requires a careful reconstruction of lateral canthus.

If lateral canthal reconstruction is improper, tears may dribble from lateral conjunctival cul de sac once fibrosis of the incision occurs.

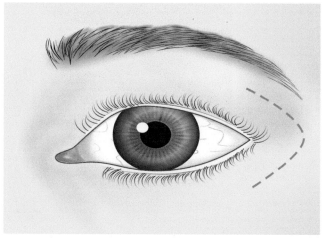

Fig. 8: Modified Krönlein incision.

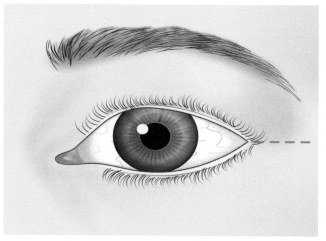

Fig. 10: Berke's incision.

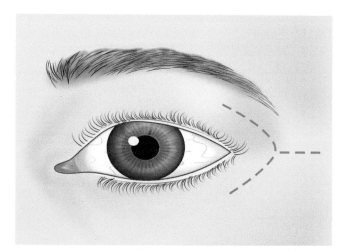

Fig. 9: T-shaped incision.

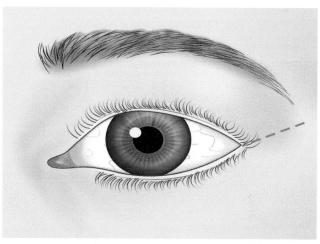

Fig. 11: Reese modification of Berke's incision.

Reese Modification of Berke's Incision (Fig. 11)

- Upward slanted incision to be concealed by the spectacles
- Incision to follow the natural fold of one of the creases of the "crow feet" to decrease the dimpling
- Limitation of the length of the incision to 30 mm or less to avoid damage to the terminal plexus of branches of temporal artery that supply the subcutaneous tissue and fascia of temporalis muscle near its insertion.

Disadvantage: Restriction of working space.

Guyton's Hairline Incision (Fig. 12)

- Incision lies just within the hairline anterior to the ear
- About 7 cm long with slight concavity forward
- 6 cm or more from the lateral orbital rim.

Disadvantage:
- Requires large skin flap
- Extensive dissection through vascular zone of the terminal branches of the temporal artery.

Kocher's Incision (Fig. 13)

Sweeping curved cut parallel to and slightly above the eyebrow extending from the midpoint of the eyebrow to the level of zygomatic arch.

Stallard Incision

The horizontal component lies along the zygomatic arch as in previous techniques but the vertical curved arm may be placed in the eyebrow, in the eyelids just inferior to the superolateral orbital margin or directly over the lateral orbital rim.

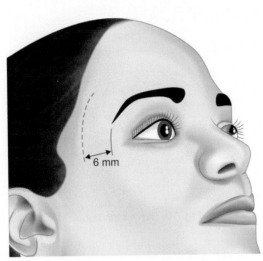

Fig. 12: Guyton's hairline incision.

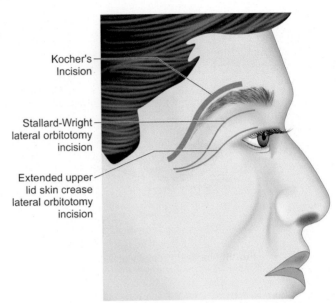

Fig. 13: Kocher's, Stallard-Wright and extended upper lid crease incisions for lateral orbitotomy.

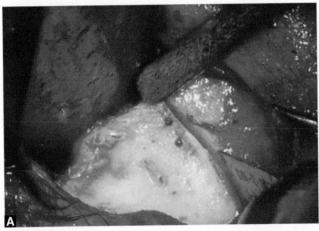

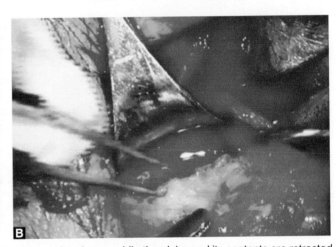

Figs. 14A and B: (A) Lateral orbitotomy: The osteotomy is created using an electric saw while the globe and its contents are retracted with a lid spatula positioned firmly by an assistant; (B) The bone flap is grasped with a rongeur and fractured outwardly to break at the thin area just anterior to the zygomatico-sphenoid suture (about 12 mm posterior to the edge of the rim).

S-shaped Stallard-Wright incision, extending from beneath the eyebrow laterally and curving down along the zygomatic arch allows good exposure of the orbital rim and interferes less with the lateral canthal tissue (Fig. 13).

The Bony Orbitotomy in Lateral Approach

- After the skin incision a curved vertical incision from well above the zygomaticofrontal suture to slightly below the level of zygomatic arch, is made on the tissue covering the lateral orbital rim
- The lateral palpebral tendon lying along this bony rim is tagged

- The periosteum is peeled and cleavage is created between the periorbita (the inner layer of the periosteum) and bone. Careful posterior dissection is required to prevent damage to the orbital branch of middle meningeal artery
- The osteotomy 3–3.5 cm wide is performed from 3 mm to 4 mm above the frontozygomatic suture till the body of the zygoma (Fig. 14A). The bone flap is grasped with a rongeur and fractured outwards to break at the thin area just anterior to the zygomatico-sphenoid suture (about 12 mm posterior to the edge of the rim) (Fig. 14B)
- The periorbita is incised in a rectangular manner
- The lateral rectus is retracted by preplaced bridle suture

- The lesion is dissected and removed while keeping watch over dilatation of pupil during surgery that may occur due to pressure on optic nerve
- The periorbita is approximated meticulously and limbs of lateral canthal tendon are reattached. The bone is positioned back. The muscle and skin are closed in layers.

Transcranial Orbitotomy

Indications: Lesions located in deep superior and apical orbit.

Complications:
- Related to craniotomy such as infection, death, and stroke
- Paresis of frontalis branch of facial nerve
- Burr holes in the forehead
- Frontal sinus mucocele
- Meningitis

- Supraorbital nerve injury and resulting numbness
- Paresis of levator and superior rectus
- Blindness due to optic nerve injury.

SUMMARY

Orbital surgery is performed for incisional biopsy, debulking or excision orbital masses. It is also required for orbital wall fracture repair and orbital decompression. After a thorough clinical and radiological examination the type of orbitotomy is chosen to keep the mass between optic nerve and the surgeon's instruments to avoid injury to the optic nerve. Cosmetically acceptable incisions like swinging eye lid, upper lid crease incision, and transcaruncular approaches are widely used. Meticulous dissection and thorough hemostasis avert catastrophic complications. However, a detailed informed consent including blindness should be taken.

Orbital Decompression

Ruchi Goel

INTRODUCTION

Orbital decompression aims at improving the volume to space discrepancy that occurs in thyroid eye disease (TED) by allowing the enlarged muscles and orbital fat to expand into the periorbital spaces with resultant relief in pressure on the optic nerve, its blood supply, and reduction in proptosis.

Four major approaches of orbital decompression:
1. Transorbital (Fig. 1)
2. Transcranial
3. Transantral
4. Transnasal.

INDICATIONS

- Urgent intervention is required in:
  - Acute dysthyroid optic neuropathy
  - Corneal decompensation
  - Acute globe subluxation.

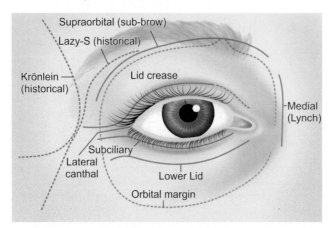

Fig. 1: Orbital incisions for transorbital decompression.

- Rehabilitation in the stable stage:
  - Proptosis causing disfigurement
  - Chronic pain/discomfort and congestion
  - Corneal exposure.

CLASSICAL APPROACH TO REHABILITATION IN STABLE STAGE

Orbital decompression

↓

Eyelid surgery

↓

Strabismic surgery

AREAS OF ORBITAL DECOMPRESSION

- Fat compartment
- Floor
- Medial wall
- Inferomedial complex
- Lateral wall.

Fat Decompression

Fat decompression decreases orbital pressure and apical compression by allowing the muscles and remaining fat to prolapse forward. Both intraconal and extraconal fat can be approached by either transconjunctival or transcutaneous route. Inferior approach is safer as it has lesser critical structures in this area and a greater volume of fat that can be removed. The proptosis reduction ranges from 3.5 mm to 5.9 mm. Also, the intraocular pressure is reduced by 3.4 mm Hg.

Complications of Fat Decompression

- Intraoperative:
    - Bleeding
- Postoperative:
    - Infection
    - Hemorrhage
    - Supraorbital anesthesia
    - Diplopia
    - The transcutaneous approach for extraconal fat removal may result in postoperative eyelid malposition.

Bony Decompression

The bony decompression involves selective removal of bones forming the walls of the orbit (Fig. 2 and Table 1).

The amount of proptosis reduction increases with the number of orbital walls decompressed (Table 2).

Preoperative CT orbit is performed for:

- Evaluation of level of ethmoid roof and cribriform plate to minimize risk of CSF leak in patients with anomalous bony anatomy
- Assessment of size of sinuses

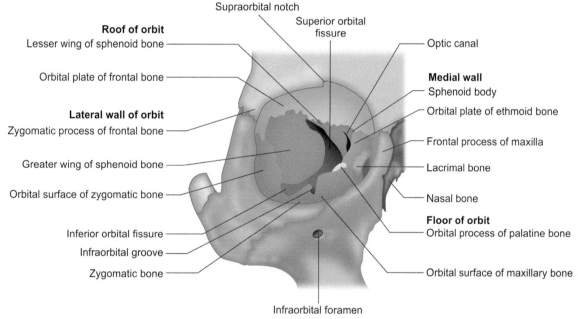

Fig. 2: Bones that form the orbit.

TABLE 1: Bone removal in floor, medial wall, and lateral wall decompression.

Floor	Original technique: Removal of the entire floor ± infraorbital nerve *Modifications:* Limitation of lateral extent to the space medial of the infraorbital nerve to preserve the function of infraorbital nerve. Sparing 10 mm of bone anteriorly under the globe to avoid hypoglobus.
Medial wall	*Anterior*—till posterior lacrimal crest *Posterior*—up to the anterior wall of the sphenoid sinus (in cases of optic neuropathy till the annulus of Zinn) *Superior*—up to frontoethmoidal suture *Inferior:* The orbital strut present inferomedially separates the medial and inferior walls. This strut is left completely or partly to avoid postoperative hypoglobus and strabismus. *Inferomedial posterior position:* The orbital process of the palatine bone is removed to allow for connection of the inferior and medial dissections in the orbital apex.
Lateral wall	The periosteum of the lateral orbital rim is incised parallel to the axis of the orbit. A subperiosteal plane is created till the tips of the inferior and superior orbital fissures are visualized. The orbital rim around the lacrimal fossa is thinned using high speed burr to improve visualization and facilitate instrumentation access. The diploe found within the greater wing of the sphenoid is entered by drilling anterior and superior to the tip of the inferior orbital fissure. The inferior orbital fissure is skeletonized and the thick bone extending from the tip of the superior orbital fissure to the frontozygomatic suture is removed.

TABLE 2: Relation between number of walls and amount of proptosis reduction.

Number of walls	Amount of proptosis reduction (in mm)
1	0–4
2	3–7
3	6–10
4	10–17

- Relative contribution of fat vs. muscle to the proptosis
- Relative location of inferior orbital nerve.

Floor and Medial Wall Decompression

Decompression of orbital floor alone is rarely performed and is usually combined with the medial wall as an inferomedial procedure.

Three main approaches to the floor have been described—transorbital, transantral, and transnasal.

Transorbital

The transcutaneous approach: An incision is made immediately below and parallel to the lash line in the lower eyelid (Fig. 3).

The transconjunctival approach: An incision is made on the palpebral conjunctival surface of the lower eyelid below the tarsus or in the fornix (Fig. 4).

Transcutaneous approach has a higher incidence of ectropion and lower eyelid retraction, relative to transconjunctival approach.

Medial wall: This is the best approach for dysthyroid optic neuropathy. The following approaches are used:
- *The Lynch approach:* An incision is made midway between the medial canthus and the nasal bridge, the periosteum is exposed, trochlea is disinserted, ethmoidal bundles are cauterized, and medial canthal tendon and the lacrimal sac are retracted to create a plane for decompression. The disadvantage is medial canthal scarring
- *Coronal approach:* An extended incision is made over the scalp, the supraorbital nerve and trochlea are repositioned. Due to high morbidity like frontal bossing, skin necrosis, alopecia, and anesthesia, it is rarely used for decompression
- *Transcaruncular approach:* The transcaruncular approach avoids cutaneous scarring and is the preferred route to access the medial wall. After splitting the caruncle, the incision is extended upward and downward to the mid orbit. It can be combined with transconjunctival or swinging eyelid techniques to access the floor and inferolateral wall.

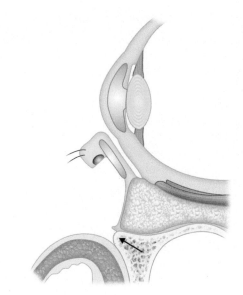

Fig. 3: The transcutaneous approach: An incision is made immediately below and parallel to the lash line in the lower eyelid.

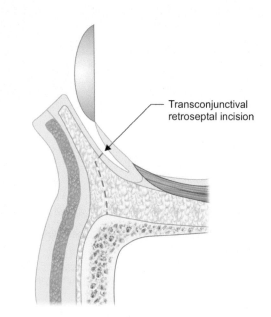

Transconjunctival retroseptal incision

Fig. 4: The transconjunctival approach: An incision is made on the palpebral conjunctival surface of the lower eyelid below the tarsus or in the fornix.

Transantral

This technique was described by Ogura and Walsh in which maxillary sinus is accessed via a Caldwell-Luc antrostomy. The complications of this approach are paresthesias, anesthesia, oroantral/gingivolabial fistula, and devitalized teeth.

Transnasal

The advantage of this technique is that it does not result in an external scar similar to transantral and transconjunctival approaches. Endoscopic transnasal decompression has become a popular technique.

The Lateral Wall

In the early 1990s, transorbital decompression of the deep lateral wall was popularized by Goldberg and associates. Incisions for lateral wall decompression:

- *Krönlein's incision:* A large curvilinear incision convexly running toward the lateral canthus from the hairline to the level of the tragus
- *Stallard and Wright's incision:* Running through the eyebrow, laterally into the crow's feet
- Berke's canthal splitting lateral linear incision
- *Lateral eyelid crease incision:* A popular approach that provides an excellent access to the lateral orbit and cosmetically superior as it is hidden in the eyelid crease and crow's feet
- *"Swinging eyelid" approach* (lateral canthotomy and lower fornix incision)
- Indirect approach via craniotomy.

Complications:
- *Intraoperative*—CSF leak, hemorrhage, and stroke
- *Postoperative*—Supraorbital and infraorbital anesthesia, alacrima, and motility disorder.

"Balanced" Decompression

Combination of lateral wall decompression through lateral eyelid crease incision and en block resection of lateral rim with drilling of the deep sphenoid is combined with a medial Lynch incision approach and external ethmoidectomy in order to eliminate floor related complications (such as hypoglobus, muscle imbalance, hypesthesia, and eyelid malposition). This achieves a proptosis reduction of 4.0 and 5.5 mm.

Four-wall Decompression

This is reserved for severe cases and includes removal of posterolateral roof resulting in more than 10 mm proptosis reduction.

CONCLUSION

To conclude, the primary indications of orbital decompression are compressive optic neuropathy and excessive proptosis. It is also done prior to strabismus surgery, for improvement of cosmesis, steroid dependence, and intractable pain. The amount of proptosis reduction is directly proportional to the number of walls decompressed. The complications of orbital decompression include diplopia, hypesthesia in distribution of infraorbital nerve, lower eyelid entropion, sinusitis, cerebrospinal fluid leak, nasolacrimal duct obstruction, retrobulbar hemorrhage, frontal lobe hematoma, and vision loss.

Enucleation, Evisceration, Orbital Exenteration and Orbital Implants

Akshay Gopinathan Nair

INTRODUCTION

Enucleation and evisceration are routine surgical procedures that an oculoplastic surgeon performs regularly. Simplistically put, enucleation is the removal of the globe from the orbit after separating all connections between the globe and the orbit, including severing the optic nerve.[1] Historically, it is said to be one of the oldest ophthalmic procedures that has been in practice.[2] Evisceration, on the other hand, is the removal of the contents of the globe while retaining the sclera and the attachments of the extraocular muscles. Both these procedures have special indications, with some overlap. Ideally, enucleation or evisceration surgery should result in adequate volume replacement achieved by implant; adequate surface area of the socket that should be lined with conjunctiva or any other mucus membrane; fornices that are deep enough to hold a prosthesis in place; good tone and strength of orbicularis oculi to hold the prosthesis within the fornices and finally satisfactory cosmetic outcome of the prosthesis in terms of external appearance and motility. An orbital exenteration is possibly one of the most disfiguring and destructive surgeries in ophthalmology. It involves removal of all the structures within the orbit—the globe, extraocular muscles, optic nerve, lacrimal gland, and orbital fat as well as the periorbita that encloses all these structures. This chapter will review the indications, surgical techniques, and complications.

ENUCLEATION

Deciding on an enucleation is a critical decision that must be reviewed and re-reviewed by the advising ophthalmologist before finally performing it. Typically, two qualified ophthalmologists must sign off on a decision to enucleate or eviscerate an eye. Many factors must be considered before advising an enucleation—the psychological condition of the patient, the visual potential of the eye, systemic ramifications of the disease for which the surgery is to be performed, any cosmetic concerns that the patient may have, and finally, the possible potential for complications.[1] The most common and most important indication for enucleation of an eye is the presence of an intraocular malignancy. Among the other indications for enucleation, a painful blind eye, prevention of sympathetic ophthalmia, phthisis bulbi, neovascular glaucoma, and endophthalmitis are the more common ones (Table 1).

TABLE 1: Table demonstrating the common indications for enucleation and evisceration along with select contraindications.

	Enucleation	Evisceration
Intraocular malignancy	Yes	No (Absolute contraindication)
Painful blind eye	Yes	Yes
Endophthalmitis	Yes	Yes
Penetrating trauma	Yes	Relative contraindication
Small phthisical eye	Yes	Yes
Panophthalmitis	No (Absolute contraindication)	Yes

Other rare indications include microphthalmia in children to improve the bony growth in children by enucleating the globe and placing a suitably sized orbital implant, in an attempt to improve overall cosmesis.[3] A relatively rare and possibly controversial indication for primary enucleation is a severe trauma leading to complete disruption of the ocular anatomy. Ophthalmologists, usually, tend to primarily repair the globe regardless of the extent of damage. Enucleation may also alleviate concern that surgery may contribute to the potential risk of sympathetic ophthalmia in the fellow eye. However, the low incidence of sympathetic ophthalmitis, early diagnosis, and improved medication have made this "prophylactic enucleation" somewhat controversial and debatable.[4]

The choice of anesthesia for enucleation is general anesthesia. General anesthesia offers pain control and hypotension—both of which are ideal for enucleation. Preoperatively, if the media is opaque, an ultrasound examination should be performed. Typically, two qualified ophthalmologists must concur on the diagnosis and the decision to perform an enucleation and the surgical consent form typically bears the signatures of the treating ophthalmologists. After confirming the eye to be operated, a 360° peritomy is the first step performed. In this chapter, a popular and our preferred technique (Figs. 1 to 4)—the myoconjunctival technique is being described.[5] Subconjunctival dissection in between the recti muscles is carried out and extended peripherally to separate Tenon's capsule from the sclera. In the myoconjunctival technique, each of the four recti is hooked, identified, and a traction suture with 4-0 silk is taken passing through the muscle, very close to the insertion of the muscle on the globe. A few millimeters away, the muscle is secured with double-armed 6-0 vicryl sutures or any other absorbable suture. The muscle is severed in between the two sutures—either with bipolar cautery or a sharp pair of scissors, leaving the traction suture on the muscle stump attached to the globe and the vicryl suture still attached to the muscle. Cutting of this muscle can be done with either a cautery or with scissors. The superior and inferior oblique muscles are typically cut without tagging. Once this is done, a lateral canthotomy may be performed to allow the globe to gently prolapse out of the socket. Some surgeons prefer to do a canthotomy in all cases and therefore do it in the beginning. A temporal approach with a curved enucleation scissors or a straight pair is preferred to cut the optic nerve. Some surgeons opt for a nasal approach using a pair of curved enucleation scissors. Gentle traction on the globe is provided using the nondominant hand which makes the optic nerve stretched. The optic nerve is strummed keeping the blades of the scissors closed to assess the position and length of the optic nerve as well as get an idea

about the distance from the orbital apex. Some surgeons prefer to place an enucleation spoon to protect the globe and provide upward traction. Severing the optic nerve is a critical step. It has been reported that longer optic nerve segments were obtained at enucleation with mildly curved scissor blades from both temporal and nasal surgical approaches. On the other hand, strongly curved scissor blades uniformly produced smaller specimens.[6] This is particularly important while operating eyes with intraocular malignancies, especially retinoblastoma. It is vital while performing enucleation in these cases to obtain a long segment of optic nerve so that the entire tumor is removed since retinoblastoma commonly spreads via extension into the optic nerve.[6] Hemostasis is achieved by pressure using gauze for at least 3–5 minutes. Once, hemostasis has been obtained, an orbital implant is introduced into the orbit, within the muscle cone—this space can be identified by the presence of orbital fat and is posterior to Tenon's capsule. Ideally an implant that is at least 20 mm in size should be placed even in children such that it stimulates normal orbitofacial growth.

The Tenon's capsule is closed in two distinct layers using absorbable sutures. In the myoconjunctival technique, the previously secured recti muscle edges are passed through the overlying conjunctiva and tied. The distance between the edge of the conjunctiva and the site of passing these sutures is approximately the same distance between the limbus and the insertions of the respective recti. Thus, the recti are attached "myoconjunctivally" to fornices on all four sides. The conjunctiva is closed in a continuous fashion using absorbable sutures. A conformer is placed and a temporary tarsorrhaphy is performed. This conformer is replaced with a prosthesis at a suitable date after ensuring the conjunctiva has healed completely. Apart from the myoconjunctival technique described here, other techniques include the imbrication technique, where the superior rectus is imbricated (overlapped and sutured) with the inferior rectus, and similarly, the medial rectus is imbricated with lateral rectus. In the integrated implant technique, where a porous implant is used, the muscles are directly sutured to the scleral cap or the mesh used to wrap the implant in a location corresponding to muscle insertion.

Enucleating the wrong is a very serious error that can be avoided by clear, repeated communication, performing a surgical "time-out, marking the eye by the performing surgeon and thorough examination of both eyes just before commencing the surgery.[1] More common intraoperative complications include orbital hemorrhage and loss of a muscle. Patients should be advised to discontinue any anticoagulant medications at least a week before surgery to minimize the risk of uncontrolled bleeding. In most cases, prolonged pressure using gauze stops bleeding in

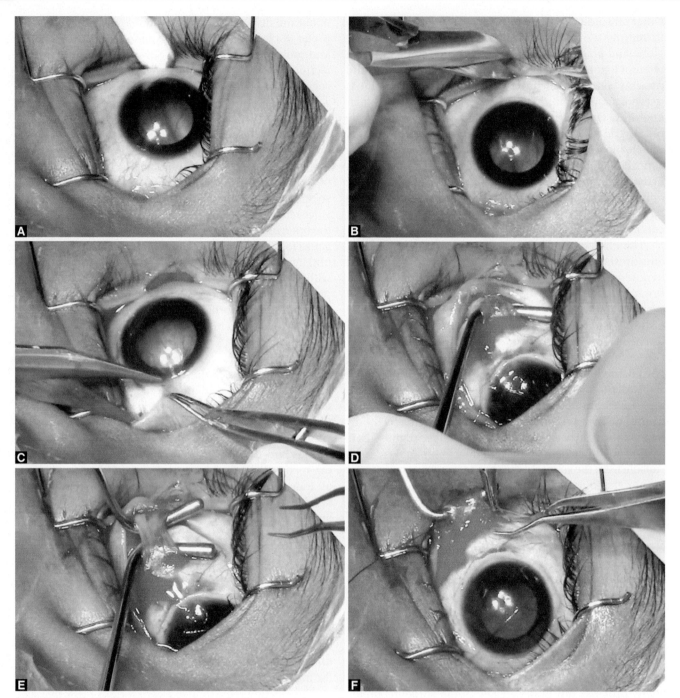

Figs. 1A to F: (A) The first step in an enucleation is to perform a thorough examination of the eye to ascertain that the correct eye is being operated upon. (B) Following this a lateral canthotomy is done. (C) Careful 360° peritomy is done. The extraocular muscles are (D) hooked and (E) isolated and (F) a traction suture is taken with 6-0 silk close to the insertion of the muscle. Here the muscle being hooked and tagged is the lateral rectus.

most cases. Other techniques include injecting anesthetic drugs with epinephrine before cutting the optic nerve and the placement of a hemostat forceps around the nerve for a few minutes prior to cutting it.[7] In some rare cases, orbital exploration may be required to identify the bleeder and coagulate it. The use of Gelfoam or bone wax is also

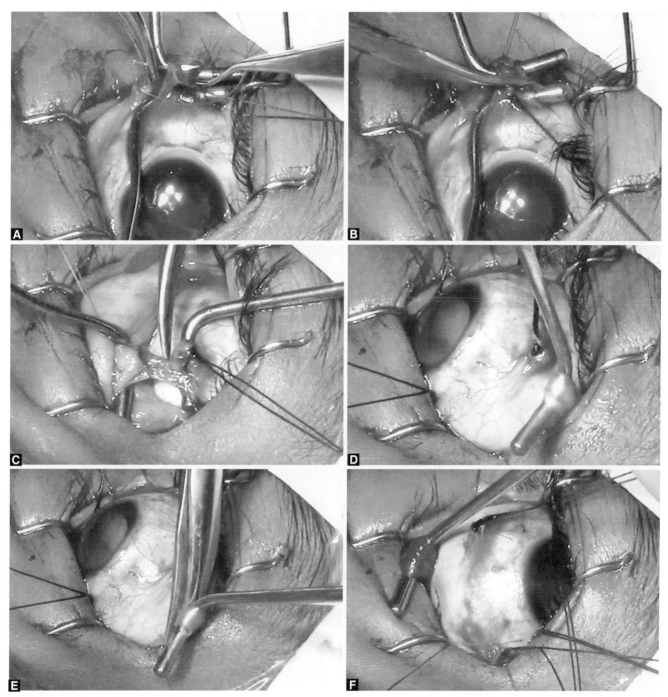

Figs. 2A to F: A tag suture is taken with a double-armed 6-0 vicryl suture about 6 mm away from the initial traction suture (A) and the muscle is cut in between the two sutures (B). (C) The same technique is performed on all the extraocular muscles. Shown here is the lateral rectus being cut. After all recti have been cut, the superior oblique is then hooked (D) and cut without tagging (E). The inferior rectus is also hooked (F) and cut.

helpful in stopping such bleeds. The loss of a muscle is an intraoperative complication that can be prevented by meticulous tagging of the muscle.

Common early postoperative complications are lid edema, hemorrhage, conjunctival prolapse, chemosis, and rarely, orbital infection. Patients often complain of

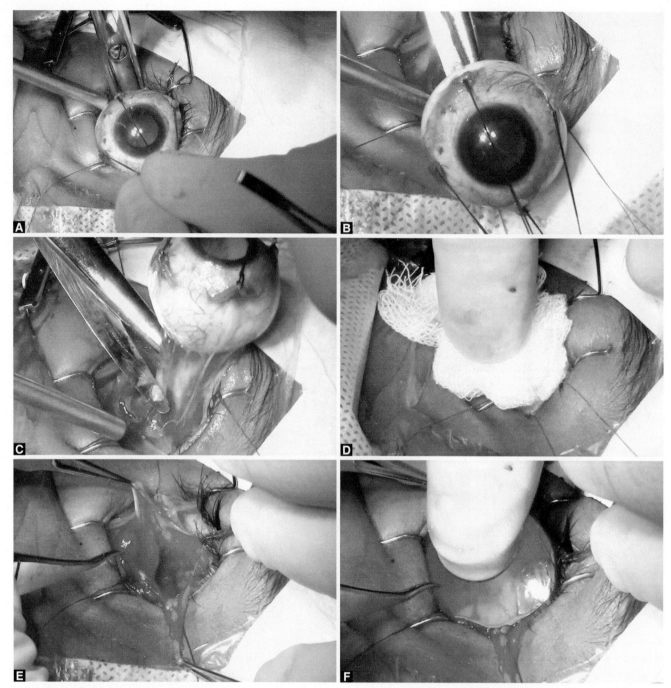

Figs. 3A to F: (A) Upward traction is provided by pulling the four silk traction sutures and this makes the optic nerve taut. (B) After strumming the optic nerve, a slightly curved scissor, which was introduced from the temporal side, is used to cut the optic nerve. (C) After severing the optic nerve, all other adnexal attachments are also cut. A gauze pack is used to stop any bleeding (D) and kept in place for a couple of minutes with application of constant pressure. The space posterior to the posterior Tenon's fascia is identified (E) and the implant is introduced within (F).

severe orbital pain and vomit. Other late complications are enophthalmos, which can occur if a small implant is placed. A superior sulcus deformity is primarily caused by loss of orbital volume and loss of tone of tissues within the orbit. It is clinically seen as a deep groove or space between the upper eyelid and orbital rim, giving the appearance of enophthalmos and ptosis.[1] A common late complication following an enucleation is postenucleation socket

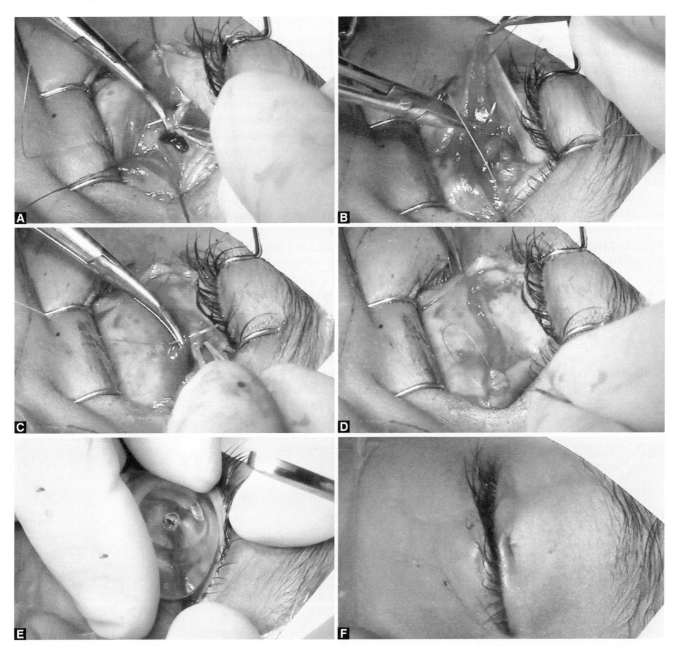

Figs. 4A to F: (A) The posterior Tenon's fascia is closed with interrupted absorbable sutures. (B) The next step is to attach the extraocular muscles to the fornix and this is done by passing the double-armed vicryl sutures out through the space between the Tenon's and the conjunctiva and attaching the muscles in the fornix. (C) The anterior Tenon's fascia is then closed with interrupted sutures. (D) The conjunctiva is closed in a continuous fashion. A conformer is placed (E) and finally a temporary suture tarsorrhaphy is performed (F).

syndrome (PESS). This term includes multiple clinical manifestations such as ptosis, enophthalmos, superior sulcus deformity, shallow anterior fornix, atrophy of orbital fat, and entropion, or ectropion of the lower lid. All of these conditions combined lead to reduction in the size of aperture and inability of the socket to hold a prosthesis. In some cases, when an orbital implant is not placed following an enucleation, over time, the conjunctiva contracts and

scars leading to a contracted socket which may not hold an orbital prosthesis. The management of contracted socket is beyond the scope of this chapter.

EVISCERATION

Evisceration of the eye is the removal of the contents of the eye, leaving the external shell—the sclera and the extraocular muscles intact. Usually, an orbital implant is placed within the scleral shell with layered closure over it. There are multiple variations in the surgical technique; the primary steps remain the same (Figs. 5 to 7). Just as it is for all ocular surgeries, it is important to recheck and verify the eye to be operated upon before placing the speculum. An evisceration can be performed under local anesthesia (peribulbar or retrobulblar anesthesia). The first step is 360° conjunctival peritomy. Injecting a small amount of local anesthetic subconjunctivally allows easy peritomy and better pain control. The conjunctiva should be handled minimally in an attempt to preserve as much conjunctiva as possible. A limbus-based stab incision is made with a blade and the entire corneal button is cut with scissors. Many surgeons prefer to leave the corneal button on. Here, the preferred technique involves removal of the button. The intraocular contents are then removed with the aid of an evisceration spoon or a scoop which is a round, flat curette. Other instruments that can create a cleavage plane in between the choroid and the sclera are a Freer's periosteum elevator. Suprachoriodal dissection is done to remove the entire intraocular contents—the choroid, retina, and the vitreous body as a whole—in toto. Meticulous removal of all uveal tissue is important; theoretically, this step decreases the potential risk of sympathetic ophthalmia.[8] After removal of all the uveal tissue, absolute alchohol is applied within the scleral shell using cotton tips dipped in alchohol. Bleeding vessels may be visible on the inner surface of the scleral shell which can be cauterized. This causes denaturation of any residual protein that might otherwise incite inflammation or present as the antigenic stimulus for sympathetic ophthalmia. Following this, the surgical field must be thoroughly irrigated with saline since any residual alcohol itself can cause postoperative inflammation, if not completely washed away. Sclerotomy permits the placement of larger implants and there are multiple variations in the methods of sclerotomy. The authors prefer to make four petals by creating linear sclerotomies in between the four recti muscles.[9] The incisions extend from the scleral rim and run posteriorly till the optic nerve head insertion. A posterior circular sclerotomy is performed around the optic nerve head to detach the nerve from the scleral petals, each of which is attached to a rectus muscle. The choice of implant and the different advantages and disadvantages of each of the different types of implant is a vast topic in itself and beyond the scope of this chapter. The authors prefer to use a nonintegrated polymethylmethacrylate (PMMA) implant within the scleral petals. Closure is in layers with overlap of the anterior edges of the petals. The Tenon's fascia and conjunctiva are closed in layers with nonabsorbable

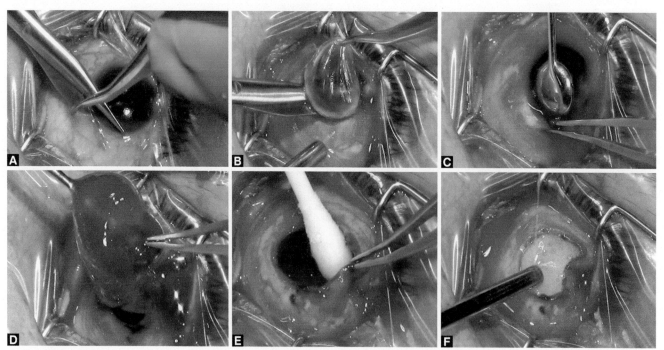

Figs. 5A to F: The first step in an evisceration is a 360° peritomy (A) followed by removal of the corneal button (B) Careful dissection (C) and removal of the intraocular contents is done (D) which is followed by application of absolute alcohol within the scleral shell to denature any residual choroidal material (E). A thorough saline wash is essential as any residual alcohol can lead to severe postoperative inflammation (F).

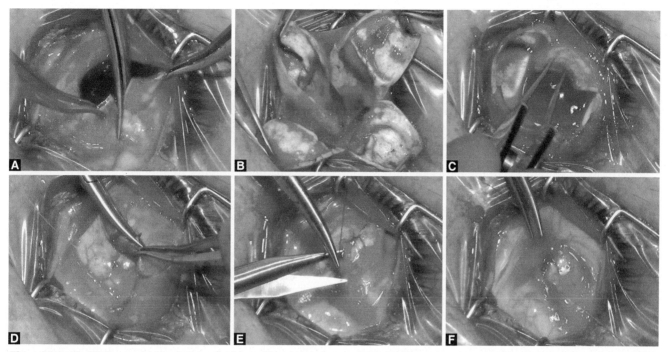

Figs. 6A to E: (A) Four scleral petals are fashioned by performing vertically linear cuts in between each of the recti muscles. (B) The vertical cuts can extend posteriorly up to the optic nerve attachment. A posterior circular sclerotomy can be performed all around the optic nerve to detach it from the sclera. The implant is placed within the four petals (C) and the petals are overlapped to and sutured to provide maximum coverage to the implant (D and E). The Tenon's fascia is closed with absorbable sutures (F).

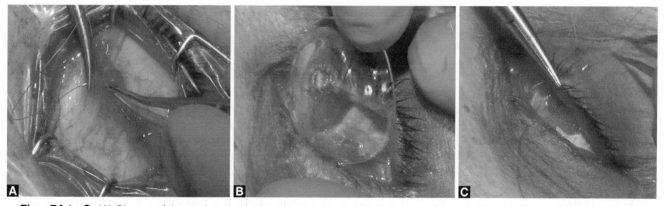

Figs. 7A to C: (A) Closure of the conjunctiva is done in a continuous fashion . A conformer is placed at the end of the surgery to maintain the fornices (B) followed by a temporary tarsorrhaphy (C).

sutures. A conformer is placed and the authors prefer to perform a temporary tarsorrhaphy. A customized ocular prosthesis is placed after 4–6 weeks.

There are many different techniques of performing sclerotomies and relaxing incisions on the sclera to accommodate larger implants. Many authors have described these techniques in literature. Lee and colleagues advocated the creation of scleral windows posterior to each of the rectus muscle insertion.[10] Jordan and Anderson described a technique that involved disinsertion of the optic nerve and the creation of small radial sclerotomies.[11] Another technique called the "scleral quadrisection" has also been described by Yang, et al.[12] Massry and Hold have described obliquely splitting the scleral cavity into two sections and releasing the flaps from their optic nerve attachments.[13] Our preferred technique is the four petal technique proposed by Sales-Sanz and Sanz-Lopez where they created four complete sclerotomies from the limbus to the optic nerve with optic nerve disinsertion. This resulted in the creation of four petals that was attached to a rectus muscle each. The petals were then brought anteriorly to cover the implant.[9] Georgescu et al. reported a novel technique which was more useful in patients with smaller globes, namely phthisis bulbi and microphthalmos. In this technique, a 5-mm wedge of sclera was excised nasally and temporally and a 360° equatorial scleral incision was made, dividing the scleral into anterior and posterior halves.[14]

Kaltreider and Lucarelli proposed an algorithm for selection of an implant size for patients undergoing enucleation, evisceration, and secondary implantation. The formula 2 mm subtracted from the axial length gives the implant diameter. However, further subtraction of 1 mm from implant diameter is required for evisceration and for hyperopia. In their pilot study, they showed that this formula allowed for 100% replacement of the volume removed, and left space for a prosthesis of approximately 1.5–2.5 mL. It also eliminated clinically unacceptable superior sulcus deformity and enophthalmos in most of the patients.[15] Alternatively, a sizer can be used intraoperatively to help in assessing the ideal size of the implant to be used.

Historically, literature shows that the most common indication for evisceration was severe penetrating ocular trauma despite the possibility of sympathetic ophthalmitis. In such cases, the rationale behind evisceration is the removal of the eye (or its contents) prior to sensitization can be a preventive measure. However, in recent times, evisceration is not the procedure of choice in severe ocular trauma. In a case with extensive disruption of the globe, often times, it is not feasible to remove all uveal tissue if an evisceration is to be done. In such cases, therefore, performing an enucleation may serve the purpose of preventing sympathetic ophthalmia better.[8] Conventionally, evisceration has been the procedure of choice for infections such as endophthalmitis and enucleation is the surgery of choice for intraocular malignancies. For other indications such as a disfigured or painful blind eye, phthisis bulbi and absolute glaucoma, surgeons show varying preferences with no clear consensus. However, one of the most important contraindications for evisceration is suspected intraocular malignancy.[16]

IMPLANTS

Following an evisceration or enucleation, it is necessary to place-in an implant in suitable cases to replace the volume of the globe within the orbit (Box 1). Apart from volume replacement, implants serve multiple roles–promoting orbito–facial growth which is crucial in children; preventing contraction of the orbital soft tissue and aiding in motility of the prosthesis. From the point of view of classification, there

Box 1: Characteristics of an ideal orbital implant.

- Should provide adequate volume replacement
- Should provide good motility transmitted to prosthesis
- Should provide adequate support to the prosthesis
- Should possess a low rate of associated complications
- Technically easy to implant into the orbit
- Biocompatibility
- Non-degradability
- Economical

are many different types of implants and therefore there exist multiple classification systems—they are classified on the basis of shape, size, material, etc. However, the most important and basic simplification is the division of implants into two groups—porous (bio-integrated) and nonporous implants, also known as inert (nonintegrated).

Nonintegrated implants do not have any provisions for attachments of the extraocular muscles. They typically have smooth surfaces and do not allow ingrowth of fibrovascular tissue. Obviously, nonintegrated implants have no direct attachment to the ocular prosthesis. The motility of the ocular prosthesis, in cases of inert orbital implants, is the movement which is transmitted from the nonporous spherical implants through the surface tension in the interface between the conjunctival surface and the posterior surface of the ocular prosthesis, as well as the movement of the fornices.

In order to allow for better motility of the prosthesis, some authors prefer to "wrap" these implants following enucleation. There are a host of materials namely donor sclera, bovine pericardium, processed human pericardium, polytetrafluoroethylene (e-PTFE), and polyglactin mesh among others.[17] The extraocular muscles can be attached to the wrapping material and this is known to increase the amount of motility. However, nonintegrated implants do not allow for any attachment or direct interaction with the prosthesis. Commonly used nonintegrated, nonporous implants are glass, rubber, silicone, steel, gold, silver, acrylic, and the most commonly used is PMMA.[18] In contrast, the porous nature of integrated implants allows fibrovascular ingrowth throughout the implant and thus also insertion of pegs that are directly connected to the prosthesis. Pegging typically is carried out 6–8 months after the initial surgery. Pegging though is not without its share of complications namely chronic conjunctivitis, discharge, infection, and pyogenic granulomas.

As mentioned earlier, the attachment of extraocular muscles to the implant or its wrapping material is believed to improve implant motility and reduce the risk of implant migration. The amount of movement transmitted from the implant to the prosthesis determines the degree of final prosthetic motility. Another less frequently used type of implants is "quasi-integrated implants", such as the Allen implant and the Iowa implant. These implants have irregularly shaped surfaces that create an indirect coupling mechanism between the implant and prosthesis. It is understood that these implants can impart a higher degree of movement to the prosthesis. Directly integrating the implant to the prosthesis, as is done in pegging for porous implants—through an externalized coupling mechanism would ideally provide the highest degree of prosthesis motility. Limited availability, relatively higher maintenance, and complications have reduced their popularity among surgeons.

Porous orbital implants are manufactured from different materials including natural and synthetic sources. These materials are hydroxyapatite, aluminum oxide, and polyethylene. Hydroxyapatite is formed from a salt of calcium phosphate that is present in the mineralized portion of human bone and is reported to be nontoxic, nonallergenic, and biocompatible.[1,19] While hydroxyapatite implants are typically spherical in shape and commercially available in many sizes; aluminum oxide and porous polyethylene implants are available in different shapes and sizes. Porous implants are thought to offer better implant movement than the traditional nonintegrated implants mainly because while placing porous implants, the extraocular muscles are directly attached to the implant. The pores also allow for fibrovascular in-growth and therefore also have a lesser rate of migration and exposure.[20, 21]

Ceramic implants have gained some popularity in recent times primarily due to a highly interconnected pore network within, that allows them to act as a passive framework for host fibrovascular in-growth. This fibrovascular intergration with orbital tissue potentially has low complication rates while increasing motility of the prosthesis when pegging is performed. The vascularization of porous implants was also thought to reduce the incidence of implant migration, implant exposure, and implant extrusion. In addition, vascularization of a porous implant is believed to increase the success rate of surgical repair or patch grafting in case of implant exposure.[1,22] However, literature suggests that porous implants were found to have higher exposure rates overall when compared to smoother synthetic implants.[23]

Multiple factors lead to complications such as implant exposure—namely infection, poor wound healing, ill-fitting prostheses—especially small or tight prostheses which lead to the development of pressure points between the implant and prosthesis and over time, can lead to a defect in the underlying conjunctiva. This subsequently can also lead to extrusion of the implant. Exposed implants themselves can also be the nidus for further infection leading to a vicious cycle that invariably ends in implant extrusion.

In some cases, small defects over porous implants may rarely close spontaneously. Most exposures require additional procedures such as the use of amniotic membrane grafts and scleral patch grafts to promote conjunctival healing. Other techniques that have been used for the treatment of implant exposure include repair using different materials such as hard palate mucosa, dermis fat graft (DFG), buccal mucosa, and temporalis fascia. Even the use of autologous serum drops to promote epithelial healing following surgeries to cover the defect has been reported with some success.[24]

The placement of an implant in an enucleation or evisceration being performed for fulminant infection is a controversial question. Traditionally, in surgery it is believed that in the presence of infections, the placement of an implant may hamper wound healing, delay infection clearance, result in implant exposure and extrusion. However, many studies have reported the contrary—some authors have reported that evisceration with primary porous implant placement is a viable treatment option for patients with endophthalmitis with very few cases of implant exposure and infection.[25] Tripathy and Rath reported that evisceration with primary placement of nonporous silicone implants in fulminant endophthalmitis/panophthalmitis provided good postoperative cosmetic outcome to the anophthalmic socket at an economical cost.[26]

ORBITAL EXENTERATION

Orbital exenteration is by far the most disfiguring surgery in ophthalmic practice. It is also practised by head and neck surgeons, ENT surgeons, and neurosurgeons. The indications for orbital exenteration are large, diffuse orbital malignancies as well as eyelid and conjunctival malignancies that have extended into the surrounding structures such as the globe and the orbit. The aim of performing an orbital exenteration is to achieve cure with tumor-free margins. Other rare indications for orbital exenteration include painful or life-threatening orbital inflammations and infections such as refractory idiopathic orbital inflammatory disease and invasive sino-orbital fungal infections (Box 2). Occasionally, this procedure may also be performed as a palliative measure. It summarizes the common indications for orbital exenteration.

Exenteration may be classified into subtotal, total, and radical or extended exenteration. A subtotal exenteration is one which does not involve complete orbital clearance. In some cases, such as an anteriorly located tumor like a large invasive conjunctival squamous cell carcinoma that invades the anterior orbit, where surgical excision of the tumor alone would not be feasible, a subtotal exenteration may be performed. In cases like this, posterior structures

Box 2: Indications for orbital exenteration.

- Primary orbital tumors
- Orbital extension of eyelid tumors
  a. Basal Cell Carcinomas
  b. Squamous Cell Carcinomas
  c. Sebaceous Gland Carcinomas
- Extraocular/Orbital extension of intraocular tumors like uveal melanoma
- Orbital extension of conjunctival tumors
- Invasive sino-orbital fungal diseases (e.g. Mucormycosis)
- Nonresponsive, recalcitrant orbital inflammatory disease (rarely)

such as the orbital fat, the stumps of the extraocular muscles, and other structures at the orbital apex are left intact. A total exenteration is the removal of all structures within the orbit up to the orbital apex. This is required in posteriorly located tumors that extend all the way up to the apex. There is no residual tissue left behind and the bony socket is left behind. A variation in surgical technique is the "eyelid sparing exenteration". Here, the eyelid margins and the tarsus are typically sacrificed leaving behind some amount of orbicularis oculi muscle and skin; the edges of which are approximated to provide a skin-lined orbital socket which is more esthetic, offers better rehabilitation option, and heals earlier. An eyelid-sparing technique can be employed in a sub-total exenteration as well as a total exenteration. Once healed well, the skin-lined sockets are resilient and can withstand orbital radiation, when required, without exhibiting necrosis. A radical or extended orbital exenteration typically involves complete removal of all orbital contents as well as adjoining structures; such as maxillectomy, ethmoidectomy; excision of the frontal sinus and nose. This is usually performed in cases of tumors that arise from the skull bones, paranasal sinuses, or cranium and invade into the orbit and orbital structures.

In cases where an eyelid-sparing exenteration cannot be performed, the surgical site is usually left to granulate by secondary intention. It could be covered with a split-thickness skin graft. Those sockets left to heal with secondary intention usually result in shallower orbits. They also have slightly prolonged healing compared with those lined with split-thickness skin graft.[27] There are various techniques used to reconstruct and fill the dead space within the orbit following an exenteration. These include muscle flaps, free flaps and tissue transfer, orbital fat, bone flaps, autologous bone, or Osseo-integration, and periosteal flaps.[27] Postoperatively, an orbital prosthesis is used which can be magnetically attached, or simply placed within the socket with the concavity offering a snug fit for the prosthesis. A spectacle mounted prosthesis is also an option. However, many patients prefer to patch the socket and cover it rather than wear an orbital exenteration prosthesis.

SUMMARY

To summarize, enucleation and evisceration surgeries have overlapping indications as the surgery of choice in painful blind eyes; but enucleation remains the procedure of choice in cases where the surgery is being performed on eyes with intraocular tumors. Wherever possible, adequate volume replacement with implants should be done. This fills the void left behind by removal of the eye and reduces the potential for volume deficit within the socket.[1] Conformers should be retained following the surgery, to avoid forniceal shortening. Factors such as the material for implants and size of implant are largely dependent on the surgeon's preferences. Orbital exenteration is a disfiguring surgery that involves the removal of the entire orbital contents and is typically indicated in advanced orbital malignancies.

REFERENCES

1. Moshfeghi DM, Moshfeghi AA, Finger PT. Enucleation. Surv Ophthalmol. 2000;44(4):277-301.
2. Beard CH. Enucleation. Ophthalmic Surgery. Philadelphia: P. Blakiston's Son & Co.; 1910. pp. 457-77.
3. Nunery WR, Chen WP. Enucleation and evisceration. In: Bosniak S (Ed). Principles and Practice of Ophthalmic Plastic and Reconstructive Surgery, Volume 2, 1st edition. Philadelphia: W.B. Saunders Company; 1996. pp. 1035-46.
4. Galor A, Davis JL, Flynn HW Jr, et al. Sympathetic ophthalmia: Incidence of ocular complications and vision loss in the sympathizing eye. Am J Ophthalmol. 2009;148(5):704-10.e2.
5. Shome D, Honavar SG, Raizada K, et al. Implant and prosthesis movement after enucleation: A randomized controlled trial. Ophthalmology. 2010;117(8):1638-44.
6. Coats DK, Paysse EA, Chu Y. Obtaining maximal optic nerve length during enucleation procedures. Arch Ophthalmol. 2000;118(1):70-3.
7. Stone W. Complications of evisceration and enucleation. In: Fasanella RM (Ed). Management of Complications in Eye Surgery. Philadelphia: W.B. Saunders; 1957. pp. 278-317.
8. Phan LT, Hwang TN, McCulley TJ. Evisceration in the modern age. Middle East Afr J Ophthalmol. 2012;19(1):24-33.
9. Sales-Sanz M, Sanz-Lopez A. Four-petal evisceration: A new technique. Ophthalmic Plast Reconstr Surg. 2007;23(5):389-92.
10. Lee SY, Kwon OW, Hong YJ, et al. Modification of the scleral openings to reduce tissue breakdown and exposure after hydroxyapatite implantations. Ophthalmologica. 1995;209(6):319-22.
11. Jordan DR, Anderson RL. The universal implant for evisceration surgery. Ophthalmic Plast Reconstr Surg. 1997;13(1):1-7.
12. Yang JG, Khwarg SI, Wee WR, et al. Hydroxyapatite implantation with scleral quadrisection after evisceration. Ophthalmic Surg Lasers. 1997;28(11):915-9.
13. Massry GG, Holds JB. Evisceration with scleral modification. Ophthalmic Plast Recosntr Surg. 2001;17(1):42-7.

14. Georgescu D, Vagefi MR, Yang CC, et al. Evisceration with equatorial sclerotomy for phthisis bulbi and microphthalmos. Ophthalmic Plast Reconstr Surg. 2010;26(3):165-7.

15. Kaltreider SA, Lucarelli MJ. A simple algorithm for selection of implant size for enucleation and evisceration: A prospective study. Ophthalmic Plast Reconstr Surg. 2002;18(5):336-41.

16. Manschot WA, van Peperzeel HA. Choroidal melanoma. Enucleation or observation? A new approach. Arch Ophthalmol. 1980;98(1):71-7.

17. Klapper SR, Jordan DR, Punja K, et al. Hydroxyapatite implant wrapping materials: Analysis of fibrovascular ingrowth in an animal model. Ophthalmic Plast Reconstr Surg. 2000;16(4):278-85.

18. Beard C. Remarks on historical and newer approaches to orbital implants. Ophthalmic Plast Reconstr Surg. 1995;11(2):89-90.

19. Perry AC. Integrated orbital implants. Adv Ophthalmic Plast Reconstr Surg. 1990;8:75-81.

20. Shields CL, Shields JA, De Potter P, et al. Problems with the hydroxyapatite orbital implant: Experience with 250 consecutive cases. Br J Ophthalmol. 1994;78(9):702-6.

21. Jordan DR, Chan S, Mawn L, et al. Complications associated with pegging hydroxyapatite orbital implants. Ophthalmology. 1999;106(3):505-12.

22. Shields CL, Shields JA, Eagle RC Jr, et al. Histopathologic evidence of fibrovascular ingrowth four weeks after placement of the hydroxyapatite orbital implant. Am J Ophthalmol. 1991;111(3):363-6.

23. Custer PL, Kennedy RH, Woog JJ, et al. Orbital implants in enucleation surgery: A report by the American Academy of Ophthalmology. Ophthalmology. 2003;110(10):2054-61.

24. Kamal S, Kumar S, Goel R. Autologous serum for anterior tissue necrosis after porous orbital implant. Middle East Afr J Ophthalmol. 2014;21(2):193-5.

25. Park YG, Paik JS, Yang SW. The results of evisceration with primary porous implant placement in patients with endophthalmitis. Korean J Ophthalmol. 2010;24(5):279-83.

26. Tripathy D, Rath S. Evisceration with primary orbital implant in fulminant endophthalmitis/panophthalmitis. Orbit. 2015;34(5):279-83.

27. Ben Simon GJ, Schwarcz RM, Douglas R, et al. Orbital exenteration: One size does not fit all. Am J Ophthalmol. 2005;139(1):11-7.

11

CHAPTER

Anophthalmic Socket: Evaluation and Management

Raj Anand

INTRODUCTION

All the structures in the orbit are meant to serve the eye; when the eye is lost, for whatever reason, the adnexal structures lose their purpose and the support; for this very reason, this socket is also known as the orphan socket. This socket undergoes certain anatomic and pathophysiologic changes which form the basis of anophthalmic socket management.

CLASSIFICATION

Broadly speaking, anophthalmia can be divided in two categories, congenital and acquired. These two types of anophthalmic socket represent two different entities with different anatomy, pathophysiology, and management.

EPIDEMIOLOGY

Congenital anophthalmia is fortunately rare with reported prevalence of 0.2–0.3 per 10,000 live births.[1,2] Growth of the bony orbit and ocular adnexal tissue is dependent on presence of eyeball;[3] therefore, absence of globe translates into a smaller bony orbit (Fig. 1) and rudimentary socket (Fig. 2). This socket may be too small to accommodate a prosthesis.

Acquired anophthalmia, in contrast, is a result of surgical intervention (enucleation or evisceration), the prevalence of acquired anophthalmia following enucleation in the western world has been reported to be 2.6 to 5 per 100,000 population.[4,5] However, the same has been estimated to be almost 100 times more common in Indian population at 33 per 10,000 population.[6] If the data for anophthalmia

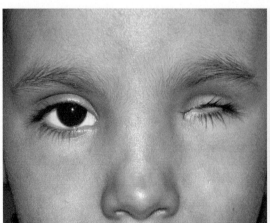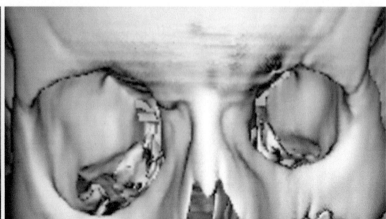

Fig. 1: Congenital anophthalmia with rudimentary adnexa (left) and smaller bony orbit (right).

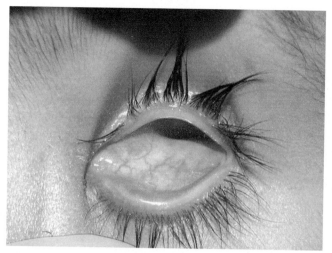

Fig. 2: Congenital anophthalmia with shallow inferior fornix and smaller socket.

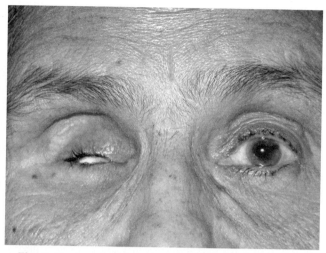

Fig. 3: Postenucleation socket syndrome deep set eye with hollow superior sulcus under the eyebrow.

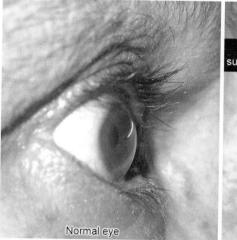
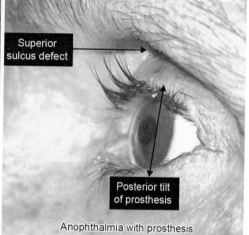

Fig. 4: Socket changes in anophthalmia left eye compared to the normal contralateral side—right eye (lateral view).

following evisceration is also added to this number we can imagine very well the large number of anophthalmic sockets that we deal with in clinical practice.

ANATOMY AND PATHOPHYSIOLOGY

Eyeball floats in the cushion of orbital fat in the midorbit and is held in place with various septa. After the eye is removed by enucleation, the socket tissues lose that support of septal tissue and tend to fall back posterior and inferior. These set of changes in the orbital soft tissue lead to what is known as "post enucleation socket syndrome" (PESS) (Fig. 3).

Figure 4 shows clinical comparison of anophthalmic socket appearance with ocular prosthesis vis-a-vis normal eye in lateral view. The vertical plane of prosthesis is tilted backward and there is hollowness under the eyebrows (known as superior sulcus defect).

These clinical changes are reflection of the deeper changes in the orbital soft tissue. A parasagittal high definition CT scan through the anophthalmic orbit and normal orbit (for comparison) shows these changes very well (Fig. 5). The extraocular muscles tend to be short and pulled posteriorly, thereby pulling the orbital soft tissues as well with them.

CLINICAL FEATURES

Acquired Anophthalmia

Clinical features of acquired anophthalmia varies to a great extent, depending on how the anophthalmia has been managed by the treating ophthalmologist—ocularist (the professional who fabricates a custom artificial eye or ocular prosthesis) team. A healthy socket after enucleation/

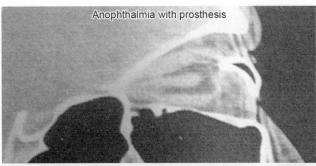

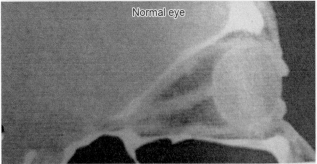

Fig. 5: Post enucleation socket syndrome changes in the deeper tissues of anophthalmic socket (as seen in the parasagittal CT scan) compared to the normal orbit.

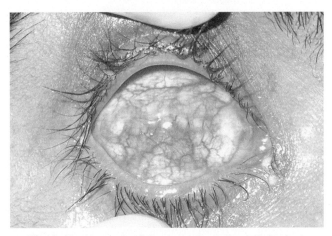

Fig. 6: Healthy socket following evisceration with implant.

evisceration with implant has smooth healthy conjunctiva-tenon layer covering the orbital implant that is central in location and gives convex contour to the socket (Fig. 6). The fornices are adequate and allow comfortable fit to prosthesis with complete movement of the lids.

A well-made ocular prosthesis over a healthy socket with implant can virtually be indistinguishable from contralateral side in appearance. The patient also is symptom free with this prosthesis; on the other extreme if the socket is not optimally treated and the prosthesis is not fitting well, this is a cosmetic blemish and the patient has

persistent complains of discharge, pain, and difficulty in retaining prosthesis (Fig. 7).

Congenital Anophthalmia

Congenital anophthalmia in contrast presents totally different picture from acquired one. The eye has not developed during fetal growth and the surrounding ocular adnexal tissues are also rudimentary (Figs. 1 and 2). The eyelids are small and the palpebral fissure is also greatly reduced in dimensions; the fornices are so shallow that it may not allow any prosthesis to be retained in the socket. Dimensions of bony orbit are also reduced because of lack of growth stimulus from developing eye (Fig. 1). This orbital bony asymmetry may lead to significant facial asymmetry in later years of life.

Contracted Socket

Contracted socket is the most frequently encountered complication associated with anophthalmia. This is defined as shrinkage and shortening of all or part of orbital tissues causing a decrease in the depth of fornices and orbital volume ultimately leading to inability in retention of the prosthesis.[7]

Evaluation of contracted socket is done to assess two clinical features—volume loss and loss of the surface area of the socket. Contracted sockets have been graded from grade 0 to grade 5 depending on the severity of contraction (Fig. 8).[8]

Grade 0   Socket is lined by healthy conjunctiva with deep well-formed fornices.

Grade 1   Shallowing or shelving of lower fornix preventing retention of prosthesis.

Grade 2   Loss of upper and lower fornices.

Grade 3   Loss of upper, lower, medial, and lateral fornices.

Grade 4   Loss of all four fornices and reduced palpebral aperture.

Grade 5   Recalcitrant variety of socket contraction after multiple prior failed attempts.

Recalcitrant variety of grade 5 contracted socket is also called a malignant socket; treating these sockets for optimal cosmetic and functional outcome is very challenging and more often than not the fibrous scar issue comes back with vengeance after surgical trauma. It may be better option for such patients to go for nonsurgical alternatives like orbital prosthesis (Fig. 9).

There are multiple factors responsible for contracted sockets. They are summarized as:

- *Etiological factors:*
  - Chemical burn
  - Radiation-induced [mostly after retinoblastoma as external beam radiotherapy (EBRT)]

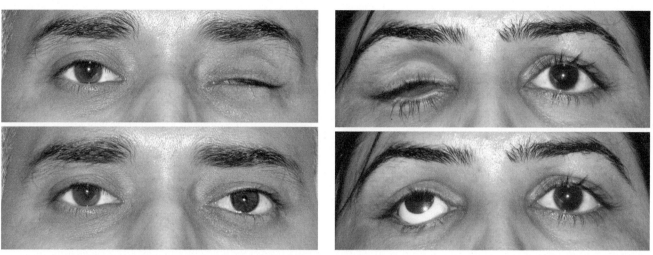

Fig. 7: Well-fitting prosthesis in a healthy socket (left), poorly fitting prosthesis in a contracted socket (right).

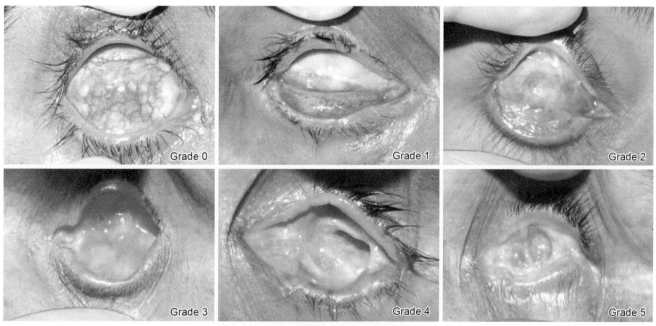

Fig. 8: Different grades of socket contraction.

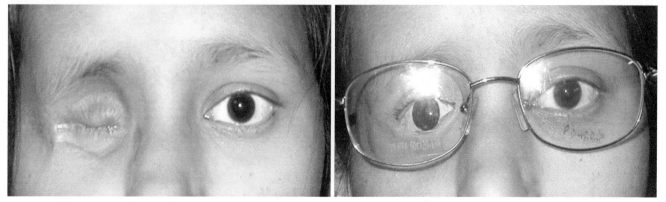

Fig. 9: Grade 5 contracted socket managed with glued on silicon orbital prosthesis.

- *Surgical factors:*
  - Excessive sacrifice of conjunctiva tenon layers
  - Suboptimal surgical technique involving extensive orbital dissection
  - Migrated orbital implants
  - Implant exposure/extrusion secondary to suboptimal tissue coverage.
- *Underlying disease factor:*
  - Cicatricial conjunctival diseases
  - Chronic inflammation and infection.
- *Prosthesis related:*
  - Not wearing a prosthesis
  - Poorly fitting prosthesis.

Dry versus wet socket:

Socket is a mucosa lined cavity and this mucosa keeps the socket surface healthy and prosthesis clean. However, there are situations where the mucosal lining is fully keratinized and contracted. In such cases skin graft in the socket may be used to treat socket contraction. This is not the ideal socket for two reasons—first, there is foul smelling keratin deposit on the skin surface that needs frequent cleaning; and second, the prosthesis remains dry and lusterless (Fig. 10).

Role of Ocular Prosthesis in Socket Health

Role of well-fitting prosthesis in maintaining socket's health is critical. There are broadly two types of ocular prosthesis available:

1. Stock artificial eye or readymade artificial eyes that is available off the shelf.
2. Customized ocular prosthesis that is fabricated by the ocularist, after taking impression of the socket and the color of the eye is carefully matched to the fellow eye.

The difference between the two types is that readymade artificial eyes are of fixed dimensions and color, and they may or may not match the individual socket. They do not have matching back surface to the socket and this leads to tear collection behind the prosthesis. This tear collection, being stagnant and warm, provides good milieu for bacterial growth and the secretion becomes purulent. This purulent collection in the socket over the period of years gradually causes repeated inflammation and subsequent contraction of the socket surface causing loss of fornices and difficulty in retention of prosthesis (Fig. 11).

In contrast, the customized ocular prosthesis has the back-surface matching with the socket surface and there is no room for tear collection and subsequent inflammation. The tear in fact is useful in keeping the prosthesis clean with every blink due to normal tear film dynamics. This is why a patient with custom ocular prosthesis can continuously wear prosthesis over prolong period of weeks to months without removing, whereas patients with ill-fitting readymade prosthesis have to remove the prosthesis frequently to clean the discharge collection behind the prosthesis (Fig. 12).

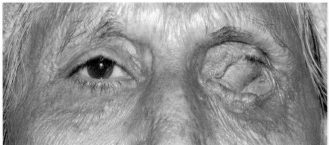
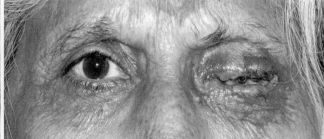

Fig. 10: Contracted keratinized socket treated with skin graft retaining conformer well.

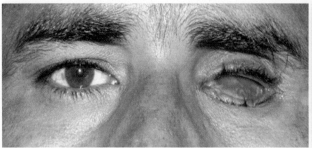
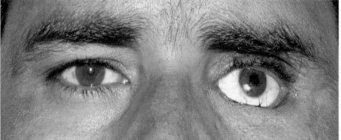

Fig. 11: Ill-fitting prosthesis over long period of time has caused shallowing of inferior fornix (left) and difficulty in prosthesis retention (right).

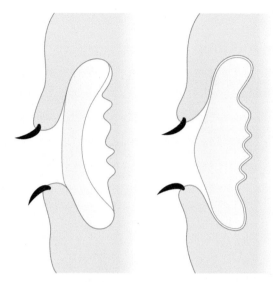

Fig. 12: Diagrammatic representation of fitting of stock eye (left) vs. custom made ocular prosthesis (right). Note the difference in the empty space behind the prosthesis that leads to discharge collection and subsequent inflammation.

Making of Customized Ocular Prosthesis

A brief outline of steps in making an ocular prosthesis is presented in Figure 13. An impression tray (made from conformer) is used to take the impression of the socket (1). Alginate paste is injected behind the impression tray (2), the paste solidifies in a couple of minutes and we get a solid alginate mold of the socket (3), based on this alginate mold, a wax model is made to assess the height of palpebral fissure and lid contour (4). A button is placed on the wax model to mark the area of iris. Iris is painted on an acrylic disk attached to a stem (5). Wax model is used to make a mold in the dye stone (6), and acrylic dough is heated under pressure to get a white acrylic model (7). Acrylic model is hand painted to match the color of the fellow eye (8). A layer of clear acrylic is added on this painted white acrylic model to keep the paint durable and surface inert (9). This model is polished with buff to make the surface smooth and shiny (10). Thereafter finished prosthesis is placed in the socket to assess for comfort and appearance (11). The art and science of making ocular prosthesis is called "ocularistry" and professional practicing this is called "ocularist".

There are different prosthesis types to meet the special requirement of a particular socket.

Hollow prosthesis—for socket with high volume deficit, they are lightweight, hence, take care of lower lid lag (Fig. 14).

Self-lubricating prosthesis—this prosthesis has a reservoir of lubricating fluid within, that is released slowly to keep the prosthesis moist when socket lubrication is not adequate.

Prosthesis with wedge—this prosthesis has a wedge on the front surface to lift the upper lid, that is drooping and patient does not want a surgical correction.

Orbital prosthesis—when the socket contraction is too severe to accommodate a prosthesis, orbital prosthesis with built-in lids and adnexal skin may be used (Fig. 9).

MANAGEMENT

Anophthalmia has implications in patient's life beyond the clinical aspect. With time, most of the patients get accustomed to mono ocular vision and can perform day to day activities without much problems.[9] However, the stigma of disfigured eye lasts forever and this has profound implications in personal, professional, and social life.

Volume loss in orbit is secondary to loss of the eyeball. 10–20% of volume loss after enucleation/evisceration with implant (compared to the contralateral orbit) is optimal. The prosthesis can easily compensate for this volume loss and the result is cosmetically pleasing. However, if the orbital soft tissue volume loss is more than 50%, prosthesis alone may not adequately compensate this and additional surgery may be required to add volume to the socket. Either a secondary orbital implant or dermis fat graft (DFG) is required to add volume to the orbit. If there is only volume loss with adequate and healthy surface in the socket, secondary implant works well (Fig. 15).

In case of volume loss along with surface area loss (as mostly seen in contracted sockets), dermis fat graft is preferred because DFG adds volume as well as surface area to the socket (Fig. 16).

The DFG is harvested from upper and outer quadrant of the buttock, measuring about 25–30 mm in size and fusiform in shape (Fig. 10). This graft is sutured in the socket after creating space under the subtenon plane in the intraconal space. The graft margin is sutured well with the host conjunctiva tenon all around to promote early epithelialization and vascularization.

Mucus membrane graft is indicated for contracted sockets with only surface area loss. Mucus membrane may be harvested from the lip mucosa or buccal mucosa and they are secured in the socket with absorbable sutures (Fig. 17).

Temporalis muscle pedicle graft is indicated for irradiated sockets with poor blood supply; free graft (like mucus membrane, dermis fat or skin graft) is unlikely to survive due to lack of blood supply; so a pedicle graft with its own blood supply is preferred (Fig. 18).

Use of appropriate surgical technique in enucleation[8-11] and evisceration[12] with orbital implants can help maintain the orbital anatomy much better. The sockets following optimal surgical technique and appropriate orbital

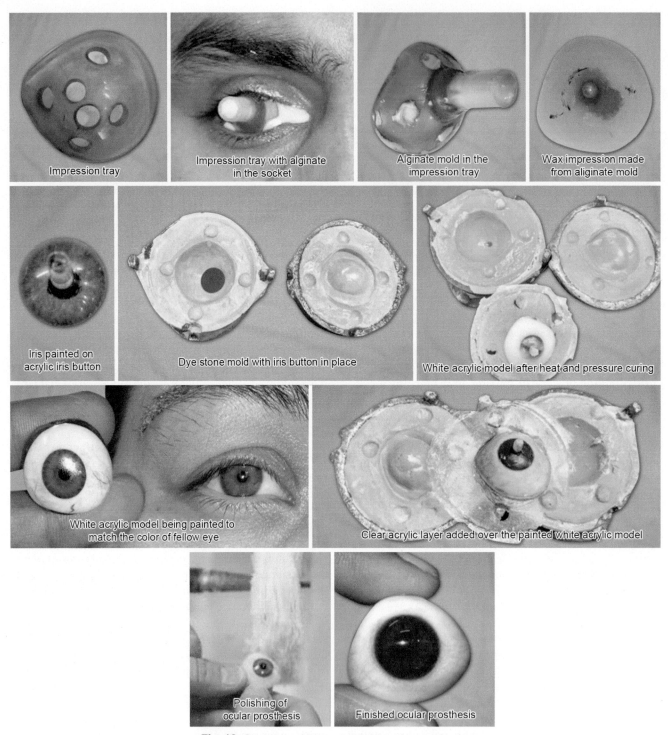

Fig. 13: Steps in making customized ocular prosthesis.

implants maintain orbital soft tissue orientation and most of these changes of PESS may be avoided. Figure 19 shows socket after enucleation and following prosthesis. Note the symmetry of eye on both sides and absence of superior sulcus defect following an optimal surgical technique and good prosthesis.

Orbital implants used after enucleation or evisceration are broadly of two types—the nonintegrated PMMA (or

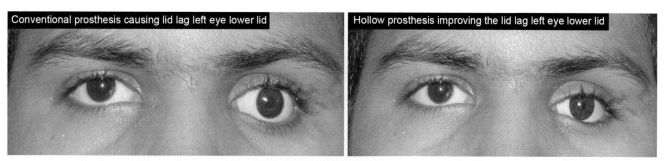

Conventional prosthesis causing lid lag left eye lower lid | Hollow prosthesis improving the lid lag left eye lower lid

Fig. 14: Hollow prosthesis correcting the lid lag in left eye lower lid.

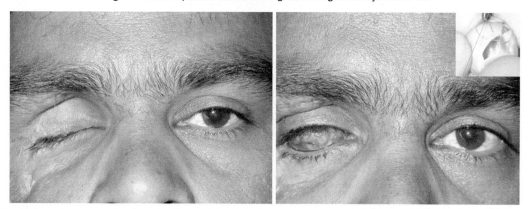

Fig. 15: Volume loss with adequate surface area reconstructed with sclera wrapped secondary orbital implant.

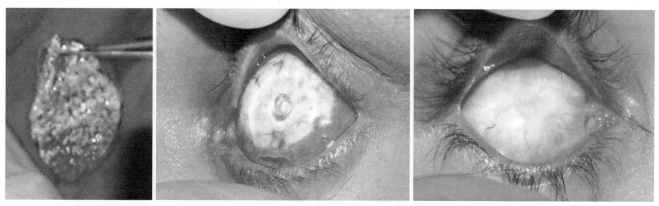

Fig. 16: Volume loss with reduced surface area in contracted socket reconstructed with dermis fat graft. Harvested dermis fat graft (left), graft in the socket secured with sutures and conformer (middle) and well-healed and epithelized graft in socket (right).

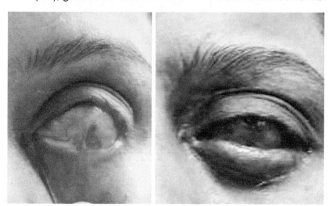

Fig. 17: Obliterated inferior fornix following chemical injury (left), fornix formation done with mucus membrane graft with retention of conformer in the socket (right).

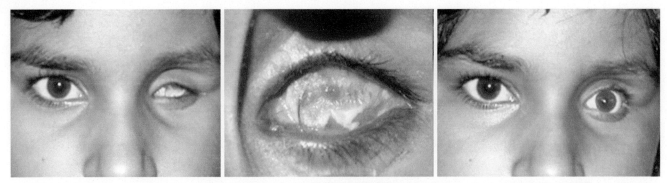

Fig. 18: Child with irradiated socket (left) following enucleation for retinoblastoma, temporalis pedicle graft in socket (middle), achieved good outcome with ocular prosthesis (right).

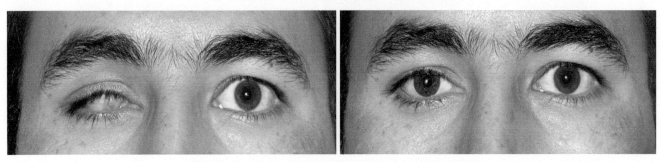

Fig. 19: Healthy socket following enucleation with implant.

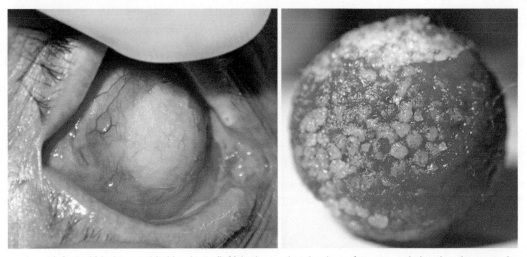

Fig. 20: Exposed and infected Medpore orbital implants (left) in the socket, implant after removal showing the posterior vascularized and anterior nonvascularized implant (right).

silicon) spherical implants and integrated implants made up of hydroxyapatite or medpore. Nonintegrated PMMA orbital implants have been found to be better tolerated than integrated implants in general.[13,14] Integrated implants have higher risk of exposure due to the rough external surface (Fig. 20).

A congenital socket is rudimentary in which all the dimensions are reduced. The socket is so small that even the smallest of prosthesis cannot be fitted and this socket needs serial expansion with progressive sized expanders before a normal size matching prosthesis can be fitted in these sockets (Fig. 21). Gradual expansion of rudimentary

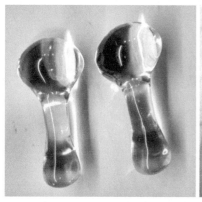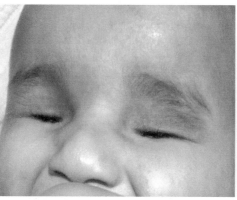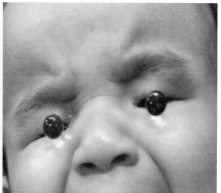

Fig. 21: Socket expanders for congenital anophthalmia (left), child with bilateral congenital anophthalmia (middle) and expanders placed in the rudimentary socket with stem to facilitate easy insertion and removal (right).

socket with progressively enlarged expanders achieves more physiologic growth and stable sockets. In contrast surgical intervention to achieve rapid dramatic enlargement is at risk of postoperative fibrosis and subsequent even stronger socket contraction.

SUMMARY

To sum up, problems associated with anophthalmic sockets have profound effect in patient's personal, professional, and social life. Appropriate team work by treating ophthalmologist and ocularist can achieve a gratifying outcome. It is always better to prevent a problem than managing a complication, optimal surgical technique during enucleation or evisceration and properly fitting ocular prosthesis goes a long way in avoiding complications in socket management. In congenital cases, the treatment in the form of socket expansion should be started as early as possible to enlarge the rudimentary socket and stimulate the growth of bony orbit.

REFERENCES

1. Shaw GM, Carmechael SL, Yang W, et al. Epidemiological characteristics of anophthalmia and bilateral microphthalmia among 2.5 million births in California, 1989-1997. Am J Med Genet A. 2005;137(1):36-40.
2. Krastinova D, Kelly MB, Mihaylova M. Surgical management of the anophthalmic orbit, part 1: Congenital. Plast Reconstr Surg. 2001;108(4):817-26.
3. Dixon AD, Hoyte DA, Rönning O. In: Fundamentals of Craniofacial Growth, 1st edition. Boca Raton, New York: CRC Press; 1997. pp. 234-5.
4. Sigurdsson H, Thórisdóttir S, Björnsson JK. Enucleation and evisceration in Iceland 1964-1992. Study in a defined population. Acta Ophthalmol Scand. 1998;76(1):103-7.
5. Erie JC, Nevitt MP, Hodge D, et al. Incidence of enucleation in a defined population. Am J Ophthalmol. 1992;113(2):138-44.
6. Vemuganti GK, Jalali S, Honavar SG, et al. Enucleation in a tertiary eye care center in India: prevalence, current indications and clinicopathological correlation. Eye (Lond). 2001;15(Pt 6):760-5.
7. Nesi FA, Lisman RD, Levine MR. Evaluation and current concepts in the management of anophthalmic socket. In: Smith's Ophthalmic Plastic and Reconstructive Surgery, 2nd edition. Missouri, United States: Mosby; 1998. pp. 1079-124.
8. Krisna G. Contracted sockets—I (etiology and types). Indian J Ophthalmol. 1980;28(3):117-20.
9. Brady FB. In: A Singular View: The Art of Seeing with One Eye, 1st edition. Oradell, NJ: Medical Economics Co.; 1972.
10. Yacoub AY. Enucleation surgery—Orbital implants and surgical techniques. US Ophthalmic Review. 2016;9(1):46-8.
11. Christmas MJ, Gordon CD, Murray TG, et al. Intraorbital implants after enucleation and their complications: A 10-year review. Arch Ophthalmol. 1998;116(9):1199-203.
12. Custer PL. Enucleation: Past, present, and future. Ophthalmic Plast Reconstr Surg. 2000;16(5):316-21.
13. Kostick DA, Linberg JV. Evisceration with hydroxyapatite implant. Surgical technique and review of 31 case reports. Ophthalmology. 1995;102(10):1542-9.
14. Shields CL, Shields JA, De Potter P, et al. Problems with the hydroxyapatite orbital implant: Experience with 250 consecutive cases. Br J Ophthalmol. 1994;78(9):702-6.
15. Remulla HD, Rubin PA, Shore JW, et al. Complications of porous spherical orbital implants. Ophthalmology. 1995;102(4):586-93.

Lid

Embryology and Anatomy of Eyelid

Ruchi Goel

EMBRYOLOGY

The development of eyelid has been divided into five phases namely eyelid formation, fusion, development, separation and maturation of eyelid structures.

- *End of 4th week of gestation:* Optic vesicle lies adjacent to the surface ectoderm (Fig. 1A).
- Surface ectoderm close to the optic vesicle thickens to form the lens placode (Fig. 1B).
- *32 days:* The lens pit indents the lens placode (Fig. 1C).
- *33 days:* The lens pit closes, the lens vesicle and optic cup press against the surface (Fig. 1D).
- The upper lid is formed by an extension from the frontonasal process (Fig. 2).
- The lower lid is formed by the maxillary process (Fig. 2).
- *37 days:* Two grooves form above and below the eye.
- Eyelid folds develop by deepening of the grooves, first below, and then above the eye (Fig. 3A).
- Eyelid folds develop into the eyelids.
- The upper and the lower eyelids meet at the outer canthus.
- The inner canthus is established a few days later.
- The two lids fuse temporarily during which the lid structures are formed with development being faster in the upper lid (Fig. 3B).
- The levator palpebrae superioris develops at 2.5 months of gestation and separates from superior rectus muscle at fourth month of gestation.

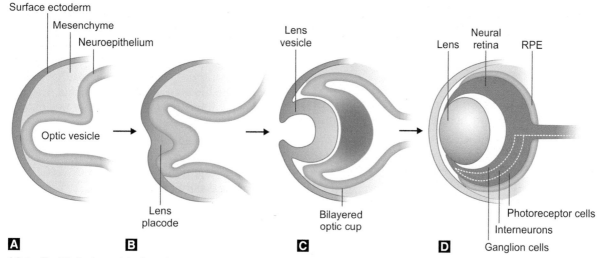

Figs. 1A to D: (A) Optic vesicle lies close to the surface ectoderm; (B) Surface ectoderm overlying the optic vesicle thickens to form the lens placode; (C) The lens placode is indented by the lens pit; (D) Lens pit is closed but the lens vesicle and optic cup lie close to the surface ectoderm pressing against the surface.

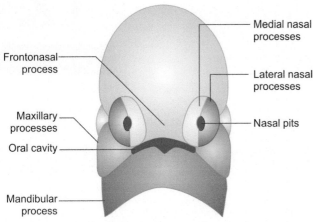

Fig. 2: The upper eyelid is formed by extension of frontonasal process and lower eyelid develops from maxillary process.

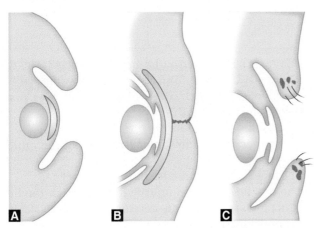

Figs. 3A to C: (A) Eyelid folds develop; (B) The two lids fuse temporarily during which the lid structures are formed with development being faster in the upper lid; (C) Separation of lids at 28th week.

• By 28th week the eyelids separate (Fig. 3C) and the earliest evidence of blinking has been observed at 33 weeks.

ANATOMY OF THE LID

The eyelids provide protective cover to the eye. The normal palpebral fissure is 30 mm horizontally and 9–10 mm vertically when open.

It consists of two lamellae:
1. *Anterior lamella*—skin and orbicularis muscle
2. *Posterior lamella*—tarsus and conjunctiva.

The structure of lid can be divided into seven layers for the sake of convenience (Fig. 4):
1. Skin and subcutaneous tissue
2. Muscles of protraction
3. Orbital septum
4. Orbital fat

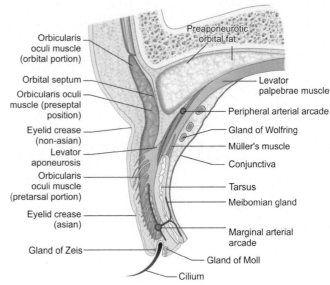

Fig. 4: Sagittal section of the lid.

5. Muscles of retraction
6. Tarsus
7. Conjunctiva.
   – *Skin*: It is the thinnest in the body and has no subcutaneous fat. The preseptal tissues are loosely attached to the underlying tissues, creating potential space for fluid collection. The upper eyelid crease is formed by the attachment of levator aponeurosis to the pretarsal orbicularis and skin.
   – *Protractors*: The *orbicularis oculi muscle* is the main protractor of the eyelid. It is divided into pretarsal, preseptal, and orbital parts.

The Pretarsal Orbicularis Muscle

• Attaches laterally to Whitnall's tubercle by lateral canthal tendon (lateral palpebral ligament).
• Medially it forms two heads that pass superficial and deep to the canaliculi. The anterior pretarsal muscle forms the anterior crus of medial canthal tendon and inserts onto the frontal process of maxilla. The posterior part also known as Horner's muscle inserts onto the posterior lacrimal crest.

The muscle of Riolan is a strip of pretarsal orbicularis present at the lid margin; forms the gray line. It may play a role in blinking, meibomian gland discharge and the position of the eyelashes.

The Preseptal Orbicularis Muscle

• Laterally forms the horizontal raphe.
• Medially inserts into the anterior crus of medial canthal tendon.

- Jones muscle forms the deep insertion of the preseptal orbicularis into the lacrimal diaphragm of the tear sac.

The Orbital Portion

- Attaches medially to medial canthal ligament, part of frontal bone and inferomedial orbital margin.
- Laterally it forms an ellipse around the orbit without interruption at the lateral canthal ligament.
- The orbital septum is a thin multi-layered fibrous tissue that arises from the periosteum over the superior and inferior orbital rims at the arcus marginalis. In the upper lid, the septum fuses with the levator aponeurosis 2–5 mm above the superior tarsal border and in the lower lid it fuses with the capsulopalpebral fascia and inserts on to the anterior, posterior and inferior tarsal surface. Thinning of septum leads to herniation of orbital fat.
- The orbital fat lies posterior to the orbital septum and in front of the levator aponeurosis (upper lid) and in front of the capsulopalpebral fascia (lower lid).
  Fat pockets:
  - *Two in upper lid*—nasal and central
  - *Three in lower lid*—nasal, central, and temporal; the nasal fat is separated from the central fat posteriorly by inferior oblique muscle.
- *Retractors:*
  Upper lid: Levator palpebrae superioris muscle (LPS) with its aponeurosis and Müller's muscle (superior tarsal muscle).

Lower lid retractors are capsulopalpebral fascia and the inferior tarsal muscle

The levator muscle originates at the apex of the orbit from the periorbita of the lesser wing of sphenoid, just above the annulus of Zinn. The muscle extends anteriorly for 40 mm and becomes tendinous at Whitnall's ligament and then continues as aponeurosis for 14–20 mm. At the transition of muscle and aponeurosis is located the superior transverse ligament of Whitnall (Fig. 5).

The Whitnall's ligament extends from fascia of the trochlea and reflected superior oblique to the capsule of lacrimal gland and lateral orbital retinaculum. It acts as a fulcrum and converts the anteroposterior pulling force of levator muscle to superior-inferior direction (The analog in lower lid is the Lockwood's ligament.).

The levator palpebrae superioris (LPS) is inserted to the anterior lower 7–8 mm of tarsus, lid skin, conjunctiva of the fornix, medial palpebral ligament and lateral palpebral ligament. The lateral horn inserts onto the lateral tubercle; the medial horn inserts onto the posterior lacrimal crest. The lateral horn divides the lacrimal gland into orbital and palpebral lobes. As the levator continues downward it divides into anterior and posterior parts. The anterior portion inserts into the septa between pretarsal muscle and skin and forms the upper lid crease. The upper eyelid fold is formed by the overhanging skin, fat, and orbicularis muscle above the crease.

The posterior portion inserts onto the anterior surface of lower half of tarsus.

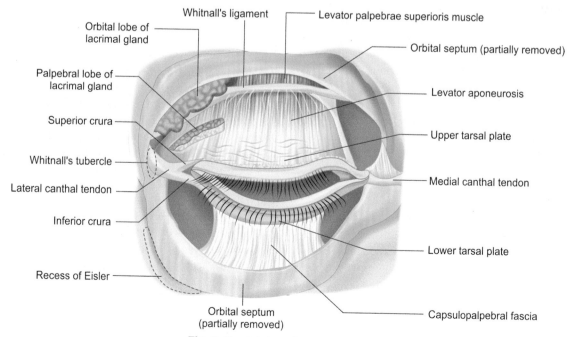

Fig. 5: Frontal view of eyelids and orbit.

The levator is innervated by the superior division of 3rd cranial nerve in the inner posterior one-third after which the nerve passes to superior rectus muscle. Ptosis with decreased upgaze implies involvement of superior division of 3rd cranial nerve.

The Muller's muscle originates in the undersurface of levator aponeurosis at the level of Whitnall's ligament, 12–14 mm above tarsus and inserts along the superior border of tarsus. It is attached to the adjacent conjunctiva posteriorly. The peripheral vascular arcade lies just above the superior border of tarsus between the levator and Muller's muscle, and helps in identification of Muller's muscle. The Muller's is sympathetically innervated smooth muscle responsible for 2 mm elevation of upperlid.

In the lower eyelid the capsulopalpebral fascia is analogous to the LPS in the upper lid (Fig. 6). It originates as capsulopalpebral head from the terminal muscle fibers of inferior rectus muscle. The capsulopalpebral head divides as it encircles the inferior oblique and fuses with the sheath of inferior oblique muscle. Anterior to inferior oblique muscle, the two portions of capsulopalpebral head join to form the Lockwood's suspensory ligament. The capsulopalpebral fascia then extends anteriorly and sends strands to the inferior conjunctival fornix. It fuses with the orbital septum and inserts onto the inferior tarsal border.

The inferior tarsal muscle, analogous to Muller's muscle runs posterior to the capsulopalpebral fascia.

- The tarsi are dense plates of connective tissue that provide structural support to the eyelids. The upper tarsal plate measures 10–12 mm vertically in the center and the lower tarsal plate measures 4 mm. The thickness is 1 mm. The tarsi are attached to the periosteum through the canthal ligaments. Located within the tarsus are meibomian glands that are sebaceous glands.

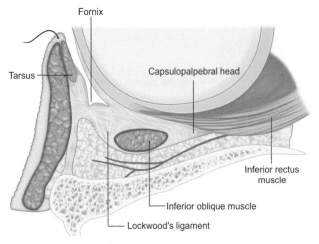

Fig. 6: Lower lid retractors.

- The conjunctiva, composed of nonkeratinizing squamous epithelium, forms the posterior layer of eyelid and contains the mucin-secreting goblet cells and accessory lacrimal glands of Wolfring (found along nonmarginal tarsal borders) and Krause (found in fornices).

Canthal tendons along with the tarsal plates maintain the palpebral fissure. The medial canthal tendon originates from the anterior and posterior lacrimal crest, fuses lateral to the lacrimal sac, and again splits into upper and lower limbs to attach to the upper and lower tarsal plates. The posterior attachment to the posterior lacrimal crest is important in maintaining the apposition of the eyelids to the globe and dipping of puncta into the tear lake.

The lateral canthal tendon attaches at the lateral tubercle on the inner aspect of the orbital rim. It splits into superior and inferior parts to attach to the respective tarsal plates.

The lateral canthal tendon is inserted 2 mm higher than the medial canthal ligament giving an upward slant. The reverse causes an antimongoloid slant.

The eyelid margin is the confluence of cutaneous stratified squamous epithelium, edge of orbicularis, and mucosal surface of conjunctiva. The margin or the free edge is called the intermarginal strip. The anterior border is rounded and the posterior border is sharp. Just in front of the posterior border, the ducts of the meibomian glands open. There are about 25 glands in upper lid and 20 in the lower lid.

The eyelashes, about 100 in the upper lid and 50 in the lower lid, originate in the anterior aspect of eyelid margin just anterior to the tarsal plate and form 2–3 rows.

The eyelashes and the meibomian glands differentiate from a common pilosebaceous unit in the 2nd month of gestation. Thus, a lash follicle may develop from meibomian gland following trauma or chronic irritation (acquired distichiasis) or an extra row of lashes may be present at birth (congenital distichiasis).

The glands of Zeis are small, modified sebaceous glands that open into the hair follicles at the base of the eyelashes; whereas glands of Moll are modified sweat glands that open in a row near the base of the eyelashes.

The grayline is the section of pretarsal muscle (Riolan) just anterior to the tarsus. This is important for operations in which the lid is split as it indicates the position of the loose, relatively avascular fibrous tissue.

The arterial supply of the eyelids comes from two main sources—(1) the internal carotid artery by way of ophthalmic artery and its branches (supra-orbital and lacrimal) and (2) the external carotid artery by way of the arteries of the face (angular and temporal). The two systems anastomose to form the marginal and peripheral arcade. The marginal arcade in the upper lid lies near to the follicles of the cilia anterior to the tarsus and the peripheral arcade

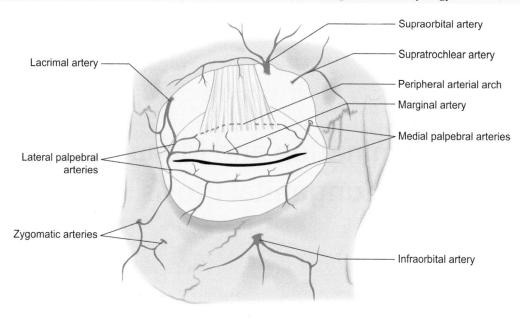

Fig. 7: Arterial supply of lid.

lies superior to the tarsus between the LPS and Muller's muscle. The lower lid has a single arterial arcade located at the inferior tarsal border (Fig. 7).

The venous drainage of the pretarsal tissues is into the angular vein medially and superficial temporal vein laterally; the posttarsal tissues drain into the anterior facial vein, orbital veins, deeper branches of anterior facial vein, and pterygoid plexus.

The lymphatic drainage from medial side, one-third of upper lid and two-thirds of lower lid drain into submandibular lymph nodes. The lateral two-thirds of upper lid and one-third of lower lid drain into the preauricular lymph node (Fig. 8).

The 3rd cranial nerve supplies the LPS, the 7th cranial nerve supplies the orbicularis muscle and the sympathetic nerve supplies the Muller's muscle. The sensory supply is by the trigeminal nerve, the ophthalmic division supplying the upper lid and the maxillary division supplying the lower lid.

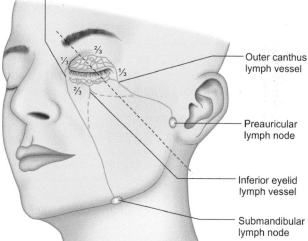

Fig. 8: Lymphatic drainage of eyelids.

Ptosis Examination and Management of Congenital Ptosis

AK Grover, Shaloo Bageja, Amrita Sawhney

INTRODUCTION

Ptosis refers to drooping of the upper eyelid. It can be congenital which is due to dystrophy of levator muscle or acquired which may be neurogenic, myogenic, involutional, traumatic, or mechanical.

Ptosis in children may be associated with refractive errors and amblyopia.

Management of ptosis requires a detailed evaluation to help in decision-making and choice of an appropriate surgical procedure.

> Pseudoptosis: It is a condition in which eyelid appears droopy due to enophthalmos or contralateral eyelid retraction.

HISTORY TAKING

The following relevant history should be elicited in all patients of ptosis:
- Time of onset
- Unilateral or bilateral
- Whether increasing, decreasing, or constant since the time of manifestation
- Family history
- Any association with:
  - Jaw movements
  - Abnormal ocular movements
  - Abnormal head posture
- History of:
  - Trauma or previous surgery
  - Poisoning
  - Use of steroid drops

- Any reaction with anaesthesia
- Bleeding tendency
- Photographic documentation.

OCULAR EXAMINATION

Visual Acuity

Best corrected visual acuity should be checked to record any amblyopia if present in cases of congenital ptosis. A cycloplegic refraction is imperative.

Head Posture

Any abnormal head posture like chin elevation which is associated with severe ptosis, must be noted as it is an important indication for surgery in children.

Any facial asymmetry, abnormal forehead wrinkles, and abnormal position of eyebrows should be looked for.

> While making eyelid measurements, frontalis muscle action should be eliminated completely by immobilizing the eyebrow with the examiner's thumb.

Palpebral Aperture

Vertical: It is measured as the difference between upper and lower lid in alignment with the center of pupil (Fig. 1). The vertical palpebral fissure width is measured in primary gaze, downgaze, and upgaze.

Normal: 9–10 mm in primary gaze.

Measure horizontal palpebral aperture to note any asymmetry between the two eyes (Fig. 2).

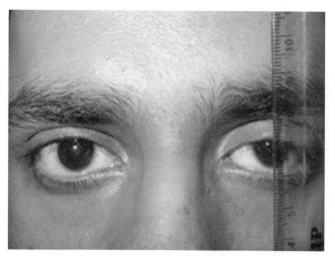

Fig. 1: Vertical palpebral fissure measurement.

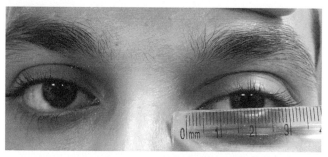

Fig. 2: Horizontal palpabral aperture measurement.

Amount of ptosis is the difference in vertical palpabral apertures in unilateral ptosis or difference from normal in bilateral ptosis.

It must be remembered that ptotic lid in congenital ptosis is usually higher in downgaze due to failure of levator to relax. The ptotic lid in acquired ptosis is invariably lower than normal lid in downgaze.

Margin Reflex Distance (Fig. 3)

The light source is held directly in front of the patient looking straight ahead. The distance between the center of the lid margin of the upper lid and the light reflex on the cornea would give the margin reflex distance (MRD 1).

If the margin is above the light reflex then MRD 1 is a positive value.

If the lid margin is below the corneal reflex in cases of very severe ptosis the MRD 1 is a negative value.

Margin reflex distance 1 (MRD 1): Normal 4–5 mm

Margin reflex distance 2 (Fig. 3): Hold the light source directly in front of the patient looking straight ahead. The distance between the center of the lid margin of the lower

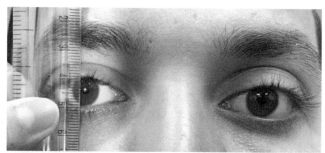

Fig. 3: Measurement of margin reflex distance (MRD) 1 and MRD 2.

lid and the light reflex on the cornea in primary gaze would give the margin reflex distance 2 (MRD 2).

*Normal MRD 2—*more than 5 mm

MRD3 as described by Putterman is the distance from the ocular (not pupillary) light reflex to the central upper eyelid margin when the patient looks in extreme upgaze. It is used to determine the amount of levator to be resected in congenital ptosis associated with vertical strabismus in whom strabismus surgery is not indicated.

B/L cases

Amount of levator resection = [Normal *MRD 3* (7 mm) – *MRD 3* of ptotic eye] × 3.

U/L cases

Amount of levator resection = [*MRD 3* of normal eye – *MRD 3* of ptotic eye] × 3.

Levator Function

It is the excursion of the upper eyelid from extreme downgaze to extreme upgaze.

It can be measured by the following methods:
- Berke's Method (lid excursion) (Fig. 4): The frontalis action is blocked by keeping the thumb tightly over the upper brow. The patient is asked to look up from down gaze and the amount of upper lid excursion is measured at the center of the lid.

It is best to have the child standing against a wall to prevent head movements when measuring the levator action.

Beard's classification of levator action
≤ 4 mm—poor levator function
5–7 mm—fair levator function
8–12 mm—good levator function
The normal levator function is between 13 mm and 17 mm

- Putterman's method: This is carried out by measuring distance between the middle of upper lid margin to the 6 O'clock limbus in extreme upgaze. This is also known as the margin limbal distance (MLD).

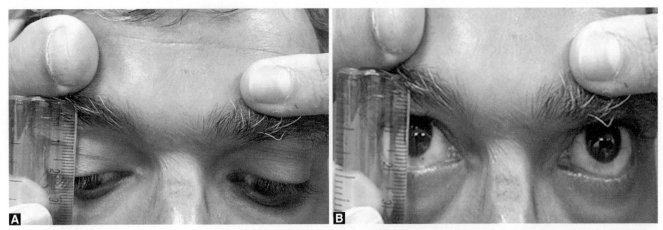

Figs. 4A and B: Measurement of levator action after blocking frontalis action with thumb: (A) Eyelid in extreme downgaze; (B) Eyelid in extreme upgaze. Levator action in this case is 15 mm.

Normal is about 9.0 mm.

The difference in MLD of two sides in unilateral cases

or

The difference with normal in bilateral cases multiplied by 3 would give the amount of levator resection required.

Iliff test: It is carried out to check levator function in infants.

The upper lid of child is everted, if the levator action is good eyelid reverts back on its own.

Margin Crease Distance (Fig. 5)

It is the distance between the center of upper lid margin to the lid crease measured in downgaze.

It helps in planning the surgical incision as proper placement of lid crease is important for symmetry.

The normal distance is between 6 mm and 8 mm in men and 8 mm and 10 mm in women.

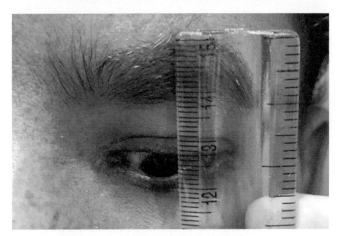

Fig. 5: Margin crease distance measurement.

> Congenital ptosis: Lid crease is faint or absent (Fig. 6)
> Aponeurotic ptosis: Lid crease recedes

Bell's Phenomenon

It is the upward rotation of eyeball on closure of the eye. Confirmation of presence of Bell's phenomenon is important before undertaking any surgical procedure to avoid risk of postoperative exposure keratopathy.

Grading of Bell's phenomenon:
Good—less than one-third of cornea is visible
Fair—one-third to one-half of the cornea is visible
Poor—more than one-half of cornea is visible.

Corneal Sensation

The presence or absence of corneal sensations should be noted. Cotton wisp test can be used for checking corneal sensations.

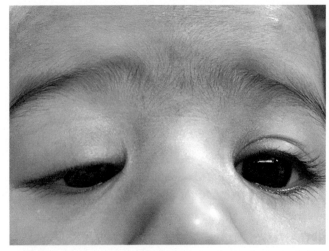

Fig. 6: Right eye congenital ptosis with brow elevation and absent lid crease.

Ocular Motility

The extraocular motility, especially the elevator muscles, should be recorded. Any association of eye movements with change in degree of ptosis should be looked for.

Tensilon Test

It is done in cases where an acquired ptosis due to myasthenia gravis is suspected.

Method:
- In adults 1 mg of neostigmine is injected I/M. If myasthenia gravis is the cause then ptosis improves in 5–15 minutes
- Alternately 10 mg/mL of edrophonium may be injected I/V. It is loaded in a tuberculine syringe and 0.2 mL injected slowly in 15–30 seconds. The needle is left in situ and rest injected slowly if no untoward incident is observed. The effect occurs in 1–5 minutes if myasthenia is the cause.

  If cholinergic reaction occurs 0.5 mg of atropine is given I/V.

Phenylephrine Test

Sympathomimetic agents like 2.5–10% phenylephrine, 0.5% or 1% apraclonidine (alpha adrenergic agonist) can be used to stimulate Muller's muscle.

Method: A drop of sympathomimetic agent are instilled in the affected eye. Any change in palpabral fissure and marginal reflex distance is noted after 5 minutes.

If adequate elevation is observed, ptosis may be corrected by Muller-conjunctival resection.

In mild cases of ptosis, positive phenyephrine test suggests that patient would respond well to Müller's muscle resection.

Ice Test

It is a simple diagnostic test and is highly specific for myasthenia gravis.
Ice pack is applied over upper lid for 5 minutes.

If the ptosis improves by more than or equal to 2 mm, test is positive.

Jaw Movements

The presence of jaw winking is assessed by moving the jaw from side to side (chewing movements) or opening and closing the mouth and observing the lid movements.

It occurs due to cross innervation between oculomotor and mandibular branch of trigeminal nerve.

Marcus Gunn Jaw winking grading:
- Mild: Less than or equal to 2 mm
- Moderate: 3–6 mm
- Severe: More than or equal to 7 mm.

Pseudoptosis

Rule out cause of pseudoptosis such as microphthalmia, anophthalmia, phthisis bulbi, hypotropia, contralateral lid retraction, brow laxity, etc.

Features of congenital ptosis
- Reduced levator function
- A weak or absent lid crease
- Lid lag on downgaze

Features of involutional ptosis
- Normal or near normal levator function
- High lid crease
- Lid drop in downgaze

MANAGEMENT OF CONGENITAL PTOSIS

Timing of Surgery

In congenital ptosis, if possible, it is advisable to wait till 3–4 years of age, as better assessment is possible and tissues are better developed to withstand surgical trauma. However, certain reports suggest that early ptosis surgery minimizes the possibility of amblyopia even in moderate cases of ptosis.

There should be no delay in surgical management in cases of severe ptosis where pupil is obstructed. The latter may cause amblyopia. In these cases a temporary procedure may be opted for followed by definitive surgery later, if necessary.

However, a silastic sling works well even in infants and may provide lasting results.

Choice of Surgical Procedure

Choice is determined by:
- Severity of Ptosis
- Levator action
- Simple ptosis or associated anomalies

Commonly Performed Surgeries

- Fasanella-Servat operation
- Levator resection/aponeurosis reattachment
- Brow suspension ptosis repair.

Indications for the Choice of Different Surgical Procedures

Ptosis	Levator action	Surgery
Mild	>10 mm	Fasanella-Servat or small levator resection
	<10 mm	Levator resection
Moderate	Good	Levator resection
	Fair	Levator resection
	Poor (rare)	Whitnall's sling or brow suspension
Severe	Fair	Levator resection or brow suspension ptosis repair
	Poor	Brow suspension ptosis repair

Surgical Techniques

Modified Fasanella-Servat Surgery

It is the excision of tarsoconjunctiva and Müller's muscle. The steps of modified Fasanella-Servat Surgery are illustrated in Figs. 7A to G.
Complications:
- Corneal abrasion
- Central peaking
- Foreign body sensation
- Suture granuloma.

Levator Resection (Figs. 8A to K)

This is the most commonly practiced surgery for ptosis correction. It may be performed by transcutaneous

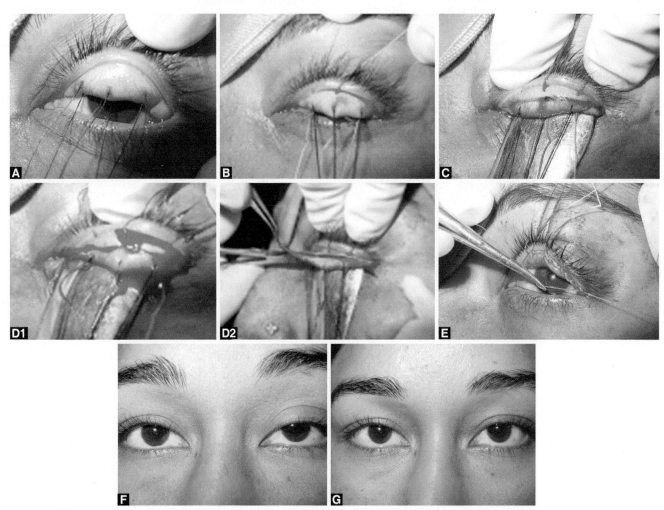

Figs. 7A to G: The steps of modified Fasanella-Servat Surgery. (A) The lid is everted and tarsal plate exposed. Three sutures are passed close to the folded superior margin of the tarsal plate at the junction of middle, lateral, and medial one third of the lid. This set of sutures helps in lifting the tarsal plate for excision; (B) Three corresponding sutures are placed close to the everted lid margin passing from fornix. The second set aids suturing by lifting and supporting conjunctival and tarsal edges during suturing; (C) Proposed incision is marked on the tarsal plate such that a relatively uniform piece of tarsus not exceeding 3 mm is excised; (D1 and D2) A groove is made on the marked line of incision with knife and is completed with the scissors or radiofrequency knife; (E) Suturing the conjunctiva taking smaller and closer bites with 8'0 polyglactin suture to prevent suture keratopathy; (F) Clinical photograph showing left upper lid mild ptosis; (G) Postoperative photograph.

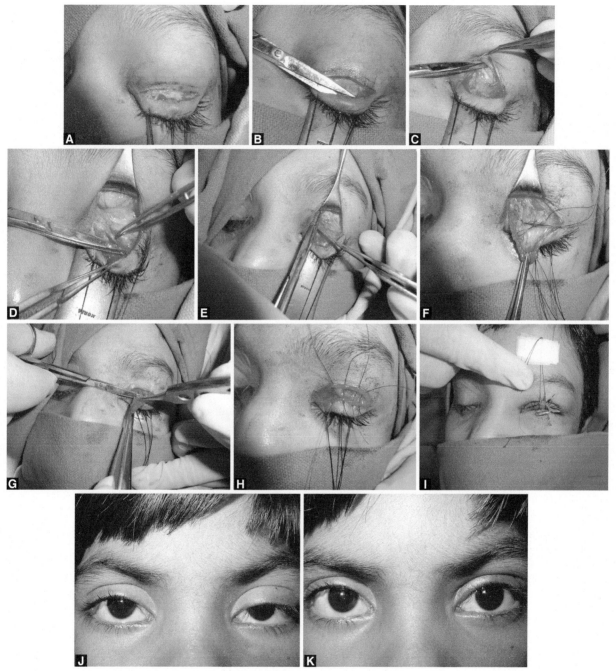

Figs. 8A to K: Everbusch technique. (A) Three sutures are passed near the lid margin to provide traction. The proposed lid crease is marked and incision through the skin and orbicularis made along the crease marking; (B) The inferior skin and orbicularis are dissected away from the tarsal plate; (C) The upper edge is separated from the orbital septum. The orbital septum is cut completely exposing the preaponeurotic fat; (D) Three partial thickness traction suture may be passed through the distal end of the aponeurosis to hold it and facilitate separation from the underlying conjunctiva. The fibers of the aponeurosis are cut from their insertion; (E) The lateral or the medial horn may be cut where it is necessary making sure not to damage the lacrimal gland or the pulley of superior oblique muscle respectively. Care should be taken that Whitnalls ligament is not damaged; (F) Three double armed polyglactin 5-0 sutures are passed through the tarsus about 2 mm from the upper border in the center and at the junction of central third with the medial and lateral thirds. These sutures are then placed in the levator and intraoperative assessment made for correction and contour; (G) The excess levator is excised. If required a strip of skin is removed from above the lid crease; (H) Four to five lid fold forming sutures are placed. The sutures pass through skin edges taking a bite through the cut edge of levator or lid forming sutures may be passed separately; (I) Skin is closed with 6'0 nylon suture and an inverse frost suture is applied to protect cornea; (J) Preoperative photograph; (K) Postoperative photograph.

route (Everbusch technique) or transconjunctival route (Blascovics technique) but the former is preferred by most surgeons because it is universally applicable and allows a good titration/assessment on the table.

1–2 mL of 2% xylocaine with 1:80,000 adrenaline is locally infiltrated in the skin-orbicularis plane.

The technique of skin approach levator resection is described in Figs. 8A to K. The amount of levator resection is judged on the table with the guidelines given below. The large and the supra maximal resections are rarely used today. It is usually preferred to use the strength provided by the Whitnall ligament and the sutures are passed at a variable proximity to Whitnall based on levator action and correction achieved on the table.

Modified Berke's guidelines (Grover, et al.)

Levator action	Recommended lid placement in congenital ptosis
2–4 mm	1 mm above the limbus
5–7 mm	1 mm below the limbus
8 mm or more	2 mm below the limbus

LPS resection can be arbitrarily termed as:
- Small 10–13 mm
- Moderate 14–17 mm
- Large 18–22 mm
- Maximal 23–27 mm
- Supramaximal > 27 mm

Complications:
- Corneal exposure
- Undercorrection
- Overcorrection
- Contour abnormality
- Defective lid crease
- Formix prolapse.

Brow Suspension Repair

Indications:
- Simple ptosis with a poor levator action
- Blepharophimosis syndrome
- Jaw winking ptosis.

Materials used:
- Synthetic materials like nonabsorbable sutures like prolene, skin clips, silicon rod, EPTFE thread, etc.
- Autologous materials like muscle strips, banked or fresh fascia lata strips have been used for suspension.

Silastic Sling

A silicon silastic sling (synthetic material) is used to connect frontalis muscle to the eyelid. It can be done as a unilateral or a bilateral procedure. Silastic sling as a unilateral procedure leads to asymmetry of eyelids in downgaze.

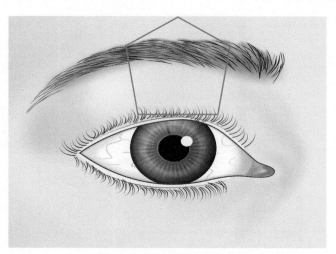

Fig. 9: Fox pentagon technique.

Indications:
- *Severe congenital ptosis*—to prevent amblyopia in a child less than 4 years of age. Bilateral fascia lata surgery is done after 4 years of age
- In cases of ptosis due to myasthenia gravis or third nerve palsy.

Method: Fox Pentagon technique (Fig. 9)
- Medial and lateral horizontal eyelid skin incisions, are made in line with medial and lateral limbus 3 mm above lid margin
- Two incisions are made above eyebrow, one vertically and little lateral to lateral eyelid mark and the second incision should be vertically up and little medial to medial eyelid mark
- A forehead mark is made between the eyebrow marks 4 mm above the eyebrow, to complete the pentagon
- Wright needle is passed through the incisions and material is pulled at a level deeper to orbicularis in the eyelid and deeper to frontalis in the forehead region
- Silicon sling is then tied and secured with polyglactin suture and buried deep into the forehead incision
- Forehead incisions are closed using nonabsorbabale suture.

Fascia Lata Sling (Figs. 10A to M)

Autologous fascia lata sling surgery is the procedure of choice in children above 4 years of age with severe congenital simple ptosis and poor levator action.

We prefer fresh autogenous fascia for suspension. Even in cases of unilateral ptosis a bilateral procedure is preferred because a unilateral surgery causes marked asymmetry in downgaze and results of bilateral surgery are more acceptable.

All cases are done under general anesthesia. Infiltration with 2% xylocaine and adrenaline is done in the region of the proposed incision in the thigh and the eyelid and the eyebrow region.

Harvesting of fascial lata: (Figures 10A to F).

Fascia lata sling suspension: Three traction sutures are passed along the lid border. Four incisions are made 3–4 mm from the lid border depending on the desired position of the lid fold. The two central incisions are on either side of the center of the lid while the other two are at the junction of middle and lateral thirds and middle and medial thirds of the lid.

The eyebrow incisions are marked next. They are made at a line perpendicular to the intersection of two incisions made laterally and two incisions made medially while the eyelid is placed in the desired normal position. A third incision is made in the middle of the first two but 3–4 mm higher than them (Fig. 10G).

The eyelid incisions are made down to the tarsus and the brow incisions are made up to the frontalis. Some blunt dissection is carried out to make pockets for the fascial knots.

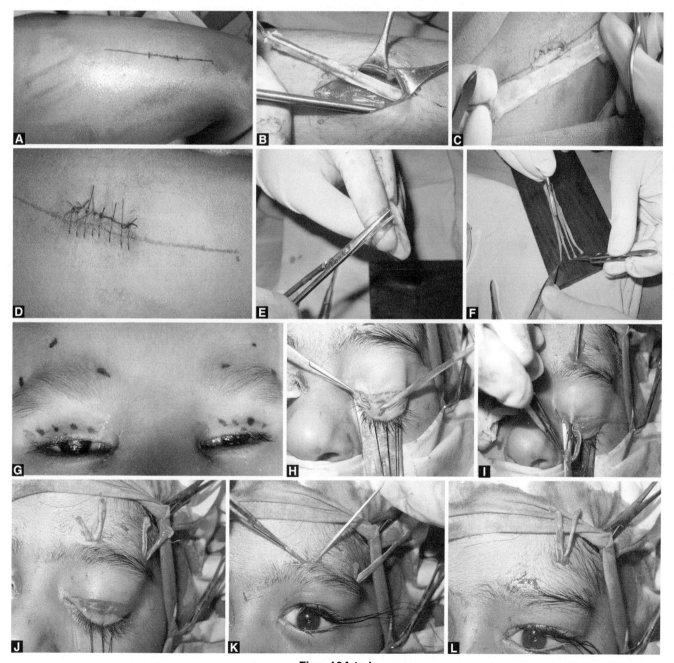

Figs. 10A to L

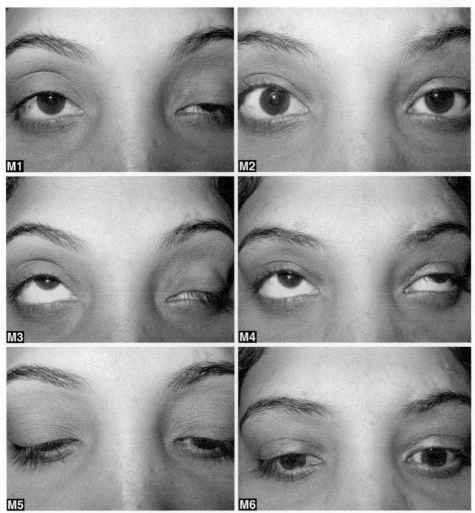

Figs. 10A to M: Fascia lata sling surgery. (A) An incision is marked along line joining the lateral condyle of femur to the anterior superior iliac spine. The marking is begun 2 inches above the lateral condyle of femur and extended up to 4 inches. The incision is given in the center 1 inch of the area that has been marked; (B) The skin incision is deepened through the fat till the glistening fascia is visible. The fascia is then cleared of the overlying tissue and underlying vastus lateralis muscle along the whole length. Two linear incisions are given 12 mm apart on the fascia along the 4 inches length of dissection using a long scissors. The superior end of the fascia is made free by making horizontal cut using a long bladed scissors while the assistants retract the skin and the subcutaneous tissue; (C) The harvested fascia lata (12 mm × 100 mm); (D) The subcutaneous tissue is closed using 4-0 polyglactin and the skin is closed using 4-0 nonabsorbable sutures; (E) The fat is trimmed from the fascia lata strip; (F) The fascia lata strip is kept on a wooden board, stretched and fixed. It is divided into four pieces each of about 3 mm width by a scalpel blade; (G) Incisions marked according to Modified Crawford technique; (H) Fascial strip is passed from the medial lid incision to central incision; (I) The two ends of a strip are then passed from the outer eyelid incisions to the outer eyebrow incision using a Wright's fascia lata needle. The needle is passed in the submuscular plain from the medial brow incision to emerge from the medial incision in the lid. The procedure is repeated on the lateral side; (J) The fascial strips are pulled up and a single tie is made so as to place the eyelid margins about 2 mm above the desired position as the lids will fall down when the knots are buried; (K) After a single tie the position and contour of the eyelid is assessed. Required adjustments are made. Presence of good lid crease is ensured at this stage. A second tie is made and secured with 5'0 polyglactin; (L) One end of fascial strip from each brow incision is pulled through the central brow incision. Knots are tied and secured; (M1 to M6) Preoperative and postoperative photographs of the patient in primary gaze, upgaze, and downgaze.

All the knots are buried in the pockets prepared earlier. The excess of skin created by shortening of the posterior lamina is judged and excised by removing a spindle of skin from the eyelid crease. Eyelid incisions require no closure.

The brow incisions and the eyelid crease incisions are closed by 6-0 nylon sutures.

Patients are prescribed oral antibiotics and anti-inflammatory agents. The bandage is removed on the first postoperative day and eye left open. The need for retention of the frost suture is assessed based on the extent of the lagophthalmos and careful monitoring of the cornea for signs of exposure. The thigh sutures are removed after 10–14 days.

Complications:
- Corneal exposure
- Undercorrection
- Overcorrection
- Granulomas.

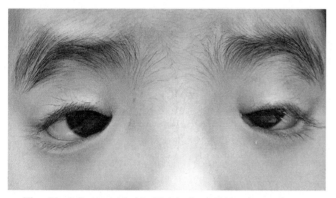

Fig. 11: A 6-year-old girl with blepharophimosis syndrome.

Complicated Congenital Ptosis

Blepharophimosis Syndrome (Fig. 11)
Surgery is often performed in two stages:
1. Stage 1 is usually done at least 3 years of age, it aims at correcting:
   - Epicanthal fold
   - Telecanthus
   - Horizontal palpebral aperture (by lateral canthoplasty).
2. Stage 2 is done 6 months after first stage to correct ptosis.
   Mustarde's double "Z" plasty or Y to V plasty (Figs. 12A and B) with transnasal wiring is done as a primary procedure. This gives a good surgical result both in terms of correction of telecanthus as well as deep placement of the medial canthus. The results are long-lasting.

Double Z plasty: The markings are made as shown in Figure 12C. The first mark is made just medial to the medial canthus (A). The proposed canthal site (B) is marked such that intermedial canthal distance is half that of interpupillary distance. The two marks are joined. All the other lines drawn are 2 mm smaller than the line AB. Two lines are drawn from A parallel to upper and lower lid margins. From the center point of AB (C), a line is drawn

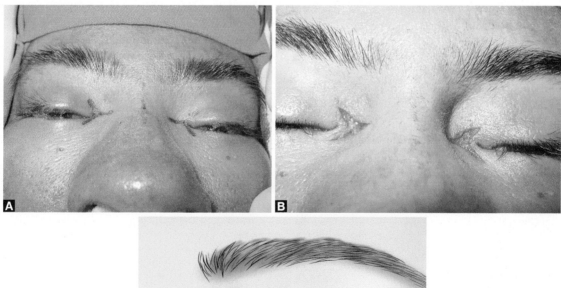

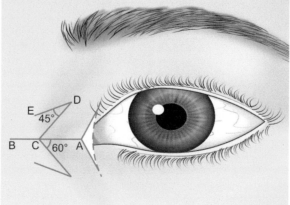

Figs. 12A to C: (A) Marking of Y-V plasty; (B) Undermining of flaps in Y-V plasty; (C) Double Z plasty.

medially at 60° both above and below (CD). Another line is drawn outward at an angle of 45° from the point of D (DE).

Lateral canthotomy and canthoplasty, where it is planned, is carried out before the skin incisions for epicanthus and telecanthus correction are made. The incisions are made through the skin down to the orbicularis. The flaps are undermind. The site of proposed canthus is cleared of all tissues up to the periosteum and the medial palpebral ligament is exposed. The periosteum is incised medial to the insertion of medial palpebral ligament (MPL) and is reflected along with the lacrimal sac.

A large bony opening 12–15 mm high and 10–12 mm wide is made as for dacryocystorhinostomy but located more posterior and superior. The edges of the bony opening are smoothened. A similar procedure is performed on the opposite side.

Medial palpebral ligament of one side is wired with 28/30 G stainless steel wire close to its attachment to the tarsus and the two ends of the wire are passed to the opposite sides through the bony opening with the aid of an aneurysm needle or a Wright's fascia lata needle (Fig. 13A). The wire is threaded into other MPL with similar double bite. The two ends are tightened and a single twist given to the wires. The position of the medial canthus is assessed from the front, above, and the sides. Once the desired position is obtained, the wire is twisted several times and cut. The ends of the wire are pushed into the bony opening. After achieving the hemostasis the incision is closed in several layers. The skin flaps may need to be trimmed before they are transposed and sutured with 6-0 silk (Fig. 13B).

Medial palpebral ligament tucking may be carried out in mild cases.

Lateral canthoplasty: The lateral canthus is crushed by a straight hemostat for a few seconds. A lateral canthotomy is performed. The bulbar conjunctiva at the lateral canthus is undermined. The apex of the conjunctiva is sutured to the proposed new position of the canthus which is short of the end of the skin incision. The skin edges distal to the new lateral canthus are apposed with 6-0 silk sutures. A similar procedure is repeated on the other side.

The bandage is removed after 24 hours and sutures are removed in 5–7 days.

Stage II: The second stage is performed after 6 months. A bilateral fascia lata sling surgery is performed.

Figures 14A to C show the preoperative and postoperative results of blepharophimosis syndrome.

Marcus Gunn Ptosis

Mild cases of jaw winking where the jaw winking is minimal can be treated satisfactorily by Fasanella-Servat operation or levator resection while severe cases or cases where jaw winking is prominent, require bilateral excision of levator aponeurosis and terminal levator with fascia lata brow suspension (Figs. 15A to C).

CONGENITAL PTOSIS WITH OCULAR MOTILITY ABNORMALITIES

The common ocular motility disorders associated with congenital ptosis include:
- Superior rectus underaction (Fig. 16)
- Monocular elevation deficit
- Congenital third nerve palsy (Fig. 17).

Management:
Stage 1—Squint surgery is done as the first stage procedure.
Aims of squint surgery in ptosis are:
- To improve the position of the affected eye in primary gaze, thereby

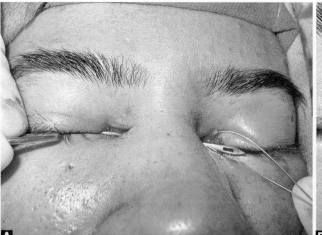
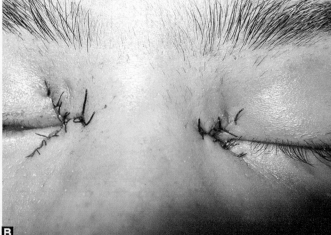

Figs. 13A and B: (A) Two ends of the wire is passed to the opposite side through the bony opening with Wright's fascia lata needle; (B) Closure in two layers, skin closed with 6'0 silk.

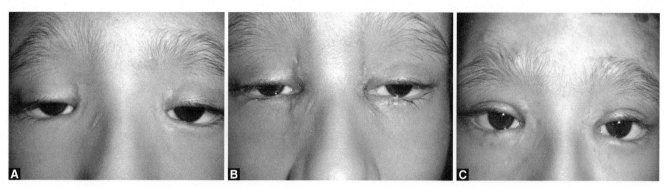

Figs. 14A to C: (A) Preoperative photograph of a child with blepharophimosis syndrome; (B) Postoperative after stage I (Y-V plasty with transnasal wiring); (C) Postoperative after bilateral fascia lata sling.

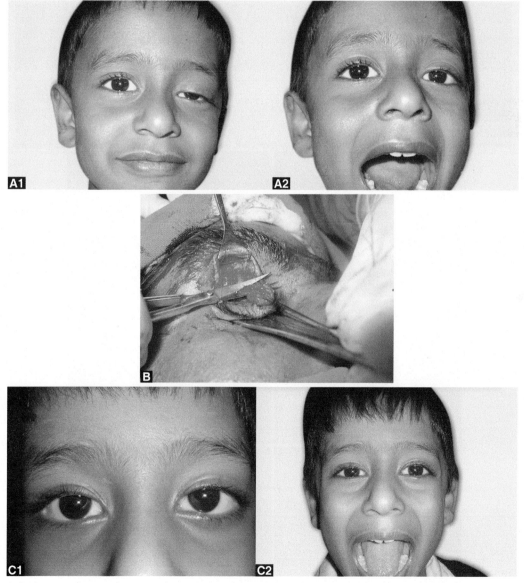

Figs. 15A to C: (A1 and A2) A 5-year-old boy with left eye severe ptosis with Marcus Gunn phenomenon; (B) Levator excision of levator aponeurosis; (C1 and C2) Postoperative photograph showing good correction and elimination of jaw winking phenomena.

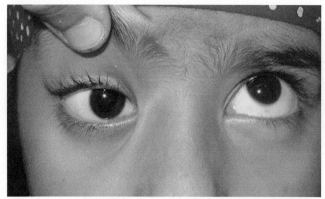

Fig. 16: Right ptosis with superior rectus dysfunction.

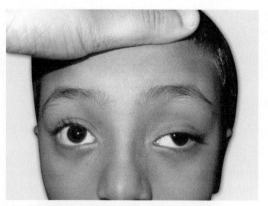

Fig. 17: Left congenital third nerve palsy.

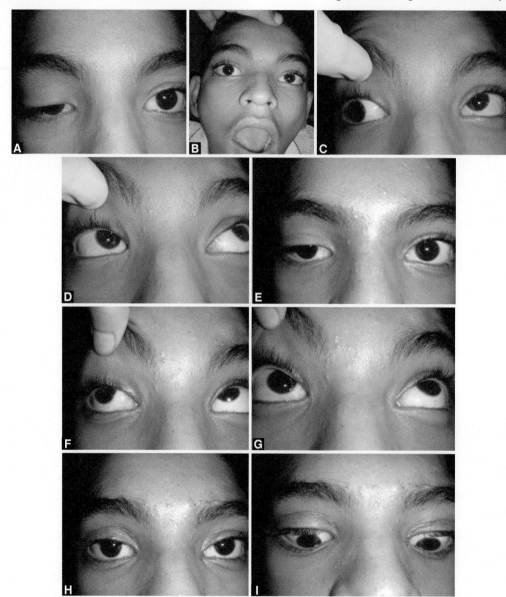

Figs. 18A to I: (A to D) Preoperative images. (A) Showing congenital ptosis with hypotropia; (B) Jaw winking; (C and D) Superior rectus underaction; (E to G) Postoperative images after stage 1 (inferior rectus recession) showing better position and motility; (H and I) Postoperative images after second stage (bilateral levator excision with fascia lata).

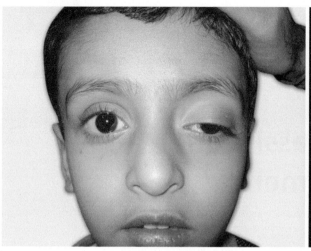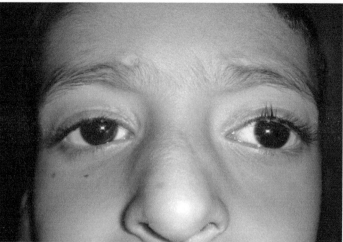

Figs. 19A and B: (A) Preoperative image showing congenital third nerve palsy with hypotropia and exotropia; (B) Postoperative image after second stage.

- – Increasing the field of binocular vision
- – Restoring esthetics
- To improve Bell's phenomenon
- Component of pseudoptosis can only be corrected after the affected hypotropic eye is aligned
- The position of eyelid can be adjusted in relation to the corrected final position of the eye.

Stage 2—The ptosis surgery is performed in the second stage after a minimum gap of 6 weeks.

Congenital Ptosis with Jaw Winking with Superior Rectus Underaction (hypotropia) (Figs. 18A to D)

Superior rectus underaction is treated by squint surgery if there is hypotropia in primary position. Ptosis with Jaw Winking is then manage by bilateral levator excision and suspension with facia lata.

Congenital Ptosis with Monocular Elevation Deficit

- If the FDT is negative:
  - – Knapp's procedure with or without horizontal muscle recession or resection can be done.

- If FDT is positive then:
  - – Inferior rectus recession with release of lower lid retractors

        or

  - – Simultaneous Knapp and inferior rectus recession can be considered

Splitting and transposition of horizontal muscle along with IR recession may be considered as simultaneous Knapp and IR recession procedure can lead to anterior segment ischemia.

Congenital Third Nerve Palsy with Hypotropia and Exotropia (Figs. 19A and B)

It can be managed in two stages:

Stage 1—IR recession with LR recession

Stage 2—Bilateral fascia lata sling.

SUMMARY

Congenital ptosis, because of its varied presentations, is a challenging condition to manage. However, a systematic evaluation leading to an appropriate choice of surgery provides extremely gratifying results, esthetically and functionally.

Acquired Ptosis: Classification and Management

Ruchi Goel, KPS Malik

INTRODUCTION

Acquired ptosis results from abnormality in lid elevators that is upper lid retractors, the levator or Müller's muscle. When the lid elevators are not involved, the condition is termed pseudoptosis. Hypotropia, microphthalmos, enophthalmos, phthisis bulbi, anophthalmos and dermatochalasis can present as pseudoptosis. In unilateral acquired ptosis, unlike congenital ptosis, the affected lid is at the same or lower level than the contralateral normal lid in downgaze (Figs. 1A and B).

CLASSIFICATION OF ACQUIRED PTOSIS

- Mechanical
- Myogenic
- Neurogenic
- Aponeurotic.

Mechanical Acquired Ptosis

- Lid and orbital tumors cause ptosis due to the increased weight of the mass (Fig. 2). Treatment includes removal of the tumor followed by correction of any residual ptosis
- Cicatricial ptosis occurs due to scarring of superior fornix and conjunctiva over the superior tarsus which may occur due to chemical burns, surgical trauma, Stevens Johnson syndrome, ocular cicatricial pemphigoid etc. Treatment is directed toward scar excision in combination with mucous membrane or amniotic membrane graft
- Blepharochalasis affects young people and presents as transient attacks of eyelid edema and erythema that usually starts around puberty. Repeated attacks result in permanent lid changes like thinning, wrinkling, discoloration of skin, lacrimal gland prolapse, orbital

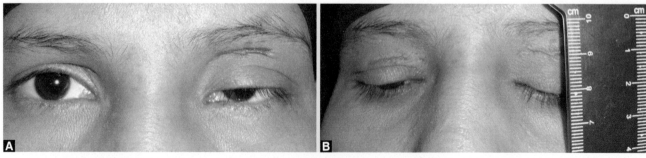

Figs. 1A and B: In unilateral acquired ptosis, unlike congenital ptosis, the affected lid is at the same or lower level than the contralateral normal lid in downgaze.

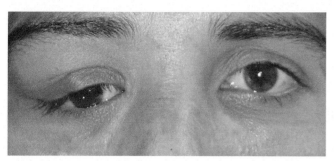

Fig. 2: Orbital mass causing mechanical ptosis of right eye.

fat prolapse or dehiscence of levator aponeurosis and canthal ligament. Recurrence may occur even after surgical management. Blepharoplasty, levator aponeurotic repair, resuspension of lacrimal gland or canthal reconstruction may be required.

Myogenic Ptosis

Chronic progressive external ophthalmoplegia (CPEO), myasthenia gravis (MG), myotonic dystrophy and oculopharyngeal dystrophy involve levator muscle or myoneural junction causing ptosis.

- **Chronic progressive external ophthalmoplegia** is mitochondrial cytopathy that may affect any age group but usually young adults. The first sign is bilateral, often asymmetric ptosis followed within years by external ophthalmoplegia. CPEO, atypical retinitis pigmentosa and complete heart block is described as Kearns Sayre syndrome. Ubiquinone (Coenzyme Q) therapy may benefit the systemic manifestations of CPEO. If stable, strabismus is treated surgically but for ptosis crutch glasses are prescribed
- **Myasthenia gravis** is characterized by weakness and fatiguability of muscles due to reduced number of available acetylcholine receptors at the neuromuscular junction. All ages may be affected with peak in young women and old men. Muscle fatigability varies from hour to hour. Muscle involvement with decreasing order of frequency are levator palpebrae superioris, the extraocular muscles, orbicularis oculi, proximal muscles of limbs, muscles of facial expression, mastication, speech and neck extensors.

Ptosis is unilateral initially and later becomes bilateral and asymmetric. If unilateral, imaging of the orbit and brain is required to rule out a mass lesion.

Worsening of ptosis occurs:
- By evening
- On repeated closure of eyelids
- On prolonged upgaze

- When opposite eyelid is elevated and held in a fixed position. Due to decreased effort required for eyelid elevation on ipsilateral side, according to Hering's law of equal innervation, the opposite side droops (See-saw phenomenon).

Cogan's eyelid twitch sign
After looking downward for 10–20 seconds when the patient moves the eyes to primary position, the upper eyelid elevates and either slowly begins to droop or else twitches before settling to a stable position caused by rapid recovery and easy fatigability of myasthenic muscle.

Eyelid retraction
In unilateral cases, retraction may occur in the opposite eye, in an attempt to elevate the ptotic lid. Persistent eye lid retraction can occur due to thyroid eye disease that is known to have an increased prevalence in MG.

Other ocular abnormalities
- There is no set pattern to extraocular muscle involvement. Oculomotor muscle dysfunction may range from involving a single muscle to complete ophthalmoplegia
- "Peek sign": On gentle eyelid closure, the orbicularis oculi muscle initially contracts achieving good eyelid apposition, and then, due to fatigue of orbicularis oculi muscle the palpebral fissure widens exposing the sclera. The patient appears to peak at the examiner
- Some degree of pupillary and accommodation dysfunction may occur.

Diagnostic testing
Clinical tests:
- The ice test is simple and has high degree of sensitivity and specificity. It is especially useful in patients where anticholinestrase agents are contraindicated due to their cardiac status or age

  The size of the palpebral fissure is measured, a surgical glove containing crushed ice is applied over the lid for 2 minutes and the palpebral fissure width is remeasured immediately after removing the ice pack. The test is positive if the palpebral fissure width increases after cooling. The improvement lasts for less than a minute.
- Improvement in palpebral fissure width can also be checked after a 30 minutes period of sleep or rest.

Pharmacological tests:
- *Tensilon test:* Tensilon is an anticholinestrase with rapid onset (30 seconds) and short duration of action (<5 minutes) that competes with acetylcholine for the enzyme acetylcholinesterase and allows prolonged action of acetylcholine at the synapse

In adults, not more than 10 mg intravenously should be injected. A test dose of 2 mg is initially given and the patient is observed for any idiosyncratic reaction or improvement in ptosis. If the improvement occurs within 2 minutes, the test is positive; if no response is seen, the remaining 8 mg of the dose is injected. If no improvement is seen within 3 minutes, the test is negative. A positive test is indicative of MG but a negative test does not rule out MG.

- *Prostigmin test:* A mixture of 0.6 mg atropine and 1.5 mg of prostigmin is injected intramuscularly. A change in ocular motility and ptosis is seen after 15–30 minutes. In children, 0.04 mg/kg body weight of prostigmin is given with a total dose not exceeding 1.5 mg.

The test is particularly useful in children because of the longer duration of action and patients with diplopia without ptosis.

Electrophysiologic tests:
Electromyography shows decremental response to repetitive supramaximal motor nerve stimulation. A rapid decrement in amplitude of 10–15% is considered abnormal.

Antiacetylcholine (anti-Ach) receptor antibody assay: Antiacetylcholine receptor antibodies are found in 90% cases with generalized MG and in 35–45% of ocular MG.

Other tests: Imaging of mediastinum for presence of thymic tumor, that may be seen in 10% patients of MG. Complete blood count, erythrocyte sedimentation rates, antinuclear antibody test and thyroid function tests are performed due to increased prevalence of other autoimmune diseases with MG.

Treatment of MG

- Pyridostigmine bromide, an anticholine esterase agent is the first line of therapy in a dose of 60 mg orally every 3-4 hours. It is to be given cautiously in cardiac and asthma patients
- Thymectomy is performed in generalized MG—
  - In all patients with thymoma irrespective of age
  - In patients with inadequate control with pyridostigmine between puberty and 50 years (no significant thymic tissue remains after middle age).
- If anticholine esterase is ineffective and thymectomy cannot be performed other drugs used are prednisolone, azathioprine, cyclosporine and mycophenolate mofetil
- Short term immunotherapy includes plasmapheresis and intravenous injection of human immunoglobin. These help in stabilizing the patient in myasthenic crisis and are also used for short term management of patients undergoing thymectomy.

Neurogenic Ptosis

Dysfunction of third cranial nerve supplying levator muscle or sympathetic innervation to Muller's muscle is included in this category.

Horner's syndrome may be congenital or acquired. It is caused by damage or interruption of the sympathetic nerve to the eye resulting in overbalance of parasympathetic supply that caused a constriction of the pupil, relaxation of all the muscles around the eye and a sinking of the eye into the orbit.

It is characterized by ptosis, miosis, and enophthalmos with or without anhidrosis. Variation in iris color does not occur in acquired Horner's. The anisocoria is more apparent in dim illumination and the affected pupil shows dilation lag when the room light is suddenly switched off.

Causes of Horner's Syndrome

First-order neuron lesions: Central disorders of the nervous system like vascular occlusion, tumors, cervical disk disease and other disorders involving the upper cervical spinal cord.

Second-order neuron lesions: Apical lung tumors (Pancoast syndrome), metastases, chest surgery, thoracic aortic aneurysms or trauma to the brachial plexus.

Third-order neuron lesions: Degenerative changes in the wall of the carotid artery or following vasospasm.

Pharmacological Tests

Cocaine blocks the re-uptake of norepinephrine released at neuromuscular junctions of the iris dilator muscle, thereby increasing the amount of norepinephrine available to stimulate the muscle. Instillation of 10% cocaine in a normal eye after 45 minutes results in dilatation of pupil but in Horner syndrome, the pupil dilates poorly because little or no norepinephrine is being released into the synaptic cleft.

Apraclonidine, a weak α_1-agonist, produces no significant effect in most normal eyes, however, in sympathetically denervated eyes, the iris dilator muscle develops adrenergic supersensitivity. Reversal of anisocoria on instillation of 0.5% or 1% apraclonidine in both eyes is diagnostic of Horner's syndrome.

Hydroxyamphetamine releases norepinephrine from the presynaptic terminal. It is used for further localization of the lesion. In a postganglionic lesion the amount of baseline anisocoria is increased following instillation of hydroxyamphetamine drops. In a preganglionic Horner syndrome, the postganglionic neuron is intact so there is no increase in anisocoria as the hydroxyamphetamine dilates the Horner pupil as much as it does the normal pupil.

Treatment for Acquired Cases

Management varies depending upon the cause and is directed towards eliminating the disease that produces the syndrome.

Aponeurotic Acquired Ptosis

It is the most common form of acquired ptosis. It mostly affects elderly but can occur in younger age following trauma, chronic ocular inflammation and blepharochalasis. There may be disinsertion from tarsus or dehiscence in the central part of the aponeurosis separating its upper or lower parts. The patient may present with a high or absent upper lid crease and good levator excursion. Superior sulcus may be deepened by superior migration of orbital septum or in cases with extensive thinning of supra tarsal lid, iris color becomes visible through the lid.

Involutional ptosis is a form of acquired aponeurotic ptosis with degenerative processes like dehiscence of medial limb of Whitnall's ligament and fatty degeneration of levator muscle.

Surgical Treatment of Ptosis

For aponeurotic ptosis, levator repair through anterior approach or Muller's muscle-conjunctival resection (MMCR) through posterior approach is used.

In levator repair, the aponeurosis is reattached to the tarsus. In bilateral surgery, the upper lid margins are placed at or 1 mm below the superior limbus in primary position; in unilateral surgery, the margin is placed 1–2 mm above the contralateral lid in primary position.

Muller's muscle-conjunctival resection is indicated in aponeurotic or Horner's syndrome ptosis with good levator function and adequate superior conjunctival fornix. The amount of resection is titrated to the improvement of ptosis on instillation of 10% phenylephrine drops.

To conclude, acquired ptosis may be mechanical, myogenic, neurogenic or aponeurotic. Aponeurotic ptosis is the most common and can be satisfactorily treated surgically. More complicated interventions are required in the diagnosis and management of other varities.

Entropion and Ectropion

Ruchi Goel, KPS Malik

INTRODUCTION

Cornea requires a uniform wet surface for optimal functioning. A sharp angle of contact of the posterior border of the lid margin results in capillarity that moistens the surface of the eye. The orbicularis oculi plays an important role in closure of eyes and functioning of lacrimal pump. The lids are held in appropriate position by horizontal pull exerted by the canthal tendons and vertical pull by retractor muscles. Aging causes laxity of all the tissues. Whether the lid margin will turn in or out depends on the interplay of forces involved in maintaining the taut position of the lids. Ectropion is the outward turning of lid margin and entropion is inward turning of the lid margin. These abnormalities can be classified as given in Table 1.

For corrective intervention it is important to ascertain the type of abnormality and the structure at fault.

WORK-UP TIPS FOR ECTROPION AND ENTROPION

- *History:* Duration and severity of symptoms; episode of facial palsy, lid trauma, previous lid surgery, trachoma, leprosy, etc.

TABLE 1: Classification of entropion and ectropion

Entropion	Ectropion
• Congenital	• Congenital
• Acquired	• Acquired
– Spastic	– Involutional
– Mechanical	– Mechanical
– Involutional	– Cicatricial
– Cicatricial	– Paralytic

- The position of the lid margin and punctum is noted in upgaze and primary position. Mild punctal ectropion of lower lid may become visible only in upgaze
- The tarsal plate is examined for thickening/thinning. A thick superior tarsus can be caused by trachoma leading to cicatricial entropion and responds well to wedge resection. A thin superior tarsus may be seen in previously operated cases where alternative surgical procedures like tarsal fracture may work well. A thinned out inferior tarsus may occur due to aging
- The lids should be examined for presence of mass lesion that may induce mechanical ectropion/entropion; any cicatricial skin changes
- The patient should be asked to close the lids tightly. This may induce an underlying spastic entropion of lower lid. It will also help in detection of facial paresis if any
- *Faria-e-Sousa method to diagnose spastic or intermittent entropion:* Topical anesthetic is instilled and the patient is instructed to look down. The central lower eyelid is pinched, and skin is rolled over the superior tarsal border and pressed against the globe. The eyelid skin is then spread against the globe and released while the patient keeps looking down. Persistence of entropion with eye movements and blinking for at least 3 minutes indicates spastic or intermittent entropion
- Ocular surface is examined to rule out hyperlacrimatory state
- The patency of lacrimal passage is checked. Watering may occur due to anatomical blockage and not due to ectropion or entropion
- *Generalized eyelid laxity:* The *pinch test* effectively determines the amount of lid laxity. Lid is lax if it can be pulled more than 6 mm away from the globe (Fig. 1). In

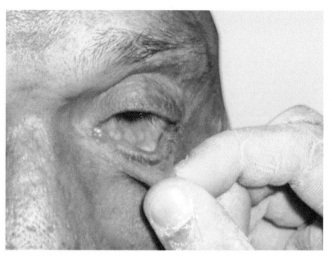

Fig. 1: Pinch test for generalized lid laxity.

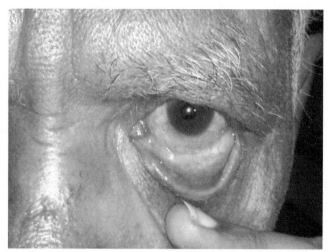

Fig. 2: Patient with vertical lid laxity having fornicial fat head.

snap back test, a downward traction is made to the lower lid and then release. On releasing, the lid reverts back to its normal position, without the aid of a blink if normal but not in presence of laxity

- *Vertical laxity:* The patient is asked to look up and then down. Signs of vertical lid laxity are:
  - Diminished lower lid excursion between extreme up- and downgaze
  - Absence of lower lid skin crease on downgaze
  - Deep inferior fornix
  - Horizontal white band inferior to the lower border of tarsal plate
  - Fornicial fat head (Fig. 2)
  - Increased passive elevation of the center of the lower lid.
- *Medial canthal tendon (MCT) laxity:* The punctum lies lateral to the caruncle at rest and should not be displaced more than 1–2 mm with lateral lid traction (Fig. 3)
- MCT laxity can be graded as follows:
  - *Mild*—if punctum gets stretched up to the limbus
  - *Moderate*—if punctum gets stretched up to pupil
  - *Severe*—if punctum can be stretched beyond the temporal pupillary border
  - *Lateral canthal tendon laxity:* The lateral canthal angle is evaluated with the lid at rest. It lies 1–2 mm medial to the lateral orbital rim and should have an acute angular contour, as a rounded appearance indicates laxity. The lateral part of the lid if pulled medially should not result in more than 1–2 mm movement of the lateral canthal angle.

ECTROPION

Ectropion is characterized by rotation of lid margin outward and is more common in lower lid. With advancing age, there is decreased resilience and laxity of periocular tissues

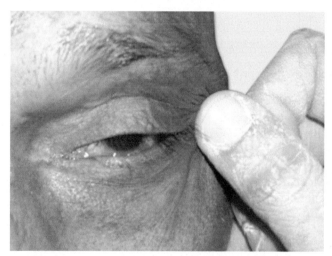

Fig. 3: Lateral lid traction to test for medial canthal laxity.

because of age-related microinfarction and secondary atrophy. This inadequate support and effect of gravity results in pronounced stretching of the lower lid, enhancing the burden on suspensory canthal tendons and resulting in ectropion. Furthermore, the constant wiping and rubbing of eyes due to epiphora, further aggravates the condition. In contrast, the upper lid ectropion usually arises due to cicatricial changes of the anterior lamella.

Grading of Ectropion

Punctum alone can be everted or the entire lid may be everted. If the whole lid looks as if turned inside out it is known as *tarsal ectropion* (Fig. 4). In a normal lid the inferior punctum is directed posteriorly against the globe and should not be visible without pulling the lid downward. Direction of the punctum away from the globe is the earliest sign of medial lid ectropion and can be graded as *mild* (unopposed on looking up), *moderate* (unopposed even

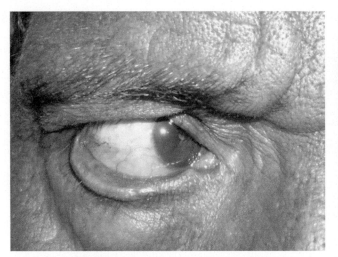

Fig. 4: Tarsal ectropion right lower lid.

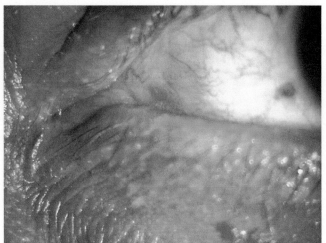

Fig. 5: Medial moderate ectropion: Punctum is unopposed in primary position.

in primary gaze) (Fig. 5), and *severe* (palpebral conjunctiva and fornix are exposed).

Management of Ectropion

Congenital Ectropion

Congenital ectropion is a rare entity, seen in premature infants due to birth trauma causing orbicularis slippage/lamellar slippage. It has also been reported in Down syndrome, blepharophimosis syndrome, and ichthyosis (Fig. 6). Manual repositioning and inversion of the eyelid with topical antibiotics and lubricating agents is required. In severe cases, skin grafting is necessary to avoid corneal scarring.

Acquired Ectropion

Involutional Ectropion

The procedure depends upon the extent of ectropion:

- *Generalized*:
  - Tarsal strip procedure (if medial canthal laxity is >3–4 mm then not to be used alone as it can cause lateral displacement of lower punctum)
  - Horizontal lid shortening (with blepharoplasty if excess skin is present)
  - "Safdarjung suture" or prolene sling.
- *Mainly medial*:
  - Medial conjunctivoplasty if there is no horizontal laxity.
  - If medial canthal tendon laxity is also present then it is combined with medial canthal tendon plication.
  - If associated with generalized lid laxity then Lazy-T procedure is used.

Lateral tarsal strip (LTS):

Tenzel described the use of the *lateral canthal tendon sling* for correction of the involutional ectropion where a new lateral canthal tendon is fashioned from the lateral tarsus by

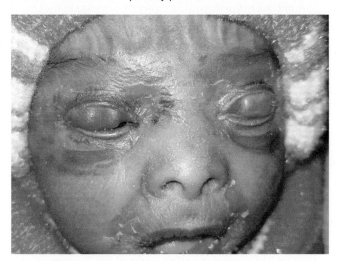

Fig. 6: Both eye upper lid ectropion in ichthyosis.

excising the surrounding anterior lamella and conjunctiva and attaching it to the lateral orbital rim periosteum through a button hole made into the upper lateral canthal tendon. Later, Anderson modified Tenzel's lateral canthal sling and called it "tarsal strip" procedure.

Lateral tarsal strip produces a horizontal lid shortening with a diagonal tightening of the orbital septum and lower lid retractors producing an effective improvement in both horizontal and vertical lid laxity.

Lateral canthotomy and transection of the inferior crus of the lateral canthal tendon is performed (Fig. 7A). The lateral canthal tendon is deepithelized of epidermis, lid margin, and lateral tarsal conjunctiva (Fig. 7B).

The eyelid is split into anterior and posterior lamellae (Fig. 7C) and a tarsal strip is fashioned from the posterior lamella (Fig. 7D). The tarsal strip is sutured to periosteum at the lateral orbital wall, adjusting the height and tension of the lateral canthus using 5-0 polypropylene suture (Fig. 7E).

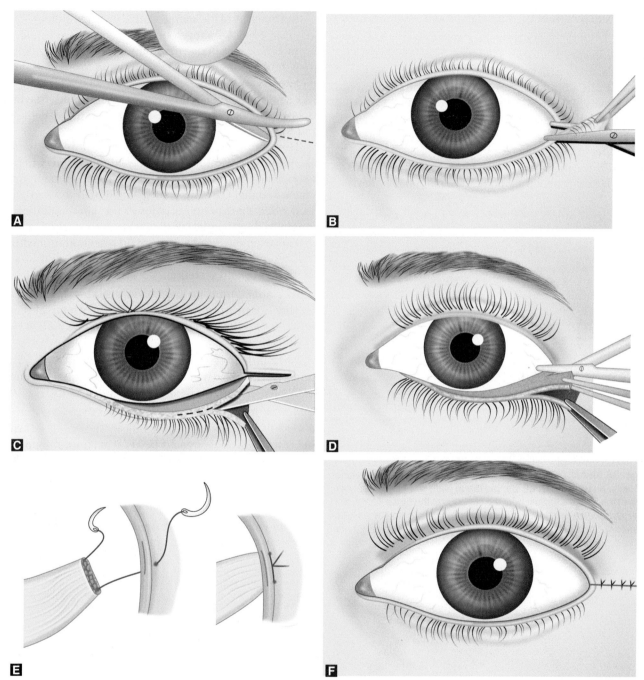

Figs. 7A to F: (A) LTS: lateral canthotomy is performed; (B) The lateral canthal tendon is deepithelized of epidermis, lid margin, and lateral tarsal conjunctiva; (C) LTS: eyelid is split into anterior and posterior lamellae; (D) LTS: A tarsal strip is fashioned from the posterior lamella; (E) LTS: tarsal strip is sutured to periosteum at the lateral orbital wall, adjusting the height and tension of the lateral canthus using 5-0 polypropylene suture; (F) A triangular shaped excess skin is excised and the wound is closed with 6-0 silk.

A triangular portion of the lower lid skin is resected and the wound closed (Fig. 7F).

Horizontal lid shortening procedures:
The horizontal shortening procedures are used for correction of horizontal lid laxity in both entropion and ectropion. The difference lies in the way the shortened lid is anchored to the periosteum or lateral canthus. In entropion, a tightening is to be produced at the lower border of tarsus (to prevent its outward rotation and subsequent inward rotation of lid margin), so additional suture bites are

taken from the lower border of tarsus and adjoining tissue (Figs. 8A and B).

Bick's procedure of horizontal lid shortening: A full thickness triangular excision of eyelid tissue is performed at the lateral canthus. The amount of resection depends on the degree of eyelid laxity. The tarsal plate is then reattached to the cut end of the lateral canthal tendon (Fig. 9).

Both Bick's procedure and LTS shorten the lid laterally. They differ in two respects:
1. In LTS, the incision is placed from the lateral canthus to the lateral orbital rim and has the potential to damage

the integrity of the lateral canthal tendon whereas Bick's avoids the LCT altogether.
2. In LTS, tarsal plate (made up of meibomian glands) is buried that may incite granuloma formation at the lateral canthus.

Bick procedure modified by Reeh, is performed, in which an inverted house shaped lid shortening is done (Figs. 10A and B).

Horizontal lid shortening can be combined with a blepharoplasty (Kuhnt-Szymanowski procedure wherein a subciliary incision is made and skin flap is made from a lateral triangle, and lid is shortened under the flap). It is used when there is excess of lower lid skin in addition to generalized horizontal laxity.

However, the disadvantage of lid resection procedures is occurence of lid notching, lid shortening, and loss of meibomian gland secretion.

Malik's Safdarjung suture: Lower eyelid suspension by passing 5-0 polypropylene suture in the pretarsal plane between the attachments of the lateral and medial canthal tendons (Fig. 11).

Medial canthal plication: Anterior limb of medial canthal tendon is stabilized by suturing it to the medial end of lower tarsal plate in patients with medial canthal laxity (Fig. 12).

Medial spindle procedure/medial Punctal eversion in absence of conjunctivoplasty: Significant horizontal lid laxity and normal MCT, is treated by vertical shortening of the posterior lamella (Figs. 13A and B).

A probe is placed in the inferior canaliculus and a diamond shaped tarso-conjunctiva and inferior lid retractors are excised from below the punctum using 11 blade and scissors. The apex of the diamond should be 4 mm below the lower punctum. The closure is performed with

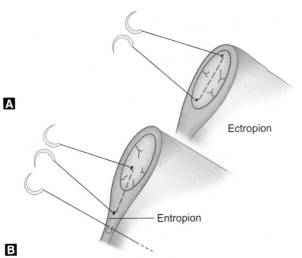

Figs. 8A and B: (A) Ectropion: A 5-0 double armed polypropylene suture is passed higher up into the tarsal plate so that the superior limb of the suture exits just near the cut edge of the upper lid margin; (B) Entropion: A 5-0 double armed polypropylene suture is passed from lower border of tarsus and capsulopalpebral fascia to anchor it to the periosteum.

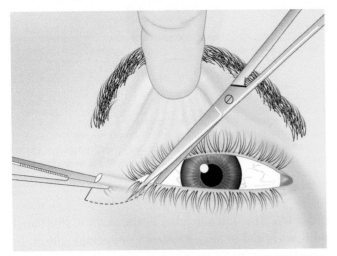

Fig. 9: Bick's procedure of horizontal lid shortening. A full thickness triangular excision of eyelid tissue is performed at the lateral canthus.

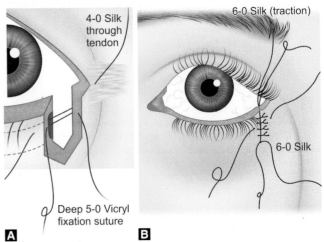

Figs. 10A and B: Bick's procedure modified by Reeh. (A) Inverted house shaped lid (pentagon) shortening of lower lid; (B) After excision of tissue wound is closed as in lid margin repair.

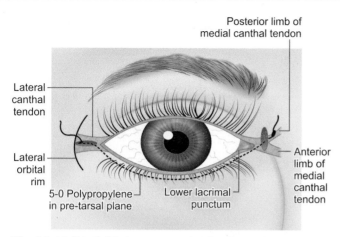

Fig. 11: Malik's Safdarjung suture. A 5-0 polypropylene suture is first tied near the attachment of lateral canthal tendon at the orbital rim, then passed in the pretarsal plane closely hugging the lower lid margin to exit medially to be tied to the medial canthal tendon and adjacent periosteum.

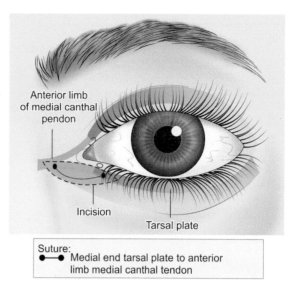

Fig. 12: Medial canthal plication.

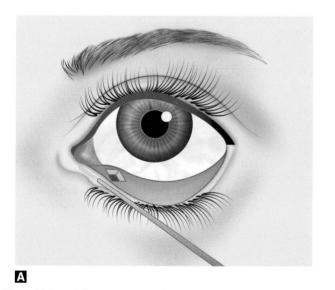

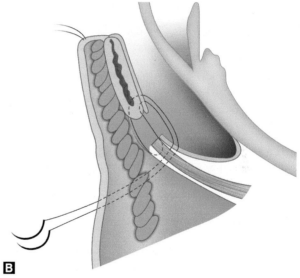

Figs. 13A and B: Medial spindle procedure. (A) A probe is placed in the inferior canaliculus and a diamond shaped tarsoconjunctiva and inferior lid retractors are excised from below the punctum; (B) The closure is performed with double armed inverting sutures.

double armed inverting sutures using 5-0 nonabsorbable sutures brought out inferiorly through the orbicularis and skin and tied on to the bolster. The sutures are left for 2–3 weeks.

The Byron-Smith Lazy-T procedure: This involves full thickness eyelid resection with excision and closure of medial spindle of conjunctiva. The term lazy "T" is derived from the fact that the final lid sutures appear like a "T" lying on its side (Figs. 14A to D).

Mechanical Ectropion
Mechanical ectropion requires excision of the mass.

Cicatricial Ectropion
Cicatricial ectropion requires lengthening of the cutaneous surface and resection of subcutaneous cicatrix. For localized scar, a Z-plasty is performed (Figs. 15A to D). For generalized scarring and shortage of skin, skin replacement with a local transposition flap or a free flap is done.

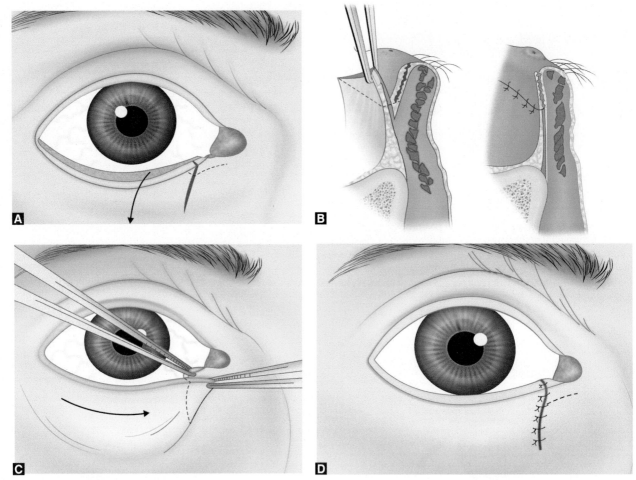

Figs. 14A to D: Lazy 'T' procedure. (A) A vertical full thickness incision is made 2 mm temporal to the punctum of the lower lid in the tarsal plate followed by a horizontal incision in the posterior lamella; (B) The edge of the tarsoconjunctiva and capsulopalpebral fascia are resected. The conjunctival wound is closed with 6-0 vicryl suture; (C) A full thickness section of eyelid is resected after overlapping the edges; (D) The skin is closed with 6-0 silk.

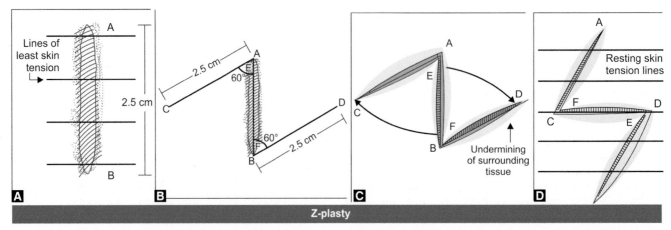

Figs. 15A to D: Z-plasty (A) Incision made along the line of the scar; (B) From each end, incisions of equal length as previous one are made at 60°; (C) The triangular flaps are dissected and underlying scar is excised; (D) The flaps are transposed and skin is sutured.

Paralytic Ectropion

In paralytic ectropion, the lower lid is supported or strengthened in form of medial canthoplasty/tarsorrhaphy, lateral tarsorrhaphy, or a cheek lift/mid face lift in longstanding cases associated with cheek ptosis. Safdarjung suture has also been found to be effective in moderate paralytic ectropion.

Medial Canthoplasty: It is performed for paralytic medial ectropion. Probes are passed in both the canaliculi and both lid margins are split as shown in the Figures 16A and B. The skin is undermined and 6-0 polyglycolic acid sutures are passed taking bite below the inferior canaliculus to above the superior canaliculus.

Medial canthoplasty with lateral canthal sling:
It is performed in paralytic ectropion with generalized lower lid laxity. The skin incision is similar to LTS procedure. The lower limb of lateral canthal tendon is cut leaving the upper limb intact. A strip of lower tarsus is fashioned and passed through a button hole created in the upper limb of the lateral canthal ligament and sutured to the periosteum of the lateral orbital rim (Fig. 17).

Tarsorrhaphy: Temporary tarsorrhaphy is performed in cases where temporary corneal protection is required as in Bell's palsy. Here the two ends of the lids are sutured without or minimal eyelid tissue so that when the tarsorrhaphy is undone the lid margins appear relatively normal.

In permanent lateral tarsorrhaphy, a shallow incision is made through the gray line at the site of proposed tarsorrhaphy in both the lids. Tissue is excised posterior to this incision to create raw surfaces opposite to each other in both the lids. The raw surfaces of both the lids are sutured together with mattress sutures tied over the bolsters on the skin of the upper and lower lids. The sutures are left for 2–3 weeks.

In another modification of permanent lateral tarsorrhaphy a gray line split is performed. Epithelium is carefully removed along the upper and lower eyelid margins. The raw surfaces are then united with absorbable sutures (Figs. 18A to C).

Fascial sling: It is performed for correction of lower lid laxity where lateral canthal sling is unsuitable as in medial canthal laxity or previous tarsorrhaphy. A strip of fascia lata is passed through the lid between the lateral and medial canthal tendons (Fig. 19).

ENTROPION

Entropion (en = in; trepin = to turn) is a turning-in of the lid margin resulting in constant irritation by the inturned

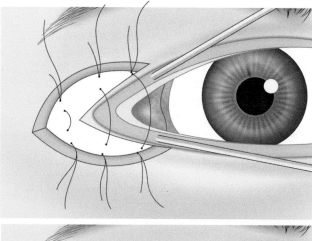

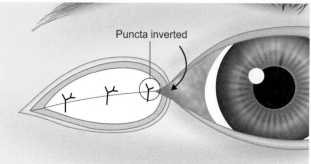

Puncta inverted

Figs. 16A and B: Medial canthoplasty. (A) Probes are passed in both the canaliculi and both lid margins are split; (B) The skin is undermined and 6-0 polyglycolic acid sutures are passed taking bite below the inferior canaliculus to above the superior canaliculus.

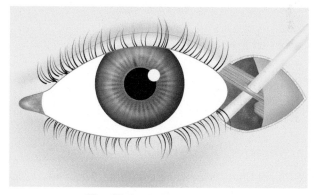

Fig. 17: Lateral canthal sling.

cilia. Patients complain of a chronic foreign body sensation, redness, watering, and discharge caused by constant rubbing of the eyelid margin, eyelashes, and skin against the ocular surface resulting in corneal abrasions and inflammation of the conjunctiva. Untreated entropion can progress to secondary corneal thinning, vascularization, and scarring. Corneal ulceration and perforation may occur in chronic cases.

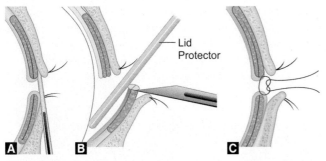

Figs. 18A to C: Lateral permanent tarsorrhaphy: (A) Gray line split; (B) Epithelium is removed along the upper and lower eyelid margins; (C) The raw surfaces are then united with absorbable sutures.

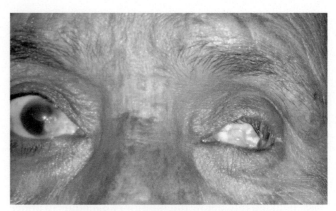

Fig. 20: Left eye mechanical entropion.

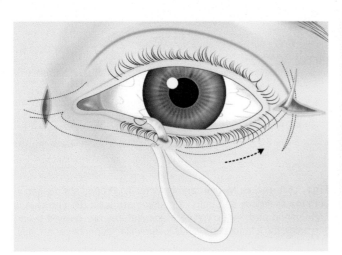

Fig. 19: Fascial sling.

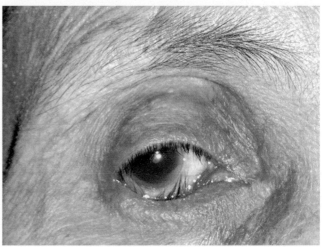

Fig. 21: Involutional entropion.

Grades of Entropion

- I: Only the posterior lid border is in rolled
- II: Inturning up to the inter-marginal strip
- III: The whole lid margin including the anterior border is inturned

Classification of Entropion

Spastic entropion is an acute condition, affecting any age and affects the lower lid following ocular inflammation. It is usually transient and is managed by temporary measures such as taping, treatment of the causative irritation and inflammation. It is managed along the lines of involutional entropion if it does not resolve.

Mechanical entropion occurs in consequence to absent lower lid support as in cases with shrunken globe (Fig. 20).

Cicatricial entropion is caused by conjunctival scarring due to chemical burns, trauma or surgery, trachoma, Stevens-Johnson syndrome, and mucus membrane pemphigoid.

Involutional Entropion

Etiology—laxity of tissues causing lamellar dissociation (overriding of preseptal orbicularis over tarsus plate), lower lid retractor weakness, loss of stiffness and inward buckling of tarsal plate causing the upper border to invert more than the lower and horizontal eyelid laxity (Fig. 21).

Congenital Entropion

Rare condition caused by disinsertion of lower lid retractors and overaction of marginal orbicularis muscle.

Epiblepharon is more common than entropion. It is a developmental anomaly characterized by the presence of a fold of skin running horizontally across the upper (epiblepharon superior) or lower lid (epiblepharon inferior). Occasionally there may be two or even three skin folds.

The main differences between these two clinical entities are:

- *The position of the lid margin:* In true entropion the lid margin is inverted along its entire length whereas in epiblepharon it is the lashes only which are pushed against the globe.

- Epiblepharon occurs relatively more commonly and tends to disappear by the end of the first year and therefore rarely requires surgery. Entropion gets aggravated with growth and always requires surgical intervention.

- In congenital entropion the tarsus is pulled out of position owing to relative overaction of the marginal fibers of the orbicularis whereas in epiblepharon it is the skin of the lid which bulges out and pushes the cilia against the globe, especially in downward gaze.

If corneal abrasions and scarring occur or there is failure to resolve by 2 years of age then Hotz type operation can be performed (Fig. 22). A thin strip of skin-orbicularis muscle is

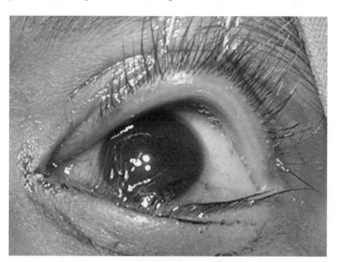

Fig. 22: Corneal abrasions and scarring caused by congenital entropion.

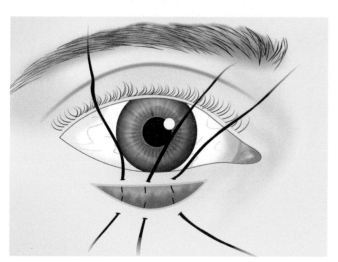

Fig. 23: Skin muscle excision for treatment of congenital entropion or nonresolving epiblepheron.

excised along the marked lower lid crease. The amount to be resected is assessed by pinching the tissues with a forceps. The wound is closed with 6-0 vicryl sutures passed from skin edge-superior orbicularis-retractor layer or tarsus-inferior orbicularis muscle-inferior skin edge (Fig 23).

Involutional Lower Lid Entropion Management

Everting sutures and adhesive strips are used for temporary relief. Even excision of horizontal strips of skin or muscle or both should be used only in mild senile entropion as the pathology is not the spasm but an actual weakening and atony of lid tissues.

Sutures

- *Quickert–Rathbun suture:* A double-armed 4-0 chromic catgut suture is placed transversely, starting just below the tarsus from the conjunctival side and exiting through the skin at a higher level
- *Iliff modification:* A 4-0 chromic catgut double-armed suture is placed from the inferior fornix to the skin in the infralash location and kept for 2 weeks (Fig. 24).

For definitive and permanent correction of involutional entropion, corrective surgery usually combines horizontal shortening of the eyelid, advancing the lower eyelid retractors, and, when needed, the creation of a full-thickness eyelid scar to prevent the preseptal orbicularis muscle from overriding the pretarsal muscle.

Weis-type procedure (transverse lid split and everting sutures): A full thickness horizontal lid incision is made 4 mm below the lash line. Three double armed 4-0 catgut sutures are passed from conjunctiva below the lid transection to the skin above it. Lid split creates a fibrous

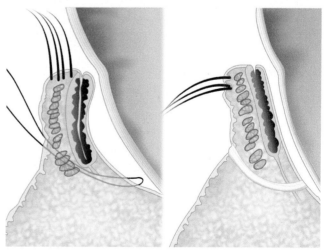

Fig. 24: Iliff modification of suture placement.

barrier to prevent upward movement of preseptal muscle and everting sutures shorten the lower lid retractors (Figs. 25A to C).

Quickert procedure: Vertical lid shortening can be also combined with horizontal shortening, a procedure known as Quickert procedure (transverse lid split, everting sutures, and horizontal lid shortening).

A vertical full thickness incision is made 5 mm from the lateral canthus till the lower border of the tarsus. A horizontal full thickness incision is placed just below the tarsus. (If the medial canthal tendon is lax, then plication is performed at this stage.) The two flaps thus created are overlapped to determine the amount of lid to be resected from the medial flap (Fig. 26A). After the resection, the flaps are sutured as in lid margin repair. The remaining closure is as in Weiss procedure (Fig. 26B).

Wheelers Orbicularis Strip Procedure

In this procedure, the horizontal lower lid laxity is corrected by exerting pressure on lower border of tarsus thus tipping the upper border outward and, also by strengthening orbicularis by shortening and overlapping. A band of orbicularis muscle is dissected from the anterior surface of the tarsal plate. It is overlapped and reattached to the tarsoorbital fascia just below the tarsus.

Hill's Modification of Wheelers Orbicularis Strip Procedure

In the original technique of Wheeler's procedure, Hill introduced creation of tissue barriers to prevent preseptal orbicularis from moving upward over the tarsus to the lid edge. The additional steps to create these barriers are (Figs. 27A to D):

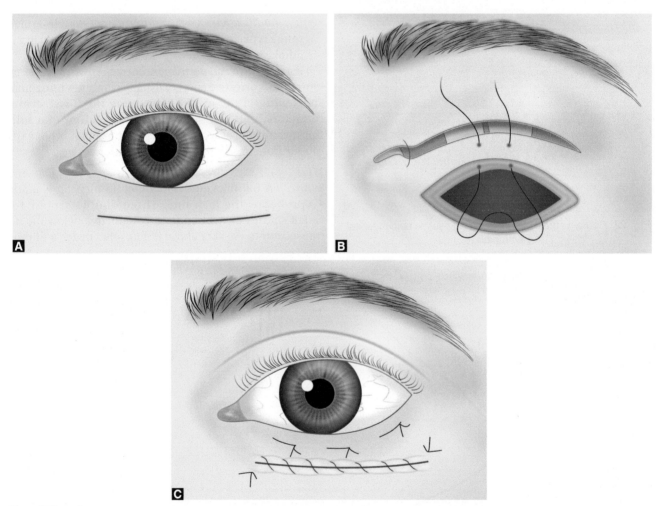

Figs. 25A to C: Weis type procedure. (A) A full thickness horizontal lid incision is made 4 mm below the lash line; (B) Double armed 4-0 catgut sutures are passed from conjunctiva below the lid transection to the skin above it; (C) Skin closed with continuous or interrupted sutures.

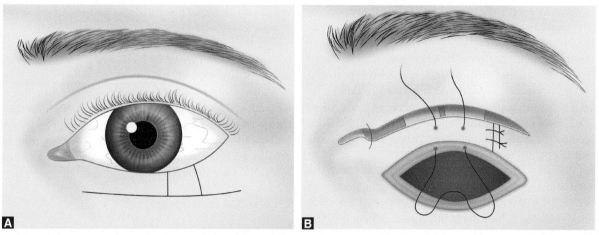

Figs. 26A and B: Quickert procedure. (A) A vertical full thickness incision is made 5 mm from the lateral canthus till the lower border of the tarsus. A horizontal full thickness incision is placed just below the tarsus; (B) The two flaps are overlapped and excess tissue is excised. The lid margin is repaired and closure is done as in Weiss procedure.

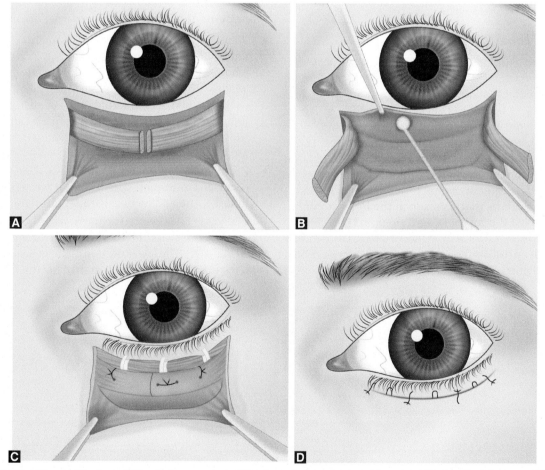

Figs. 27A to D: Hill's modification of Wheeler's procedure: (A) A linear incision is made throughout the length of the lower lid 2 mm from the lid margin. A 5 mm wide band of pretarsal orbicularis fibers is dissected free from the tarsus and skin; (B) Curettage is performed from the anterior surface of the tarsus and the under surface of the skin; (C) The band of orbicularis is overlapped and attached to the lower border of the tarsus by 4-0 plain gut-mattress sutures. Two wing sutures are placed in the orbicularis band on either side of central suture to prevent riding up of the preseptal orbicularis muscle onto the anterior surface of the tarsus; (D) The skin is closed with 6-0 interrupted silk sutures.

(1) To create an inflammatory reaction and cause the skin to adhere to the tarsus, vigorous curettage of the anterior surface of the tarsal plate and of the undersurface of the skin overlying the tarsus is performed. (2) Instead of suturing the shortened strip of orbicularis muscle to the lower edge of the transorbital fascia below the tarsus, he sutured it to the tarsal plate. This prevents rotation of lower border of tarsal plate outward and its upper margin from tipping inward. It also prevents the preseptal orbicularis from riding upward toward the lid margin.

Fox (1951) described another modification in which the lid is split and a wedge (apex upward) of tarsus is excised from the center of the tarsal plate (Fig. 28A and B). This was combined with the tightening of the skin and muscle of the lower lid through a skin incision below the lateral canthus.

The procedures described under the section of ectropion correction for management of lid laxity such as LTS and horizontal lid shortening techniques are used for entropion correction as well.

Plication of Lower Lid Retractors

In cases with inferior lid retractor weakness, tucking of inferior lid retractors (Jones, Reeh and Wobig) is performed alone or in combination of LTS as a primary procedure or secondary to failure of Quickert procedure. It can be performed from both skin and conjunctival side. The inferior lid retractors are identified and sutured to the anterior edge of lower border of tarsus (can also be used for ectropion correction where the inferior lid retractors are inserted on the posterior edge of lower border of tarsus).

A horizontal skin incision is made at the lower border of the tarsal plate; the preseptal and pretarsal muscles are separated to expose the lower border of tarsus. Dissection is continued deep to the preseptal muscle and inferior orbital septum is divided. The orbital fat bulges out on division of septum. The lower lid retractors lie behind the orbital fat. The fat is retracted, the retractors are held with a forceps, the patient is asked to look up and down. Holding of the retractors is confirmed by feeling of a tug on movement of the globe downward.

A 5-0 nonabsorbable suture is passed in the center through the lower skin edge-through lower lid retractors 8 mm below the tarsus through lower border of tarsal plate and out through upper skin edge (Fig. 29). Two more sutures are placed in a similar way on either side. The sutures are removed after 10 days.

Cicatricial Entropion

Cicatricial entropion of lower lid is easier to treat as compared to that of upper lid as the lower lid lies below the limbus and has limited corneal involvement and tarsal deformity.

Management of Lower Lid Cicatricial Entropion

- *Tarsal fracture:* It is performed for mild cicatricial entropion. A horizontal incision is made through the whole width of the tarsal plate just below the center to expose the deep surface of the pretarsal muscle. Three double armed 5-0 silk sutures are passed from the lower fragment of the tarsal plate to exit on the skin just below the lash line over bolsters (Figs. 30A and B). The sutures are removed after 10 days.

- *Posterior lamellar graft:* It is performed in severe cicatricial entropion with lower lid retraction of more than 1.5 mm and recurrence after tarsal fracture.

The lower lid is everted by traction sutures through the gray line. A transverse incision is made through the tarsal plate (Fig. 31A). The lower portion of the tarsus is separated from the orbicularis muscle. A graft of full thickness buccal

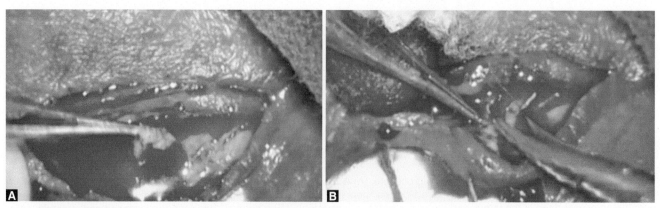

Figs. 28A and B: Modified Wheeler's procedure. (A) Microscopic view: A band of orbicularis is fashioned, retracted and a wedge of tarsus is excised with the apex upwards; (B) Microscopic view: Shortening of lower border of tarsus induced on suturing results in tipping out of the lid margin.

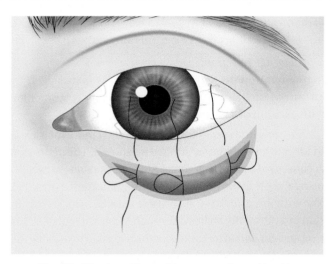

Fig. 29: Plication of lower lid retractors from skin side.

mucosa, donor sclera, or tarsal plate from opposite lid is sutured between the cut edges of the tarsal plate (Fig. 31B).

Management of Upper Lid Cicatricial Entropion

In upper lid, basis of all procedures for cicatricial entropion is eversion of lid margin by sectioning the tarsus horizontally so that lower segment turns up and ciliary margin is pulled upward (Table 2).

Anterior lamellar repositioning:
Mild cases are corrected by anterior lamellar repositioning and suturing the anterior lamella to the tarsus at a higher level.

A lid crease incision is made and anterior tarsal surface is exposed. The dissection is continued till the lash roots. A 6-0 absorbable suture is passed from the skin just above the lashes into the tarsal plate at a higher level to exit at the skin 2 mm away but at the same level as the original suture

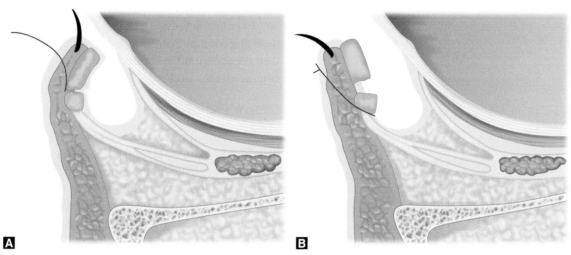

Figs. 30A and B: (A) Lower lid cicatricial entropion; (B) Lower lid cicatricial entropion correction by tarsal fracture.

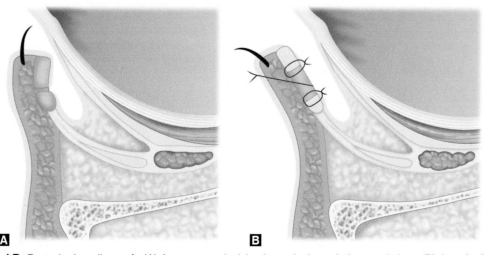

Figs. 31A and B: Posterior lamellar graft. (A) A transverse incision is made through the tarsal plate; (B) A graft of full thickness buccal mucosa, donor sclera or tarsal plate from opposite lid is sutured between the cut edges of the tarsal plate.

just above the lashes. Three such sutures are passed and left for 6 weeks. The skin fold produced due to repositioning is trimmed and the wound closed (Figs. 32A to C).

In *Jaesche-Arlt's operation*, the lid is split along the gray line up to a depth of 3–4 mm, starting just lateral to the punctum to the outer canthus. A 4 mm wide crescentic strip of skin is then removed 3 mm above the lid margin. Suturing the skin results in eversion of the lash line.

In *modified Burrow's operation*, a horizontal incision is made in the region of sulcus subtarsalis, 2–3 mm above lid margin, along the entire length of the eyelid, cutting the conjunctiva and tarsus but not the skin. The temporal end of the strip is then incised by a vertical incision. The eye

is then kept bandaged in such a way so as to keep the lid everted till healing takes place. This directs the lashes away.

Tarsal wedge resection:

Marked entropion with thickened tarsus is managed by Streatfeild Snellen procedure (anterior lamella repositioning with excision of a wedge of tarsal plate).

The gray line is split for 1–2 mm. A lid crease incision is made and anterior tarsal surface is exposed. The dissection is continued till the lash roots. A wedge of tarsus is excised using a blade at the point of maximum thickening of tarsus. Three double armed 6-0 absorbable sutures are passed from skin just above the lashes—through lower cut end of tarsus to upper cut end of tarsus to exit through skin just above the lash line 2 mm apart and tied over bolsters (Figs. 33A and B).

Modified Ketssey's operation (Transposition of the tarsoconjunctival wedge) involves creation of a horizontal incision along the whole length 2–3 mm from the lid margin involving conjunctiva and tarsal plate. Mattress sutures are then passed from the upper cut end of the tarsal plate to emerge on the skin 1 mm above the lid margin.

Lid Split ± Mucous Membrane Graft

The lid is split at the gray line into anterior and posterior lamella. The posterior lamella is advanced. Three double armed 5-0 absorbable sutures are passed through the upper fornix, conjunctiva—through the skin in position of the prospective skin crease. The recessed edge of the anterior lamella is sutured to the advanced tarsus to leave 4 mm of exposed raw surface to granulate. Alternatively, the exposed tarsal surface may be covered with amniotic membrane graft or buccal mucosal graft (Figs. 34 and 35).

TABLE 2: Management of upper lid cicatricial entropion.

Grade of cicatricial upper lid entropion	Procedure of choice
Mild	Anterior lamellar reposition Jaesche-Arlt's operation (Rarely done) Modified Burrow's operation (Rarely done)
Moderate/severe	Thick tarsus: Tarsal wedge resection
	Thin tarsus: Modified Ketssey's operation (similar to tarsal fracture) Lid split ± mucous membrane graft
	Keratinization of tarsoconjunctiva: Rotation of terminal tarsus
	Moderate lid retraction: Posterior lamellar advancement
	Severe lid retraction: Posterior lamellar graft or tarsal excision

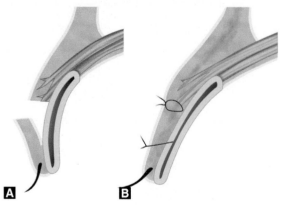
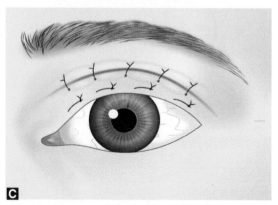

Figs. 32A to C: Anterior lamellar repositioning. (A) A lid crease incision is made and anterior tarsal surface is exposed; (B) A 6-0 absorbable suture is passed from the skin just above the lashes into the tarsal plate at a higher level to exit at the skin 2 mm away but at the same level as the original suture just above the lashes; (C) The excess skin fold produced due to repositioning is trimmed and the wound closed.

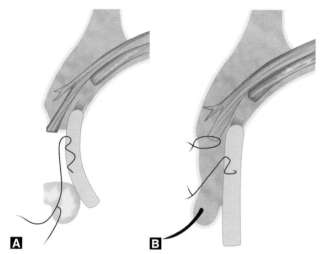

Figs. 33A and B: (A) Wedge resection: Three double armed 6-0 absorbable sutures are passed from skin just above the lashes-through lower cut end of tarsus-upper cut end of tarsus to exit through skin just above the lash line 2 mm apart; (B) Wedge resection: Final appearance.

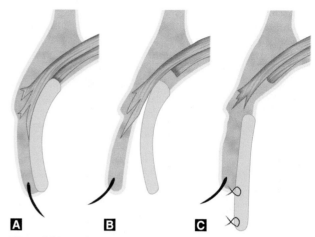

Figs. 34A to C: (A) Upper lid cicatricial entropion; (B) Anterior and posterior lamellar separation; (C) The posterior lamella is advanced and anterior lamella is sutured on top of it leaving 4 mm of tarsus exposed.

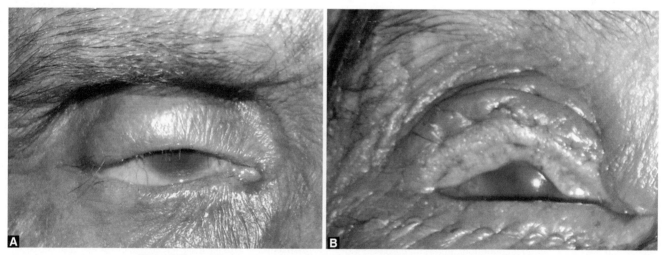

Figs. 35A and B: (A) Preoperative appearance of upper lid cicatricial entropion; (B) Upper lid entropion corrected by lid spit and posterior lamellar advancement.

Trabut type procedure (rotation of terminal tarsus with posterior lamella advancement) is used to make a new lid margin in cases with keratinization of tarsoconjunctiva.

The upper lid is everted and incision is made through the tarsus 2–3 mm from the posterior lid margin. The lid is split to allow advancement of the upper portion of tarsus inferiorly. The lower portion of tarsus is cut and rotated 180°. The posterior lamella is advanced to create the new lid margin. The rotated segment of tarsus is sutured to the advanced portion of tarsus (Figs. 36A and B). Three double armed 5-0 absorbable sutures are passed through the upper fornix—conjunctiva—through the skin in position of the prospective skin crease.

Posterior lamellar graft:
A horizontal incision is made in the tarsal plate. The terminal tarsal remnant is freed and everted. A plane is created between the posterior surface of upper lid retractors and the proximal tarsal segment. A nasal mucoperichondrium graft is sutured with 6-0 absorbable suture to the two portions of the tarsus and also to the overlying orbicularis and skin (Fig. 37).

Tarsal excision:
This is a rarely performed procedure in which the tarsus is excised and the conjunctiva and lid retractors are recessed and held with sutures to the overlying skin.

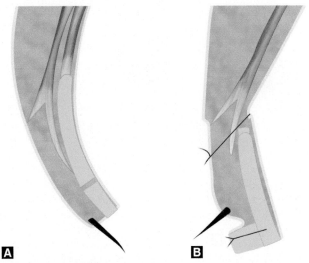

Figs. 36A and B: (A) Trabut procedure: The lower portion of tarsus is cut; (B) The cut portion of tarsus is rotated 180° and sutured to the advanced posterior lamella.

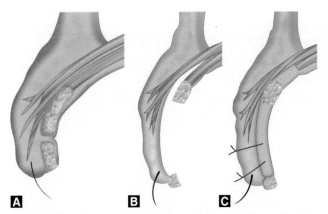

Figs. 37A to C: Posterior lamellar graft: (A) A horizontal incision is made in the tarsal plate; (B) A plane is created between the posterior surface of upper lid retractors and the proximal tarsal segment; (C) A nasal mucoperichondrium graft is sutured with 6-0 absorbable suture to the two portions of the tarsus and also to the overlying orbicularis and skin.

Trichiasis:

Trichiasis is the misdirection of the cilia that results in their rubbing against the cornea. It may involve a few lashes or the entire lid margin. It can be caused by trachoma, spastic entropion, blepharitis, pemphigoid, injury scars, chemical burns, operations, destructive operations, and inflammations like Steven–Johnson syndrome.

Symptoms are irritation, pain, lacrimation, redness, and reflex blepharospasm. This may lead to recurrent corneal erosions, opacities, vascularization, ulcers, and eventually threaten vision. Isolated cilia can be epilated as a temporary measure. For permanent cure, destruction of hair follicle by electrolysis, radiofrequency, argon laser ablation, and cryosurgery can be performed. Generalized trichiasis requires anterior lamellar repositioning surgeries.

- *Electrolysis: A* 30-gauge electrode is used to deliver low current to each hair follicle. A flat positive pole is applied to the temple, while the negative, a fine steel needle, is introduced into the hair follicle and a current of 2 mA is used

  The negative pole is determined by placing the terminals in saline. The strength of the current is gauged by the rate of evolution of hydrogen gas in the saline. Bubbles are seen at the puncture site and the eyelash is easily wiped out with a cotton swab if treatment is adequate. *Disadvantages:* High recurrence rate, adjacent normal lashes are damaged, lid notching, and focal madarosis.

- *Radiofrequency:* The radiofrequency signal is delivered through a partially insulated needle tip inserted along the shaft of the cilia to the cilia base. The energy is delivered at very low power setting for about a second on cut mode. On removal of the needle tip the lash is easily extracted

- *Trephination:* It is a new technique that is safe and much faster and results in lesser complications and scarring. In this procedure a Sisler ophthalmic microtrephine 1.0 mm is used to cut the lash follicles

- *Diode laser (810 nm):* The diode laser treatment of trichiasis has been found to be effective and requires 4–5 treatments 4–6 weeks apart. The pulse length used is approximately 50 ms, and the energy intensity is approximately 50 J/cm^2

- *Cryotherapy:* It is used for segmental trichiasis. The involved area is frozen for approximately 25 seconds, allowed to thaw, and then refrozen for 20 seconds (double freeze-thaw technique). Permanent destruction of follicles can be achieved with freezing the follicles to the temperature of –20°C. Lashes are mechanically removed after the treatment

  Disadvantages: Persistent edema, loss of skin pigmentation, notching of lid margin, and interference with goblet cell function.

- *Argon laser ablation:* This procedure is not very effective and is useful for few aberrant cilia. Topical anesthesia is instilled and patient sits at the slit lamp. The lid margin is rotated outward, and the laser is aimed at the hair shaft. A total of 12–30 shots are fired per lash with settings of power 1,000–1,500 mW; spot size of 50–100 μm; and duration of 0.1–0.2 s.

The complications of this procedure are very similar to complications of electrolysis. The reported recurrence rate for electrolysis and argon laser ablation is 12–41%.

Distichiasis:

Distichiasis is an extra row of eyelashes arising from the meibomian orifices. It may be congenital or acquired following cicatrizing conjunctivitis associated with chemical injury, Steven-Johnson syndrome, and ocular cicatricial pemphigoid. Mild cases may be treated as for trichiasis. Severe cases require lamellar eyelid division and cryotherapy to the posterior lamella. In another procedure, a 2 mm strip of the posterior lamellar portion of the lid including the aberrant lashes is excised horizontally across the lid. The denuded surface of the margin is covered with a full thickness mucous membrane graft.

Madarosis:

Madarosis is decrease in number or complete loss of lashes that may be caused by trachoma, lepromatous leprosy, generalized alopecia, psoriasis, myxoedema, burns, radiotherapy, etc.

Poliosis:

Poliosis is premature whitening of eyelashes or eyebrow hair. It may be associated with Waardenburg syndrome, Vogt-Koyanagi-Harada syndrome, or chronic anterior blepharitis.

Hypertrichosis:

Hypertrichosis is an excess number of lashes (polytrichosis) and or abnormally long and luxuriant lashes (trichomegaly). It may be caused by phenytoin, cyclosporine, and latanoprost.

SUMMARY

Entropion and ectropion are commonly encountered lid margin abnormalities. They can be congenital or acquired. The involutional changes occurring in the lower lid can result in either ectropion or entropion depending on the tilt in balance of horizontal and vertical forces supporting the lower lid. The procedures for tightening the lower lid are common to both. In entropion correction, the tightening is aimed at the lower border of tarsus whereas in ectropion correction the upper border is tightened.

In the upper lid, the cicatricial entropion is frequently seen. The treatment depends on the grade of entropion, the thickness of tarsus, presence of lid retraction, and keratinization at lid margin.

Eyelid Retraction

Ruchi Goel, KPS Malik

INTRODUCTION

Upper eyelid retraction is defined as an abnormally high positioned lid in the affected eye in primary gaze.[1,2] This results in exposure keratopathy and aggressive appearance. It can be congenital or acquired.

CONGENITAL EYELID RETRACTION

Unilateral congenital eyelid retraction, cyclical oculomotor paralysis and spasm, congenital hyperthyroidism, Duane's syndrome, and Marcus–Gunn jaw winking are some of the types of congenital eyelid retraction.

Acquired lid retraction[3] can be classified as:

- *Mechanical:*
  - Retraction due to anterior displacement of globe as in severe myopia, buphthalmos, proptosis, cherubism, and craniosynostosis
  - Contact lens irritation/migration.
- *Neurogenic:*
  - Pretectal syndrome that occurs following damage to supranuclear posterior commissure. The bilateral symmetric lid retraction is termed "Collier's sign" or "posterior fossa stare". Due to upward gaze palsy, in an effort to maintain the globe in primary position, excessive innervation flows to superior rectus and also levator muscle. The retraction disappears on down gaze. Posterior commissure may be involved in stroke, tumor, infections, multiple sclerosis, closed head injury, etc.
  - *Seventh nerve paralysis:* Loss of orbicularis tone results in unopposed action of levator and Muller's muscle
  - Aberrant regeneration of cranial nerve III following misdirection of sprouting axons following trauma, aneurysm or tumor
  - Fisher's syndrome where bilateral symmetric upper lid retraction occurs along with bilateral external ophthalmoplegia, ataxia, and areflexia
  - Contralateral ptosis and pseudoretraction due to Hering's law. Visually occluding the nonretracted eye results in return of the retracted eye to its normal position.
- *Cicatricial:*
  - Posttraumatic retraction occurs due to scarring of eyelid structures
  - Postsurgical retraction follows upper eyelid skin excision, levator resection (ptosis overcorrection), and Müllerectomy
  - Postchemical or postthermal burn
- *Dysthyroid:* Eyelid retraction (Dalrymple`s sign) is seen in one-third to–two-thirds patients of Graves' disease. It is characteristically greatest at the outer third of the eyelid (Fig. 1). Factors responsible for dysthyroid eyelid retraction are hyperthyroidism, increased sensitivity of Muller's muscle to adrenergic stimulation, proptosis, secondary levator muscle-superior rectus muscle overactivity to overcome inferior rectus restriction, levator muscle fibrosis, and adnexal fibrosis
- *Hepatic cirrhosis*
- *Drug-induced*: Apraclonidine, prostigmine, and corticosteroids.

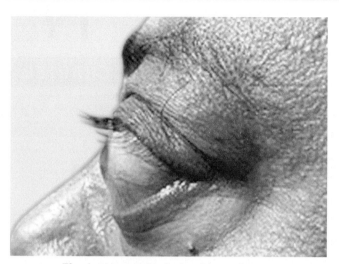

Fig. 1: Lid retraction in thyroid eye disease.

TREATMENT

In neurologic, metabolic, and pseudo eyelid retraction, treatment is directed toward the etiology. In retraction associated with marked synkinesis, levator muscle disinsertion is combined with tarsofrontalis suspension. Retraction associated with facial nerve palsy may be treated by Müller's muscle excision and lateral tarsorrhaphy (in retraction <2 mm); lid loading with gold weight; temporalis muscle transfer; levator recession.

Retraction following cicatricial changes in skin is managed by release of scar followed by Z plasty or skin grafting.

Dysthyroid eyelid retraction: Surgery is performed in the inactive phase of the systemic disease and when the retraction has been stable for months. The choice of surgery depends on the amount of retraction:

- *Less than or equal to 2 mm retraction without marked adhesion of levator muscle to orbital septum:* Müller's muscle excision by posterior approach, levator tenotomy, and small lateral tarsorrhaphy

- *More than 2 mm retraction/retraction with levator-septal adhesions:* Anterior approach levator muscle recession, division of adhesions and Müllerectomy.

Levator lengthening may be performed by placement of a spacer that can be natural (cadaveric sclera) or synthetic between upper border of tarsus and inferior recessed edge of levator muscle.

Full thickness blepharotomy can be used for moderate to severe retraction. A cutaneous lid crease incision is followed by incision of orbicularis muscle, levator muscle, Muller's muscle, and conjunctiva.

Pharmacological modulation:

- Disruption of adrenergic action of norepinephrine on Müller's muscle can be achieved by topical agents like thymoxamine hydrochloride, guanethidine sulfate, and propranolol. Guanethidine eye drops 2% or 5% twice to four times a day is used. Local side effects of guanethidine include miosis, burning sensation, conjunctival hyperemia, and punctal keratitis

- Induction of ptosis by injection of Botulinum toxin type A. It interferes with acetylcholine release from motor end plate terminal. Botulinum toxin type A, 1.2–2.5 units is injected into tissues lying 25 mm posterior to the mid-portion of superior orbital rim and between belly of levator muscle and orbital roof. Demerits are prolonged ptosis, failure to reverse retraction due to tethering of levator to orbital septum, vertical diplopia due to diffusion into superior rectus, and temporary relief.

REFERENCES

1. Cruz AA, Ribeiro SF, Garcia DM, et al. Graves upper eyelid retraction. Surv Ophthalmol. 2013;58(1):63-76.
2. Piggot TA, Niazi ZB, Hodgkinson PD. New technique of levator lengthening for the retracted upper eyelid. Br J Plast Surg. 1995;48(3):127-31.
3. Khan JA, Woog JJ. Upper eye lid malpositions: Retraction, ectropion and entropion. In: Albert DM, Miller JW (Eds). Albert & Jakobiec's Principles and Practice of Ophthalmology. Canada: Elsevier; 2008. pp. 3411-8.

CHAPTER

17

Blepharospasm and Hemifacial Spasm

Neha Rathie, Ruchi Goel

BENIGN ESSENTIAL BLEPHAROSPASM

Benign essential blepharospasm (BEB) is characterized by bilateral involuntary contractions of the orbicularis oculi muscles leading to intermittent or sustained eyelid closure and is classified as a form of focal dystonia. The commonly involved muscles are corrugator superciliaris and procerus. Secondary blepharospasm may occur as a result of ophthalmic conditions such as dry eye, iritis, or some neurologic condition such as stroke.

Epidemiology

Mostly occurs in middle and old age with a peak incidence in the fifth to sixth decade of life. Women are twice as commonly affected than men.

Etiology

The etiology for blepharospasm is poorly understood. It is argued to be a result of an organic neurologic disorder but the exact anatomic lesion remains undetermined. Various neurological conditions found to be associated with blepharospasm include lower pontine mass, thalamic infarct, putaminal hemorrhage, and frontal cortical infarct.

Clinical Presentation

Blepharospasm is seen as periods of increased blinking bilaterally. The increased frequency of spasms (every 20s approximately) results in making the patient functionally blind. There may be inability to open the eyelids between spasms. Stress, fatigue, and bright light may deteriorate the condition. Improvement occurs with rest and sleep.

Patients may have concomitant dry eye or inflammatory conditions such as blepharitits, meibomitits, iritis, corneal ulcer, etc. and hence should be thoroughly looked for in the ocular examination.

Differential Diagnosis

Parkinson's disease, psychic blepharospasm, tardive dyskinesia, habitual spasms, and the use of antipsychotic drugs.

Investigations

Essential blepharospasm is mainly diagnosed clinically. Imaging modalities such as CT scan and MRI may be done if some neurological disease is speculated.

HEMIFACIAL SPASM

Hemifacial spasm is characterized by involuntary intermittent tonic and clonic contractions of the muscles innervated by the facial nerve. It starts with fasciculation of periocular orbicularis oculi and surrounding muscles and spreads to muscles of facial expression including platysma. The patient may present with severe unilateral squint with/out a drawing up of one corner of the mouth, or as disseminated unilateral facial twitching.

Epidemiology

Like blepharospasm, hemifacial spasm also has onset in the fifth to sixth decade of life.

Etiology

The etiology for hemifacial spasms has been mostly attributed to vascular compression of the facial nerve near its origin in the brain stem. It is also seen as sequelae to Bell's palsy, facial nerve injury (e.g. airbag deployment, physical assault, etc.), demyelinated lesions such as multiple sclerosis and also brain vascular insults such as transient ischemic attack and lacunar infarcts.

Clinical Presentation

Hemifacial spasm presents as a unilateral condition that involves the entire face on one side and may continue during sleep. It may be associated with mild facial weakness.

Differential Diagnosis

Myokymia, facial tics, facial dystonia, hemimasticatory spasms, and facial myoclonus.

Myokymia is a continuous unilateral localized fasciculation within the orbicularis that occurs in normal individuals and is initiated by stress and fatigue. It is usually transient and nonprogressive.

Facial tics are habitual and usually benign. These occur mostly in childhood and can be suppressed voluntarily.

Investigations

Magnetic resonance imaging should be performed in patients where there is irritation of facial nerve to rule out posterior fossa lesions that need surgical treatment.

Magnetic resonance arteriography can be done to rule out vascular compression of the facial nerve.

TREATMENT

Medical treatment, botulinum toxin type A injections, and surgical interventions are the treatment options for hemifacial spasm and blepharospasm.

Medical Treatment

In cases of hemifacial spasms with vascular compression, microvascular decompression of the facial nerve (Janetta procedure) can be performed. Severe complications such as hearing loss, otitis media, permanent facial palsy, epilepsy, and even death can occur following this procedure. A wide variety of medications has been used to treat blepharospasm, including muscle relaxants (baclofen, benzodiazepines), analgesics, antihistamines, antidepressants (tricyclics, monamine oxidase inhibitors), anticholinergics (orphenadrine, trihexyphenidyl),

antiepileptics (phenytoin, carbamazepine), lithium, antiparkinsonian agents (amantadine, carbidopa, levodopa), and serotonin antagonists (cyproheptadine).

Botulinum Toxin

Because of unsatisfactory effects of medical treatment options and risk of serious complications of surgical interventions, botulinum toxin type A injections have become the therapy of choice for both disorders. It interferes with acetylcholine release at the presynaptic nerve terminal and causes a temporary muscle paralysis and denervation atrophy that abolishes abnormal movements. It is a simple procedure with a success rate of more than 90%.

Reconstitution of Botulinum toxin type A injection: Botulinum toxin is available as single use 50/100 units/200 units per vial. Sterile, nonpreserved 0.9/sodium chloride injection is added to obtain 5 units/0.1 mL (2 mL sodium chloride added to 100 unit vial). Not more than 5U are injected per site.

Injection Technique

Step 1—After examination the sites of spasm are carefully recorded.

Step 2—The toxin is injected in the preselected sites in the periocular region using a 30-gauge needle. Injections are given first in the orbicularis oculi muscle, the procerus and corrugator muscles, and the frontalis muscle (Fig. 1). The injections in the orbicularis muscle are superficial and those in the procerus and corrugator superciliaris are deeper. Injections are avoided in the medial aspect of lower lid to avoid tearing from lacrimal pump dysfunction and in the central upper lid to avoid postinjection ptosis. Additional

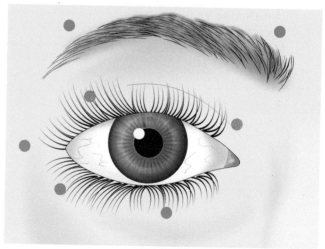

Fig. 1: Sites of injection of botulinum toxin type A in treatment of blepharospasm.

sites in cases of hemifacial spasms are the nasal fold, upper lip, chin, and other musculature of face except the retractor muscle (prevention of drooping of mouth).

Doses

Sensitivity to botulinum toxin varies among patients so the doses of injections can be modified according to the patient's response starting with the least dose.

In hemifacial spasm, 25–30 U are required on each side of face whereas higher doses are required in blepharospasm cases.

Duration of Action

Paralysis of injected muscles starts in 24 hours and lasts approximately 3–4 months. The average duration between injections is approximately 4 months as new nerve terminals and new synapses peak during 5th–10th week.

Complications

Local side effects—usually occur as a result of paralysis of periocular musculature.

- Ptosis:
  - Usually mild
  - Occurs in less than 10% of patients
  - Transient
  - Can be avoided by giving superficial injections and avoiding injections in the central part of the upper lid.
- Lagophthalmos:
  - Due to orbicularis paralysis
  - Can lead to dry eye
  - Artificial tears are given prophylactically in the postinjection period.
- Ectropion:
  - Usually mild
  - Occurs due to orbicularis paralysis
  - May lead to epiphora.

- Pain
- Hematoma
- Drooping of angle of mouth—can be prevented by avoiding injections in the retractor muscles in the corner of the mouth.

Systemic side effects: No major systemic side effects have been reported although some abnormalities of neuromuscular transmission may occur at remote sites as muscle weakness.

Development of an antitoxin may result in decreased effectivity over the time requiring larger doses up to 70 U.

Surgical Management

- Orbital myectomy—usually reserved for:
  - Cases in which botulinum toxin is ineffective
  - Injections are required too frequently
  - As a part of another procedure, e.g. blepharoptosis repair
  - Involves complete removal of orbicularis oculi, corrugator superciliaris, and procerus muscles.
- Facial nerve avulsion—no longer recommended due to high rate of complications.

SUMMARY

To conclude, benign essential blepharospasm and hemifacial spasm are facial dystonias characterized by involuntary contraction of facial muscles. BEB is a bilateral condition whereas hemifacial spasm is usually unilateral. In hemifacial spasm, unlike BEB, the spasms are present during sleep. BEB is essentially a clinical diagnosis. MRI is required to look for ectatic vessel or cerebellopontine angle lesions. Medical treatment, botulinum toxin type A injections, and surgical interventions include surgical myectomy (for BEB) and neurosurgical decompression of facial nerve.

18

CHAPTER

Congenital Abnormalities of the Eyelid

Samreen Khanam, Ruchi Goel

INTRODUCTION

Congenital abnormalities of the eyelid have a wide spectrum of clinical presentation and are often associated with systemic problems. In many patients, it is pertinent to institute ocular protective methods before definitive evaluation and management. A thorough examination by the pediatrician for systemic abnormalities is also mandatory. The congenital abnormalities of the eyelid can be broadly classified as:

- Malformations of the eyelid
- Abnormalities of the margin and position of eyelids
- Abnormalities of the palpebral fissures
- Abnormalities of the distance between the eyelids.

MALFORMATIONS OF THE EYELID

Ablepharon and Microblepharon

Ablepharon is characterized by a complete congenital absence of the eyelids. It is a rare abnormality and is associated with syndromes such as ablepharon-macrostomia syndrome. In microblepharon, there is abnormal shortening of the lids in vertical direction. Failure of lid fold development and neural crest cell migration are the pathogenic mechanisms proposed.

Preservation of the ocular surface is important and reconstruction of the lids can be attempted in suitable cases.

Cryptophthalmos

There is failure of development of the palpebral aperture. In complete forms, the skin continues from the forehead to the cheeks. In incomplete forms, a rudimentary lid and conjunctival sac may be seen (Fig. 1). This condition has

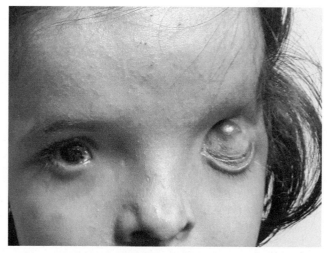

Fig. 1: Incomplete cryptophthalmos left eye.

been frequently found to be associated with an autosomal recessive disorder called Fraser's syndrome. Some investigators have found that Vitamin A deficiency during gestation has a role in its pathogenesis.[1,2]

The underlying globe is usually microphthalmic with varying degrees of anterior segment abnormalities. Treatment is difficult and usually unsuccessful.

Coloboma of the Eyelids

These are partial or full thickness defects in the eyelids, usually triangular in shape with base at the lid margin. Upper lid coloboma is usually seen at the junction of the medial and the middle one third of the eyelid (Fig. 2). It may be associated with Goldenhar Syndrome.

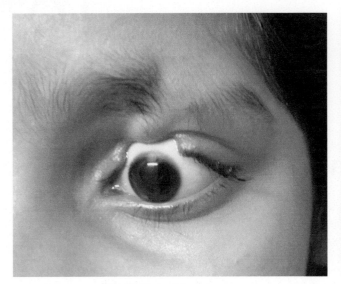

Fig. 2: Upper lid coloboma.

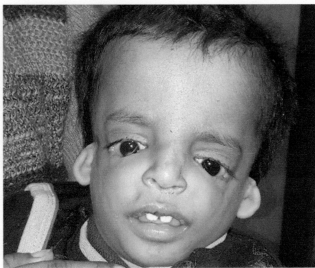

Fig. 3: Treacher Collins syndrome with bilateral slanting palpebral fissures laterally, lower lid coloboma, small malformed pinnae and dental anomalies.

Goldenhar syndrome (oculo-auriculo-vertebral dysplasia or hemifacial microsomia) comprises clinical manifestations that may include craniofacial, vertebral, cardiac, renal, and central nervous system anomalies. There are developmental defects of the first and second branchial arch. The classical features are ocular anomalies, including microphthalmia, anophthalmia, epibulbar dermoid (or lipodermoid) tumors, and eyelid colobomas; aural defects, such as preauricular tags, anotia, microtia and hearing loss; and vertebral abnormalities, such as scoliosis, hemivertebrae, cervical fusion, and mandibular hypoplasia. There is marked asymmetry due to unilateral facial involvement.

Lower lid colobomas usually occur at the junction of the middle and the lateral third of the lid. They are often associated with Treacher Collins syndrome (Fig. 3).

(Treacher Collins syndrome or mandibulofacial dysostosis: Symmetrical and bilateral diminution of craniofacial structures derived from the first and second pharyngeal arch. The palpebral fissures are short and slope laterally downward. The lower lid is colobomatous with deficient eyelashes medially. The lateral margins of the orbits may be defective, and the orbits are hyperteloric. The pinnae may be malformed, crumpled forward, or misplaced. Intelligence is usually normal. Difficulties in swallowing and feeding occur due to musculoskeletal underdevelopment and a cleft palate. Conductive hearing loss and impaired vision may occur as a consequence to underdeveloped lateral orbit and extraocular muscles.)

Lid colobomas may be associated with retinal colobomas. Amniotic bands may also mechanically lead to lid colobomas. Surgical reconstruction is necessary in most cases and is determined by the size and location of the defect, and the presence of trichiasis.[3]

ABNORMALITIES OF THE MARGIN AND POSITION OF THE EYELID

Ankyloblepharon

It is characterized by partial or complete adhesions between the margins of the superior and the inferior eyelids. It can be seen in association with clefting abnormalities of the lips or as an isolated finding. In external ankyloblepharon, the lids are fused at the lateral canthus; while in internal ankyloblepharon, they are fused at the inner canthus. Ankyloblepharon filiforme adnatum is characterized by strands of tissue that connect the upper and the lower lid margins.[4]

Epiblepharon

It is a redundant fold of eyelid skin most commonly present on the lower lid of infants.[5] It occurs due to failure of extension of lower lid retractor to the orbicularis and subcutaneous tissue and excess of skin and orbicularis muscle. It accentuates in downgaze, a feature that distinguishes it from congenital entropion.

Epiblepharon usually resolves spontaneously as the child grows older, but can sometimes cause the lashes to turn inward and rub against the cornea. It is more common in Asians. Some patients may need suture correction.

Congenital Entropion

This is much less common than epiblepharon and involves inturning of the lid margin. It has been attributed to disinsertion of lower lid retractors and overaction of marginal orbicularis muscle (Fig. 4).

If the corneal epithelium is compromised, early intervention is recommended. Surgical options include transverse blepharotomy, everting sutures or a Hotz type procedure involving excision of ellipse of skin and orbicularis.

Epicanthal Folds

These are folds of skin that are present in the medial canthal area. Four different types have been described (Fig. 4):
1. *Epicanthus superciliaris:* The fold of skin extends from above the brow to the lateral aspect of nose.
2. *Epicanthus tarsalis:* The skin fold extends from the lateral side of the upper lid to the medial canthus.
3. *Epicanthus palpebralis:* There is a fold of skin at the medial canthus that is symmetrically distributed between the upper and the lower lid (Fig. 5).
4. *Epicanthus inversus:* The fold of skin originates in the lower and extends upward up to the medial canthus.

Epicanthal folds are common in people with Asian ancestry and Down's syndrome. Most cases do not require any surgical correction. The surgical procedures employed include Mustarde's double Z plasty, Spaeth's Z plasty, and Y-V plasty.

Congenital Ectropion

Congenital ectropion is a rare condition. Severe congenital ectropion can be seen in cases with icthyosis. Lower lid ectropion may be present in patients with blepharophimosis syndrome.

Congenital Ptosis

This is a relatively common condition. The typical forms are clinically characterized by poor levator function, absent or faint lid crease and lid lag in downgaze (Fig. 6). The underlying pathology is a maldeveloped and fibrotic levator muscle. There is a high prevalence of strabismus, refractive error, and amblyopia in these patients. Congenital

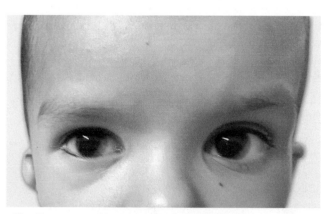

Fig. 5: Right lower lid congenital entropion and left epicanthus palpebralis.

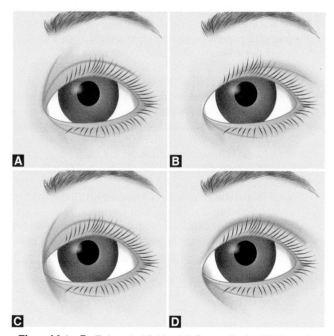

Figs. 4A to D: Epicanthal folds. (A) Superciliaris; (B) Tarsalis; (C) Palpebralis; (D) Inversus.

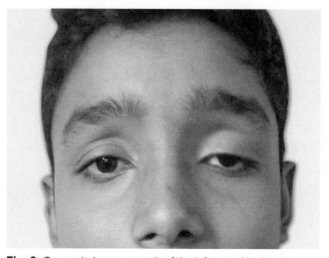

Fig. 6: Congenital severe ptosis of the left eye with absent upper lid crease.

ptosis can be corrected using the frontalis sling procedure with fascia lata or synthetic material like silicon or levator resection depending on the amount of levator action.

Congenital Horner's syndrome and congenital 3rd nerve may also present with congenital ptosis.

ABNORMALITIES OF THE PALPEBRAL FISSURES

Euryblepharon

There is enlargement of the palpebral aperture with outward and downward displacement of the lateral canthus. It may be seen as an autosomal dominant trait, in association with other craniofacial abnormalities or as an isolated finding.[6]

Blepharophimosis Syndrome

It is a clinical spectrum comprising blepharophimosis, ptosis, epicanthus inversus, and telecanthus (BPES) (Fig. 7). It may be an inherited trait or be present as an isolated finding. BPES has been discussed in detail in another chapter of this book.

Abnormal Orientation of Palpebral Fissure

Up-slanting of palpebral fissure is seen in Down's syndrome. Down-slanting of the fissure is also seen.

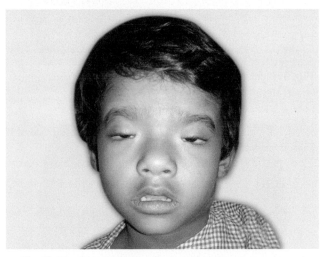

Fig. 7: Blepharophimosis, ptosis, epicanthus inversus, and telecanthus syndrome.

ABNORMALITIES OF THE DISTANCE BETWEEN THE EYELIDS AND ORBIT[7]

Hypertelorism

Increased inner canthal distance (ICD) and outer canthal distance (OCD).

Hypotelorism

Decreased ICD and OCD. Decreased distance between the medial walls of the orbits. Usually associated with craniofacial and skull abnormalities such as craniosynostosis and holoprosencephaly.

Telecanthus

The distance between the inner canthi (ICD) of the two eyes is increased. It can be:

- *Primary telecanthus:* The ICD is increased but the OCD and the interpupillary distance (IPD) are normal.
- *Secondary telecanthus:* Increased IPD along with hypertelorism.

Dystopia Canthorum

Increased ICD and lateral displacement of the lacrimal puncta. It is a specific feature of type1 Waardenburg syndrome.

REFERENCES

1. Brodsky I, Waddy G. Cryptophthalmos of ablepharia: A survey of the condition with a review of the literature and the presentation of a case. Med J Aust. 1949;1:894.
2. Levine RS, Powers T, Rosenberg HK, et al. The cryptophthalmos syndrome. AJR Am J Roentgenol. 1984;143(2):375-6.
3. Casey TA. Congenital colobomata of the eyelids. Trans Ophthalmol Soc UK. 1976;96(1):65-8.
4. Vastine DW, Stamper RL. Ankyloblepharon. In: Fraunfelder FT, Roy FH (Eds). Current Ocular Therapy, 3rd edition. Philadelphia: WB Saunders; 1989. pp. 1-835.
5. Johnson CC. Epicanthus and epiblepharon. Arch Ophthalmol. 1978;96(6):1030-3.
6. Keipert JA. Euryblepharon. Br J Ophthalmol. 1975;59(1):57-8.
7. Dolfus H, Verloes A. Developmental abnormaities of the lids. In: Taylor D, Hoyt GS (Eds). Pediatric Ophthlmology and Strabismus, 3rd edition. Edinburgh: Elsevier Saunders; 2005.

Inflammatory Disorders of the Eyelid

Samreen Khanam, Ruchi Goel

INTRODUCTION

Blepharitis is an inflammation of the eyelids. It is a common clinical condition seen in ophthalmic practice, and is frequently associated with dry eye and acne rosacea. It is anatomically divided into anterior blepharitis, which involves the lid margin and the lashes, and posterior blepharitis which involves the meibomian glands. However, these can be present as overlapping diseases (Flowchart 1). The presentation may be acute or chronic.

Features suggestive of chronic blepharitis are (Fig. 1):
- Presence of eyelid margin thickening
- Telangiectasia (prominent blood vessels on the eyelids) and posteriorly located meibomian glands
- Atrophy of the meibomian glands
- Location of the debris indicates disease duration in cases of anterior blepharitis. It takes approximately 12 weeks for lashes to grow. So, if the debris is located at the tip of the lashes as well as at the base, it indicates chronic anterior blepharitis. Presence of debris or collarettes only at the base, suggests acute blepharitis.

ANTERIOR BLEPHARITIS

It may be staphylococcal or seborrheic.
- *Staphylococcal blepharitis:* It is caused by abnormal cell-mediated immune response to the components of the cell wall of *Staphylococcus aureus* and is more common in patients with atopic dermatitis. Clinical features:
    - Hard scales and crusting are present at bases of the lashes.
    - Mild papillary conjunctivitis is common.
    - Scarring, notching, and trichiasis in long-standing cases.
- *Seborrheic blepharitis:* It has a strong association with generalized seborrheic dermatitis.
    - Soft gray white scales on the eyelids and lashes.

Flowchart 1: Classification of blepharitis.

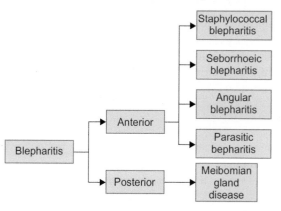

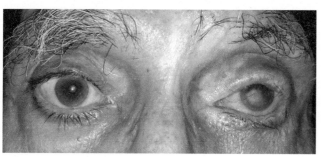

Fig. 1: Left upper lid chronic blepharitis showing rounding of posterior lid margin, loss of meibomian gland orifices, and telangiectasia.

Management

Warm compresses, lid cleaning, and scrubbing with a cotton bud dipped in dilute solution of baby shampoo or sodium bicarbonate (3%). Topical erythromycin/bacitracin and oral doxycycline are given in resistant cases. Low potency steroids are indicated for papillary conjunctivitis.

POSTERIOR BLEPHARITIS/MEIBOMITIS

It is a chronic inflammation of the meibomian glands. Alterations in the properties of meibomian gland secretions prevent expression of the meibum. Clinically, there is:
- Enlargement, irregularity, inspissation, and plugging of the gland orifices (Fig. 2)
- Keratinization of the meibomian gland duct. Thick, cheesy, toothpaste-like secretions on attempted gland expression
- Dry eye, tear film instability.

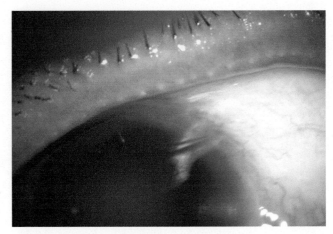

Fig. 2: Enlargement, irregularity, inspissation, and plugging of the gland orifices.

Management

Lid scrubs, lid massage, warm compresses, and topical antibiotics such as bacitracin or erythromycin. Oral doxycycline 100 mg BD for 1 week and then daily for 6–24 weeks is recommended in resistant cases. Newer options include intraductal meibomian gland probing, oral omega 3 fatty acids, and Lipiflow™. Lipiflow™ is a new instrument designed to heat the obstructed glands and create compression aimed at "milking" the meibomian glands during a 12-minute, in-office treatment (Fig. 3). Smoking cessation is essential. Tear substitutes are helpful for dry eye management.

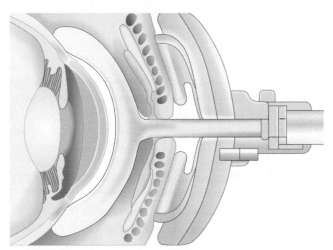

Fig. 3: Lipiflow™ works on the principle of vectored thermal pulsation technology.

PARASITIC BLEPHARITIS

Demodicosis is an infestation of the eyelash follicles by the mite *Demodex folliculorum*. Patients present with itching, pain, and burning of the eyelids. There is semi-transparent tube like crusting of the skin around the lashes. Management is with lid scrubs and topical bacitracin / erythromycin ointment.

Phthiriasis is caused by infestation by *Pthirus pubis*, a parasite of the hair of the genital region. Symptoms consist of itching and burning, and pearly white nits attached to the lashes can be seen on slit lamp examination.

Management

- Mechanical removal of nits, although tedious maybe attempted
- Local application of 1% yellow mercuric oxide ointment four times a day for 14 days
- Delousing of clothing, bedding, and personal items
- Permethrin 1%/Lindane shampoo for other affected parts of the body.

ANGULAR BLEPHARITIS

It is clinically characterized by scaling, erythema, fissuring, and maceration at the lateral and/or medial canthus. There may be associated papillary conjunctivitis and mucopurulent discharge. *Causative organisms: Moraxella lacunata* (most common) and *Staphylococcus aureus*.

Management

Lid scrubs, massage, warm compresses, topical bacitracin/erythromycin. Oral doxycycline/erythromycin for resistant cases.

HORDEOLUM EXTERNUM (STYE)

It is an acute staphylococcal infection of the eyelash follicle and the glands of Zeis located at the base of the lashes (Fig. 4). It is more common in children and young adults. Clinically, there is a tender swelling of the lid margin with abscess formation. Multiple lesions may be present simultaneously involving the entire lid margin.

Management

Warm compresses, topical/oral antibiotics, and epilation of the lash involved.

CHALAZION/MEIBOMIAN CYST

It is a chronic sterile lipogranulomatous inflammation of the meibomian glands (Fig. 5). Patient presents with a gradually enlarging painless nodule on the eyelid. Secondary

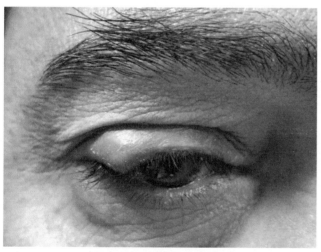

Fig. 4: Hordeolum externum.

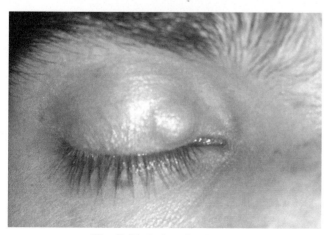

Fig. 5: Chalazion of upper lid.

infections may occur resulting in acute presentation (Hordeolum internum).

Pathology

Obstruction of the ducts of the meibomian glands results in retained sebaceous secretions. Histology shows features of chronic granulomatous inflammation with multinucleated giant cells and epithelioid cells. A chalazion at the lid margin may occur due to isolated involvement of the gland of Zeis. There may be an associated granuloma of the conjunctiva. Risk factors include co-existing blepharitis and uncorrected refractive error.

Management

- Small, asymptomatic chalazia resolve spontaneously and maybe left untreated. Conservative management with lid massage, warm compresses, expression of the contents, and topical steroids is beneficial in some patients
- Intralesional steroids lead to resolution in most cases. A dose of 0.1–0.2 mL of triamcinolone acetonide with lignocaine is injected into the lesion. A repeat injection can be given after 1–2 weeks. Injection from conjunctival approach is preferable to avoid local skin depigmentation and fat atrophy
- Incision and curettage from the conjunctival side using a chalazion clamp. Vertical incision is given through the tarsal plate, avoiding damage to the adjoining glands. Skin incision, when given, should be horizontal for better cosmesis. Suture should not be used to close the wound.

Systemic tetracycline has been advocated for the prophylaxis of recurrent chalazia in patients with acne rosacea.

Sebaceous cell carcinoma is notorious for masquerading as recurrent chalazia. Therefore, biopsy is advisable in such cases to rule out malignancy. Involvement of lid margin causing loss of eyelid architecture with eyelashes is suggestive of malignancy.

IMPETIGO

It is a skin infection that typically affects children and may involve eyelids along with the face. The infection is highly contagious and is caused by *Staphylococcus aureus* or *Streptococcus pyogenes*. Clinically, there are thin-walled blisters with golden yellow crusting on rupture. Fever, malaise, and lymphadenopathy are also seen. Topical and oral antibiotics are curative.

HERPES SIMPLEX

Eyelid lesions in herpes simplex consist of single or multiple pinhead-sized vesicles containing a clear or seropurulent fluid. Rupture of the vesicles leads to crusting and subsequent healing without scarring. Papillary conjunctivitis and keratitis may accompany the lid lesion. Diagnosis is made clinically and topical antivirals are curative.

Recurrence occurs due to reactivation of the virus lying latent in the ganglionic cells of sensory nerves. Oral acyclovir prophylaxis may be needed in such cases.

HERPES ZOSTER

The lesions in herpes zoster ophthalmicus may occur due to reactivation of the latent varicella zoster virus in the ophthalmic division of the 5th cranial nerve. Clinically, there are erythematous maculopapular eruptions, which form vesicles, ulcerate, and crusts. Cicatrization can lead to lid margin abnormalities like entropion, ectropion, trichiasis, canalicular, and punctal stenosis. Involvement of the tip of the nose (Hutchinson's sign) is associated with a higher incidence of ocular involvement.

Management

- Oral acyclovir 800 mg five times a day or valacyclovir 1 g TDS
- Topical/systemic antibiotics are given to decrease secondary bacterial infection
- Cool saline or aluminum sulfate and calcium acetate compresses can be given for local comfort.

MOLLUSCUM CONTAGIOSUM

Molluscum contagiosum is a ds-DNA poxvirus causing multiple waxy round umbilicated papules on the eyelids. It is more common in young children and young adults, and is transmitted by direct contact or fomites. Extensive lesions can be seen in immunocompromised patients.

Secondary chronic follicular conjunctivitis can occur due to shedding of the virus into the tear film.

Management

Spontaneous resolution occurs in many cases in a few months. Treatment options include shaving, cauterization, cryotherapy, and curettage. Topical and intravenous cidofovir may be needed in recalcitrant and disseminated cases.

Facial Nerve Palsy

Taru Dewan, Kanika Jain

UNDERSTANDING THE PROBLEM

Anatomy and Functions of Facial Nerve

- Facial nerve is a mixed nerve having motor and sensory root (nerve of Wrisberg). Motor nucleus of facial nerve is situated in the pons. Upper part of the nucleus which innervates forehead muscles receives fibers from both the cerebral hemispheres. Lower part of nucleus which supplies lower face gets only crossed fibers from one hemisphere. Thus the upper motor neuron palsy or cervical facial palsy is characterized by palsy/paresis of lower half contralateral side of the face. In lower motor neuron palsy, both upper and lower halves of one side are involved (Fig. 1)
- Function of forehead is preserved in supranuclear lesions because of bilateral innervation

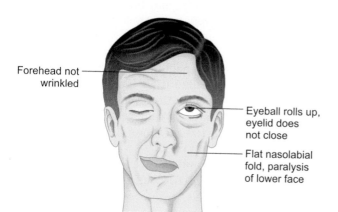

Forehead not wrinkled

Eyeball rolls up, eyelid does not close

Flat nasolabial fold, paralysis of lower face

Fig. 1: Left lower motor neuron facial palsy.

- Facial nucleus also receives fibers from thalamus and provides involuntary control to facial muscles. The emotional movements—smiling and crying are thus preserved in supranuclear palsies
- Facial nerve leaves the brainstem at pontomedullary junction, travels through posterior fossa, and enters internal acoustic meatus. At the fundus of meatus, the nerve enters bony facial canal, traverses the temporal bone, and comes out of the stylomastoid foramen and divides into terminal branches.

Branches of Facial Nerve

- Greater superficial temporal nerve—arises from geniculate ganglion and carries secretomotor fibers to lacrimal gland and those of the nasal mucosa
- Nerve to stapedius muscle—arises at the level of second genu
- Chorda tympani—it carries secretomotor fibers to submandibular and sublingual glands and carries taste sensation from anterior two-thirds of tongue
- Posterior auricular nerve—supplies muscles of pinna and communicates with auricular branch of vagus
- Muscular branches to stylohyoid and posterior belly of digastric
- Peripheral branches (supply all muscles of facial expression)—temporal, zygomatic, buccal, mandibular, and cervical branches.

What is Facial Palsy

It is the paralysis of the structures innervated by the facial nerve. There can be multiple etiologies due to a relatively long and convoluted course of facial nerve (Table 1). The most common is Bell's palsy, a disease of unknown etiology that is diagnosed by exclusion.

Bell's Palsy

It is a sudden onset, unilateral facial nerve paralysis which is considered idiopathic in nature. A viral etiology (Herpes simplex, Herpes zoster, Varicella zoster virus) has been suspected as a precursor inciting factor.[1,2]

Ramsay Hunt Syndrome

This is syndromic occurrence of facial paralysis, herpetiform vesicular eruptions, and vestibulocochlear dysfunction. These patients have a greater risk of hearing loss than those with Bell's palsy and the course of disease is more painful with a lower recovery rate.

Lyme disease—In this disease, 10% develop facial paralysis, of which 25% present with bilateral palsy.

Disability Correlates with the Loss of Function

- Inability to close the affected eye can lead to lagophthalmos, dry eye, and exposure keratitis
- Excessive lacrimation due to pooling of tears in the eye due to lacrimal pump dysfunction
- Hyperacusis and pain in the ear
- Loss of taste sensation
- Loss of facial expressions
- Dribbling of saliva, water, and food from the angle of mouth
- Synkinesis—crocodile tears (gustatory lacrimation—Bogorad's syndrome), Frey's syndrome (gustatory sweating) may develop later in some cases
- Impairment of speech.

TABLE 1: Etiology of facial palsy.

Etiology:
• Idiopathic (Bell's palsy)
• Trauma
• Infectious
• Metabolic
• Pregnancy
• Neoplastic
• Toxic
• Iatrogenic
• Dystrophia myotonica
• Mobius syndrome
• Melkersson–Rosenthal syndrome
• Hereditary hypertrophic neuropathy

WHEN TO INTERVENE?

Management options of facial nerve palsy can be categorized into:
- Immediate—find the cause and institute therapy to aid recovery
- Short-term—prevent disability while awaiting recovery
- Long-term—rehabilitation of residual disability.

HOW TO INTERVENE?

At each stage the approach towards management may be:
- Pharmacological
- Surgical
- Non pharmacologic measures—physical therapy.

The options can be employed individually or in combination depending upon the duration of palsy, severity of signs (lagophthalmos and corneal exposure), and patient factors.

Pharmacological Management

- The most widely accepted treatment for Bell's palsy is corticosteroid therapy. According to the American Academy of Neurology (AAN) 2012 guidelines, steroids are likely to be effective and increase the likelihood of recovery of facial nerve function in new onset Bell's palsy.[1,2] These guidelines are supported by those from the American Academy of Otolaryngology—Head and Neck Surgery Foundation (AAO—HNSF), 2013. The guidelines recommend use of corticosteroids within 72 hours from onset of symptoms. The dose of prednisolone for the treatment of Bell's palsy is 1 mg/kg or 60 mg/day for 6 days, followed by a taper, for a total of 10 days. Caution should be exercised in patients with tuberculosis, immunocompromised state, pregnancy, active infection, sepsis, peptic ulcer disease, diabetes, and renal or hepatic dysfunction. Antiviral agents (acyclovir, valacyclovir) may be considered if a viral etiology is suspected, but only in combination with steroids[3]
- Evaluation of the use of antiviral drugs in Bell's palsy has shown limited benefit of these drugs,[4,5] with three randomized controlled trials having demonstrated no benefit from them.[6-8] However, given the evidence suggesting that a large percentage of Bell's palsy cases may result from a viral infection—herpes simplex virus (most common viral etiology), varicella zoster virus (VZV),[9,10] the use of antiviral agents may be reasonable in certain situations. According to AAN 2012 guidelines, benefit from antivirals has not been established and, at best, is likely to be modest.[1,2] Acyclovir is administered at a dosage of 400 mg orally five times daily for 10 days. If

VZV is suspected, higher doses may be needed—800 mg orally five times daily. Valacyclovir, though expensive, has better compliance due to twice a day dosing. Dose of valacyclovir is 500 mg twice a day for 5 days. If VZV is suspected, higher doses of 1 gram three times a day can be used. If antiviral agents are used, they should be initiated in conjunction with steroids. Further studies will be needed to determine which population will most benefit from antiviral therapy

- Management of dry eye with topical ocular lubrication (with artificial tears during day and lubricating ointment at night) to prevent and treat complications of corneal exposure. Punctal plugs, temporary or permanent may be helpful if dryness of cornea is a persistent problem. Occlusion of eyelids is by using tape or by applying a patch for 1–2 days to heal corneal abrasion. Topical antibiotics can be used to prevent or treat corneal ulceration.

Surgical Management of Facial Nerve Palsy

The surgical options for the management of facial nerve palsy may be instituted at different stages. Some may be done early to prevent complications while awaiting recovery, or may be more curative designed to improve functioning, or some done later still to address cosmesis and function once the condition has stabilized.

- Botulinum toxin injections
- Facial nerve decompression
- Subocularis oculi fat (SOOF) lift
- Implantable devices—gold weights—placed into eyelids
- Tarsorrhaphy—temporary/permanent
- Transposition of the temporalis muscle
- Facial nerve grafting
- Direct brow lift
- End to end anastomosis of the severed ends of facial nerve.

Surgical repair is done by using a single or combination of procedures as mentioned above.

Botulinum Toxin Injections

Botulinum toxin can be injected transcutaneously or subconjunctivally at the upper border of the tarsus and aimed at the levator muscle to produce complete ptosis to protect cornea from exposure.[11]

Facial nerve Decompression

Performing facial nerve decompression surgery is controversial. It may be considered in patients with complete Bell's palsy that has not responded to medical therapy and with greater than 90% axonal degeneration

as shown on facial nerve EMG within 3 weeks of the onset of the paralysis.[12,13] The site of lesion/pathology must be localized on MRI on the basis of which the segment of facial nerve and the route of decompression is decided. Maxillary segment is decompressed externally and labyrinthine segment, geniculate ganglion is decompressed with a middle cranial fossa craniotomy. Best surgical results are obtained when the procedure is done within 14 days after onset of paralysis.

Subocularis Oculi Fat Lift

The SOOF is deep to the orbicularis oculi muscle and superficial to the periosteum below the inferior orbital rim. SOOF lift is designed to lift and suspend the midfacial musculature. This procedure may also elevate the upper lid and angle of mouth to improve facial symmetry. It is commonly performed in conjunction with a lateral tarsal strip procedure (lateral canthotomy and cantholysis are performed followed by removal of anterior lamella and lateral tarsal strip is shortened and then attached to periosteum at lateral orbital rim) to correct horizontal lower lid laxity.

Implantable Devices

Implantable devices in upper lid are implanted to restore the dynamic lid closure in cases with severe, symptomatic lagophthalmos associated with poor Bell phenomenon, and decreased corneal sensation. The weights allow upper eyelid to close with gravity when the levator palpebrae are relaxed. Gold or platinum weights, a weight adjustable magnet or palpebral springs can be inserted into eyelids. Pretarsal gold weight implantation is most commonly performed. Implants are inert and composed of 99.99% pure gold or platinum. Sizes range from 0.6 mg to 1.8 mg. Complications include migration or extrusion of implant, inflammation, allergic reaction, and decreased effect of weights after some time.

Tarsorrhaphy

Tarsorrhaphy decreases horizontal lid opening by fusing the eyelid margins together, increasing precorneal lake of tears, and improving coverage of eye during sleep. Permanent tarsorrhaphy is performed if nerve recovery is not expected. It may be performed laterally, centrally, or medially. The lateral procedure is the most commonly performed, however, it can restrict the monocular temporal field of vision. Central tarsorrhaphy offers good corneal coverage but precludes vision and is cosmetically unacceptable. Medial or paracentral procedure, performed lateral to lacrimal puncta, offers good lid closure without affecting the visual field and is cosmetically acceptable.

Transposition of the Temporalis Muscle

Transposition of temporalis muscle is done to provide lid closure by using fifth cranial nerve. Strips from muscle and fascia are placed in upper and lower lids as an encircling sling. Patients can initiate eyelid closure by chewing or clenching their teeth.

Facial Nerve Grafting

Facial nerve anastomosis can be used in cases with permanent facial nerve paralysis to help restore relatively normal function of orbicularis oculi muscle to help in the closure of eyelids. Nerve graft can be taken from greater auricular, lateral cutaneous nerve of thigh, or sural nerve.

Brow Lift

Brow ptosis can be improved with direct brow lift. It should not be performed in cases with corneal decompensation or poor Bell's phenomenon.

Nonpharmacologic Measures—Physical Therapy

Physical therapy in the form of facial exercises,[14] neuromuscular retraining,[15] and acupuncture[16] results in faster recovery and reduced sequelae with no adverse effects.

Follow-Up of Patient

The patient should be followed up regularly for improvement, deterioration, or any response to treatment every 2–3 weeks. If the paralysis is not resolving or is progressive in nature, a thorough neurological and ENT workup is required.

SUMMARY

- Facial palsy can have multiple etiologies.
- Immediate measures include use of steroids, antivirals, and lubricants along with neurology and otolaryngologist consultation after required imaging and investigations. Facial decompression is performed in appropriate cases.
- Short-term measures are tarsorrhaphy and lubricants for eye along with physiotherapy while awaiting recovery.
- Long-term measures are surgical interventions to improve cosmesis and function once the spontaneous recovery ceases.
- Facial retraining forms an important part of treatment.

Exposure keratopathy and dry eye are major concerns to the ophthalmologist while cosmetic disfigurement bothers the patient. Both are important issues to be addressed.

REFERENCES

1. Anderson P. (2012). New AAN Guideline on Bell's Palsy. Medscape Medical News. [online] Available from: https://www.medscape.com/viewarticle/774056. [Last Accessed January 2018].
2. Gronseth GS, Paduga R; American Academy of Neurology. Evidence-based guideline update: Steroids and antivirals for Bell palsy: Report of the Guideline Development Subcommittee of the American Academy of Neurology. Neurology. 2012;79(22):2209-13.
3. Baugh RF, Basura GJ, Ishii LE, et al. Clinical practice guideline: Bell's palsy. Otolaryngol Head Neck Surg. 2013;149(Suppl 3):S1-27.
4. Murphy TP. MRI of facial nerve during paralysis. Otolaryngol Head Neck Surg. 1991;104(1):47-51.
5. Allen D, Dunn L. Acyclovir or valacyclovir for Bell's palsy (idiopathic facial paralysis). Cochrane Database Syst Rev. 2004;(3):CD001869.
6. Sullivan FM, Swan IR, Donnan PT, et al. Early treatment with prednisolone or acyclovir in Bell's palsy. N Engl J Med. 2007;357(16):1598-607.
7. Engström M, Berg T, Stjernquist-Desatnik A, et al. Prednisolone and valacyclovir in Bell's palsy: A randomized, double-blind, placebo-controlled, multicenter trial. Lancet Neurol. 2008;7(11):993-1000.
8. Sullivan FM, Swan IR, Donnan PT, et al. A randomized controlled trial of the use of acyclovir and/or prednisolone for the early treatment of Bell's palsy: The BELLS study. Health Technol Assess. 2009;13(47):iii-iv,ix-xi,1-130.
9. Holland NJ, Weiner GM. Recent developments in Bell's palsy. BMJ. 2004;329(7465):553-7.
10. Hato N, Yamada H, Kohno H, et al. Valacyclovir and prednisolone treatment for Bell's palsy: A multicenter, randomized, placebo-controlled study. Otol Neurotol. 2007;28(3):408-13.
11. Seiff SR, Chang J. Management of ophthalmic complications of facial nerve palsy. Otolaryngol Clin North Am. 1992;25(3):669-90.
12. Julian GG, Hoffmann JF, Shelton C. Surgical rehabilitation of facial nerve paralysis. Otolaryngol Clin North Am. 1997;30(5):701-26.
13. Gilden DH. Clinical practice. Bell's palsy. N Engl J Med. 2004;351(13):1323-31.
14. Teixeira LJ, Valbuza JS, Prado GF. Physical therapy for Bell's palsy (idiopathic facial paralysis). Cochrane Database Syst Rev. 2011;(12):CD006283.
15. Cardoso JR, Teixeira EC, Moreira MD, et al. Effects of exercises on Bell's palsy: Systematic review of randomized controlled trials. Otol Neurotol. 2008;29(4):557-60.
16. Chen N, Zhou M, He L, et al. Acupuncture for Bell's palsy. Cochrane Database Syst Rev. 2010;(8):CD002914.

Eyelid and Canthal Reconstruction

Ruchi Goel, KPS Malik

INTRODUCTION

Eye lid reconstruction is performed with the aim to restore a mucous membrane lined, semirigid skeleton with a cutaneous covering that resumes normal functioning, and is cosmetically acceptable.

The assessment is done in terms of defect in the anterior and posterior lamellae and the procedure is chosen according to the extent of lid defect (Table 1). Due to laxity of skin, defects are easier to repair in older patients.

Small defects can be directly approximated. Additional 5–10 mm mobilization can be achieved by lateral canthotomy and lysis of inferior crus of lateral canthal tendon.

Medium sized defects are dealt by lateral semicircular rotational flap, the sliding tarsoconjunctival flap, and the free autogenous tarsoconjunctival graft.

Large lower lid defects are managed by sharing tarsoconjunctival bridge flap from upper lid (Hughes procedure) with an overlying skin graft or myocutaneous rotational or advancement flap.

The Mustarde semirotational cheek advancement flap is another technique to repair large lid defects.

Large upper lid defects are repaired by lid sharing techniques like Cutler-Beard, eye lid switch flap of Mustarde, or a modified "reverse" Hughes procedure.

TABLE 1: Assessment of defect size.

Size of the defect	Young patient (tight lids)	Older patient (lax lids)
Small	25–35%	35–45%
Medium	35–45%	45–55%
Large	>55%	>65%

If more than 3 mm superior tarsus remains following tumor resection, it can be advanced inferiorly to reconstruct the upper lid margin in a single stage procedure.

Lateral canthal defects that are less than one-third of upper and lower eyelid margin are closed by suturing the lateral ends of upper and lower tarsal plates to the periosteum just inside the lateral orbital rim. Larger defects require tarsoconjunctival flaps for reconstruction.

For *medial canthal defects*, tarsoconjunctival flaps in both the upper and lower lid are advanced and tarsal attachments are secured in the area of desired medial canthal tendon near the superior aspect of posterior lacrimal crest.

Recognition and appropriate repair of canalicular injury is important in all medial eyelid defects.

Infilterative anesthesia should always be used with lignocaine and epinephrine 1:100,000, irrespective of whether local or general anesthesia is used.

Skin flaps are preferred over skin grafts due to the following reasons:
- Maintenance of the original color of local tissue
- Less shrinkage (10% vs. 25–50% for grafts)
- Provision of inherent blood supply
- Volume and surface contour restoration by subcutaneous tissue.

Factors limiting blood flow to local cutaneous flap are:
- Extensive previous surgery/irradiation
- Lines of tension
- Aggressive pressure dressing
- Hematoma formation
- Infection.

Incisions should be placed within or parallel to the various facial "lines" that develop from specific orientation of collagen and elastin fibers modified by the effects of gravity and facial muscle contraction.

Skin incisions should be parallel to the lid margin in the upper lid. In the lower lid, incisions are placed perpendicular to the margin to avoid lid laxity and ectropion formation. Local cutaneous flaps can be classified as sliding, advancement, rotation, or transposition (Table 2 and Fig. 1). Z Plasty is a transposition flap technique in which the flaps are designed to change the direction of the scar so that it lies in the same direction as the skin lines. The scar is excised in an elliptical fashion, which then forms the common central member. Two interdigitating triangular flaps are outlined with a common central member in the line of contracture and the two arms of equal length are extended 60° from opposite ends of the central member. After transposition,

the central member of the resultant Z will be at right angle to the original central member (scar).

GRAFTS

- Full thickness skin grafts are composed of epidermis and the entire dermis. They can be obtained from ipsilateral/contralateral upper lid skin (in case of lower lid defects), skin from retroauricular area, supraclavicular area, inner aspect of arm, or nasolabial fold (Figs. 2 to 4)
- For construction of tarsus, upper two-thirds of superior tarsal plate, auricular cartilage (Fig. 5), hard palate mucosa, nasal septal cartilage, or nasal alae can be used
- Conjunctiva is substituted by superior bulbar conjunctiva, oral mucous membrane, nasal mucous membrane, or amniotic membrane.

TABLE 2: Local cutaneous flaps.

S. no.	Type	Features
1	Sliding flap	Area is undermined and moved over its subcutaneous base to primarily close a skin defect.
2	Advancement flap	Is three sided, after undermining, sliding skin flap is advanced to cover an adjacent skin defect.
3	Rotation flap	Undermined strip of skin that is rotated into an adjacent defect.
4	Transposition flap	Undermined skin and subcutaneous tissue is elevated and transposed to a nonadjacent skin defect.

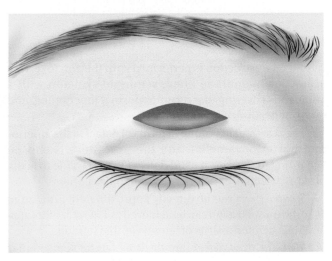

Fig. 2: Full thickness skin graft from upper lid.

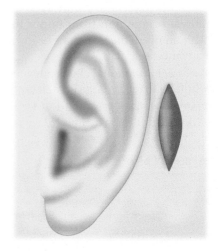

Fig. 3: Postauricular full thickness skin graft.

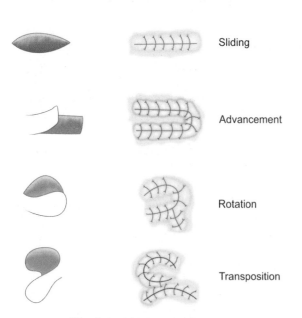

Sliding

Advancement

Rotation

Transposition

Fig. 1: Local cutaneous flaps.

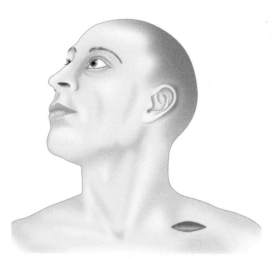

Fig. 4: Supraclavicular full thickness skin graft.

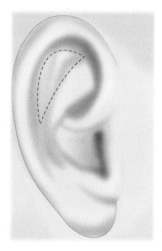

Fig. 5: Auricular cartilage graft-surface marking.

COMMONLY USED SURGICAL TECHNIQUES

Direct Closure

A full thickness, vertical, and pentagon-shaped defect with point near the conjunctival fornix is created to minimize tarsal buckling and eyelid margin notching. Three vertical mattress sutures are passed at gray line, posterior lid margin, and anterior lid margin. Initial bite of the suture is placed at the gray line about 3 mm from the cut end. This is the deep bite. The needle emerges at 3 mm from the cut end on the other side at an equal depth. A return bite 1.5 mm from cut end is taken to finally emerge 1.5 mm from cut end on the side where the suturing was initially started. On tying the suture, slight eversion of the lid margin after repair must be achieved to prevent wound contracture on subsidence of edema. The ends of the gray line and posterior lid margin suture are kept long to allow inclusion in the in knot of the anterior lid margin suture to prevent accidental corneal rub. The tarsal plate is closed with partial thickness bites using vicryl suture and finally skin is sutured using 6,0 silk (Figs. 6A and B).

Tenzel's semicircular flap is used for both upper and lower lid defects, 40–60% of the original lid margin. It can be combined with periosteal flap or supplemental ear cartilage to reconstruct the posterior lamella. A semicircular musculocutaneous flap, 18 mm horizontally and 22 mm vertically beginning at the lateral canthus, extending upward for lower lid defect and downward for upper lid defect is created. Cantholysis of the corresponding crus of canthal tendon is performed (Figs. 7 and 8).

Pedicle Flap from Lower Eye Lid Margin to Upper Lid (Fig. 9)

Upper eyelid margin can be reconstructed with intact lashes from lower eyelid margin. A full thickness pedicle is taken

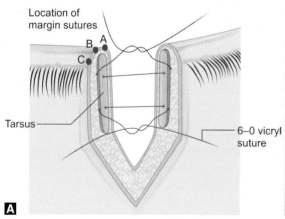

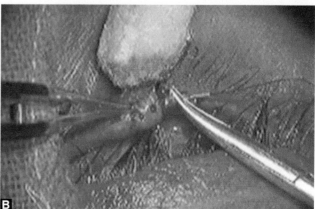

Figs. 6A and B: (A) Eyelid defect showing placement of tarsal sutures and location of margin sutures. A—posterior lid margin, B—Gray line of lid margin, C—anterior lid margin; (B) Direct closure.

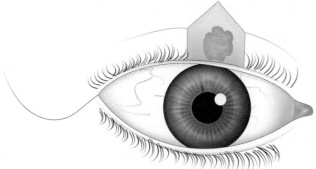

Fig. 7: Semicircular musculocutaneous flap vertically beginning at the lateral canthus, extending upward for lower lid defect and downward for upper lid defect.

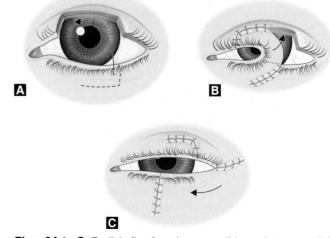

Figs. 9A to C: Pedicle flap from lower eye lid margin to upper lid.

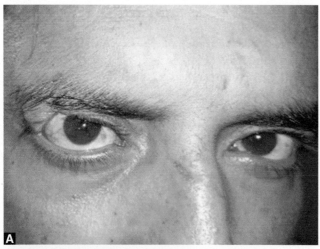

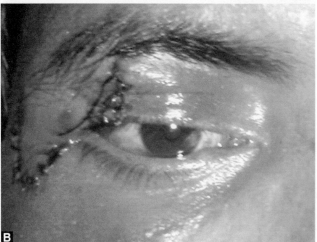

Figs. 8A and B: Right upper lid coloboma repaired using Tenzel's semicircular flap: (A) Preoperative clinical photograph; (B) Postoperative appearance.

from the central portion of the lower lid margin. The flap should be 5 mm in height to include the marginal artery and should be rectangular in shape. The end of the flap is then rotated and margin to margin attachment is made. In the second stage, the base of the flap is separated from the lower lid, rotated to the upper lid and the lower lid defect is closed with or without cantholysis.

Tarsoconjunctival bridge flap (Hughes procedure), a lid sharing procedure, is used for lower eyelid defects more than50% of the horizontal length of the eyelid. Tarsoconjunctival bridge flap from the upper eyelid is used for the reconstruction of posterior lamella. It is covered by a full thickness skin graft (Fig. 10). The flap was earlier left in place for 4–6 weeks prior to second-stage separation. Some surgeons advocate flap division at 2 weeks. In the modified Hughes procedure, the marginal upper lid tarsus is spared and levator muscle aponeuorsis is removed from the tarsoconjunctival flap. This reduces the rate of upper lid complications, such as upper lid retraction, trichasis, and entropion.

The *Cutler beard procedure* is used for large central defects of the upper eyelid. A full-thickness segment of lower eyelid tissue is passed under an intact bridge of the lower eyelid margin and is sutured into the defect in the upper eyelid (Fig. 11). In the second stage done 6–8 weeks later, the flap is divided. It is not suitable for one eyed/amblyogenic age. In Inverse Cutler Beard upper lid is utilized to repair the lower lid colobomas.

The *Hewes flap* was first described by Eva Hewes and is a one-stage technique to reconstruct the lower eyelid using a tarsoconjunctival flap transposed from the upper eyelid and hinged at the lateral canthal tendon. An advantage of the Hewes flap is that occlusion of the eye is not required (Fig. 12).

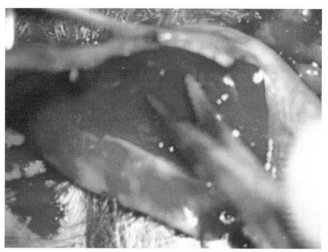

Fig. 10: Hughe's procedure: The lid is everted and tarsoconjunctival bridge flap from the upper eyelid is fashioned to reconstruct the posterior lamella of the lower lid.

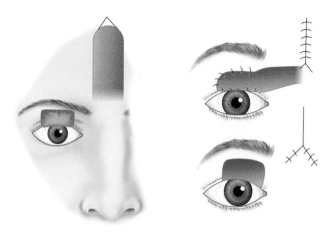

Fig. 13: Median forehead flap.

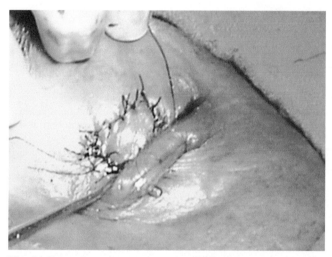

Fig. 11: Cutler Beard procedure: A full-thickness segment of lower eyelid tissue is passed under an intact bridge of the lower eyelid margin and is sutured into the defect in the upper eyelid.

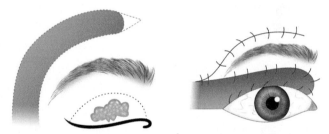

Fig. 14: Temporally based flap from suprabrow is used to supply tissue to upper lid and sometimes lower lid.

Median forehead flap is used for anterior lamellar reconstruction for massive tissue loss in upper lid (Fig. 13). The base of the flap is separated at 8 weeks. The disadvantage is a thick donor skin which is less mobile.

Temporal forehead (Fricke) flap: Temporally based flap from suprabrow is used to supply tissue to upper lid and sometimes lower lid (Fig. 14).

Mustarde cheek rotational flap is used for vertically deep lower lid defects. A semicircular flap beginning at the lateral canthus and extending to the area immediately adjacent to the auricular tragus is dissected with the superior limit of the semicircle at or above the brow to prevent sagging of the lateral lid margin (Fig. 15). A large superiorly based triangle with medial edge at the nasolabial fold is outlined. The medial triangle is excised. The posterior lamella graft is placed and the rotational cheek flap is mobilized nasally. The demerits are excessively long scar line on face, excision of a large triangle of normal skin, and the adynamic nature of the reconstructed lower lid (Fig. 16).

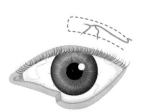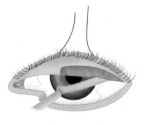

Fig. 12: Hewes flap. Reconstruction of the lower eyelid using a tarsoconjunctival flap transposed from the upper eyelid and hinged at the lateral canthal tendon.

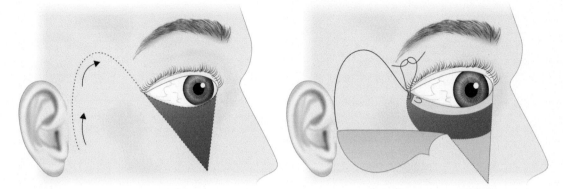

Fig. 15: Mustarde cheek rotational flap is used for vertically deep lower lid defects.

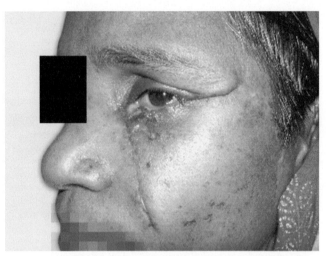

Fig. 16: Long vertical scar after Mustarde rotational cheek flap.

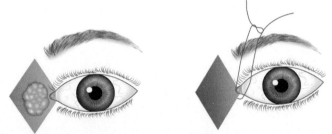

Fig. 17: Medial canthal defects should be diamond shaped if possible. Tarsal remnants of both the lids are attached to the posterior reflection of the medial canthal tendon.

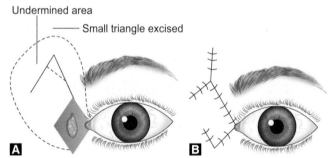

Figs. 18A and B: Glabellar forehead flap.

Medial Canthal Reconstruction

Attachment of the edge of the lid remnants to the posterior reflection of the medial canthal tendon to restore the direction of medial canthal angle is of utmost importance. Defect should be fashioned in the shape of diamond (Fig. 17). The skin defect can be closed by one of the following methods:

- *Laissez faire:* Excised medial canthal area left to heal by granulation, especially when periosteum is intact and the excision of an equal amount or more above, rather than below the medial canthal ligament
- A full thickness postauricular skin graft
- Use of a glabellar forehead flap (Figs. 18A and B)

SUMMARY

To conclude, planning of eyelid reconstruction begins with assessment of the extent of the defect. Techniques such as direct closure, Tenzel's semi-circular flap are used for both upper and lower lid. Hughes procedure, Inverse Cutler beard procedure, Mustarde cheek rotational flap, and Hewes procedure are used for lower lid reconstruction. Cutler beard and pedicle flap from lower lid margin are used for upper lid reconstruction. Flaps are preferred over grafts.

Facial Rejuvenation: Blepharoplasty, Brow Ptosis Correction, and Nonsurgical Methods

Kasturi Bhattacharjee, Samir Serasiya, Deepika Kapoor

FACIAL REJUVENATION

Facial rejuvenation is a term used to describe cosmetic surgical or nonsurgical procedures aiming to restore the youth of the facial structure or reverse aging changes such as wrinkles over face, sagginess of eyelid, prolapse of orbital fat around the lids, and drooping of eyelids, eyebrow and face. The contributions by an ophthalmic plastic surgeon in facial rejuvenation is rapidly increasing, "Blepharoplasty" being a very commonly performed cosmetic eyelid surgery worldwide. With that, the trend of using botulinum neurotoxin for nonsurgical cosmetic face rejuvenation is on the rise. Thus basic knowledge of the dynamics of oculofacial aging and the principles of surgical and nonsurgical facial rejuvenation are essential. This chapter aims to cover all relevant anatomy, surgical procedures, nonsurgical procedures, and brow ptosis.

- ◆ Applied anatomy
- ◆ Nonsurgical procedures
  - – Botulinum toxin
  - – Dermal fillers
  - – Laser skin resurfacing
- ◆ Surgical procedures
  - – Upper eyelid blepharoplasty
  - – Lower eyelid blepharoplasty
  - – Mid face lift
- ◆ Brow ptosis

APPLIED ANATOMY

A thorough understanding of the anatomy of the face is of utmost importance before undertaking any oculofacial surgery as it helps the surgeon in meticulous planning and assessment preoperatively and also guides them during the surgery.

Eyelids

For ease of understanding, the eyelids can be divided into the following structural layers:
- • Anterior lamella:
  - – Skin and subcutaneous connective tissue
  - – Orbicularis oculi muscle
- • Posterior lamella:
  - – Tarsus
  - – Conjunctiva
- • The eyelid skin is the thinnest in the body (Epidermis is only three to four layers thick; overall epidermis-dermis is <1 mm in thickness). It is loosely adhered to the underlying connective tissue, giving rise to a potential space for fluid accumulation or edema of the eyelids.
- • The orbicularis oculi muscle lies beneath the skin. It has two parts:
  1. Orbital part
  2. Palpebral parts:
     i. Pretarsal portion
     ii. Preseptal portion

Orbital portion helps in forceful closure of the eyelid. Pretarsal fibers of orbicularis are adhered to the underlying tarsal plate and they play a role in involuntary closure of the eyelids. Excision of these fibers may lead to postoperative lagophthalmos. Loosely anchored preseptal fibers are excised during the blepharoplasty surgery to gain access to the underlying orbital septum. In the aging face, as the orbital and preseptal fibers of the orbicularis muscle separate, a tear trough deformity occurs.

Orbital septum, a continuation of the periosteum beyond the arcus marginalis, is a thin sheet of fibrous tissue. It restrains the medial (white) and central (yellow) fat pads in the upper eyelid while medial, central, and lateral fat pads in the lower lid (Fig. 1).

> **The fat pads of the eyelids:**
> The upper eyelid has two fat pads: The medial and the central fat pads.
> The embryonic origin of medial fat pad is from neural crest cells while central fat originates from mesoderm, which is responsible for the color disparity.

> The lower eyelid has three fat pads the medial, central and the lateral fat pads However during lower lid blepharoplasty care should be taken to avoid any injury to the inferior oblique muscle which lies between the central and the medial fat pads in the lower lid. Any injury to the inferior oblique muscle leads to postoperative diplopia.

Levator muscle (LPS) with its aponeurosis and Müller's muscle (superior tarsal muscle) form the muscles of retraction in the upper lid. Its counterparts in the lower lid are capsulopalpebral fascia and inferior tarsal muscle. The anterior fibers of the LPS insert into the eyelid skin, forming the lid crease. The levator aponeurosis lies immediately below the central fat pad, making it prone to accidental injury during the upper lid blepharoplasty.

The tarsal plate: It is the structural framework of the eyelids and is composed of thick fibrous tissue. The tarsal plate height in the upper lid varies from 8 mm to 10 mm while that in the lower lid is around 4 mm. Medially and laterally the tarsal plate is attached to the periosteum with the help of canthal tendons. Each tarsal plate has multiple vertically oriented meibomian glands within it.

Conjunctiva: It is composed of nonkeratinizing squamous epithelial cells and forms the posterior most layer of the eyelids. Beyond the fornix it is continuous with the bulbar conjunctiva.

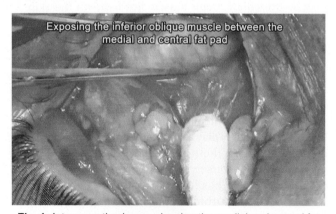

Fig. 1: Intraoperative image showing the medial and central fat pad and the inferior oblique muscle.

TABLE 1: Differences between Asian and non-Asian eyelid.

Anatomic features	Non-Asian eyelid	Asian eyelid
Preaponeurotic fat pad location	Preseptal, more superior	Pretarsal and Preseptal, more inferior and anterior
Levator-septum fusion point	Supratarsal	Between the tarsal plate and eyelid margin
Tarsal plate Height	9–10.5 mm	6.5–8.0 mm
Origin of medial lid crease	Medial eyelid	Medial canthus
Presence of lid crease	100%	50%

The prominent differences between Asian and Non-Asian eyelids are summarized in Table 1.

NONSURGICAL PROCEDURES

- Botulinum toxin
- Dermal fillers
- Laser skin resurfacing

Botulinum Toxin

Botulinum toxin, known to the world as a potent neurotoxic protein derivative, has many applications in the modern day clinics. The first ever clinical use of botulinum toxin was done by an ophthalmologist, Dr. Alan Scott, who injected it in human extraocular muscles to treat strabismus in 1970s. Since the last three decades, its functional and cosmetic uses have been increasing owing to its safe and effective outcome.

> **Characteristics:**
> - Produced by *Clostridium botulinum*, an anaerobic Gram-positive spore forming bacteria.
> - Eight different serotypes named A, B, C1, C2, D, E, F, and G.
> - Type A—most commonly used in clinical practice, most powerful and longest acting.
> - Composed of heavy and light polypeptide chains linked by a disulfide bond.
> - Synthesized as an inactive single peptide chain with a molecular mass of 150 kD.

Mechanism of Action

Botulinum toxin acts by inhibiting the release of acetylcholine (Ach) at the neuromuscular junction.

Normally, at the junction, when action potential depolarizes the axon terminal, Ach is released from the synaptic cleft. A transport protein, named SNARE (soluble N-ethylmaleimide-sensitive factor attachment protein receptor) complex, facilitates this process. The SNARE proteins are responsible for fusion of vesicle of Ach with nerve cell membrane.

Mechanism of action

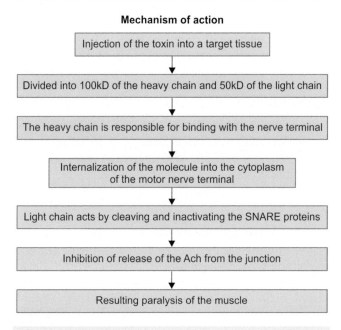

Mechanism of recovery:
The inhibitory effect continues for 2 to 6 months. Following that, the reversal of the muscle action occurs by following mechanisms:
♦ Restoration of the SNARE protein complex.
♦ Axonal sprouting
♦ Endplate elongation

Indications

Since its first use in strabismus, Botox has been tried for various clinical and esthetic conditions. FDA approved the use of botulinum toxin in December 1989, for the treatment of strabismus, blepharospasm, and spastic lid disorders of facial nerve, e.g. hemifacial spasm. Since then, it has been used for following conditions:

- *Esthetic indications:*
  Botulinum toxin injection causes relaxation of small facial muscles, which in turn leads to disappearance of the wrinkles and fine lines producing a facial rejuvenating effect. Following are the common facial esthetic indications:
  - Glabellar lines or frown lines
  - Orbicularis rhytides or crow's feet

  Off label esthetic indications:
  - Transverse forehead lines
  - Bunny lines—transverse lines over nasal bridge
  - Marionette lines—downward turning of the lateral corners of the mouth
  - Nonsurgical brow lift
  - Perioral lines
  - Platysmal bands
  - Facial sculpting in masseter hypertrophy.

- *Therapeutic indications:*
  Relaxation of the spastic muscles following botulinum injection relieves patients of their symptoms. Common therapeutic uses are as follows:
  - *Essential blepharospasm:*
    The initial dose of 2.5 units injected into the medial and lateral pretarsal orbicularis oculi of the upper and lower lids. Additional 2.5 units are also injected into the corrugators, depressor supercilii, and procerus. Moreover if the spasm is severe 1.25 units are injected below the eyebrow in the medial and the lateral part of the orbital orbicularis oculi muscle fibers. Total dose ranges from 20 to 25 units on each side.
  - *Hemifacial spasm and Meige syndrome:*
    After ruling out organic causes, botulinum toxin can be used to relieve the involuntary facial muscle contractions. Each facial site is injected with 5–10 units in the mid face region. A higher dose of 10–20 units is required for platysma muscle. One should start from a lower dose in the beginning and gradually increase up to 5 units to avoid any facial muscle asymmetry.
  - *Chronic migraine:*
    Patients having debilitating migraine (15 or more days each month with a headache lasting four or more hours each day) are ideal candidates for botulinum toxin injection.
  - Cervical dystonia
  - Various types of strabismus.

  Off-label therapeutic uses:
  - Reflex brow elevation after ptosis repair
  - Chronic headache other than migraine and tension headache not responding to conventional therapy
  - Thyroid eye disease—to reduce upper lid retraction and glabellar furrows
  - Temporary chemical tarsorrhaphy for treating corneal ulceration following fifth or seventh nerve palsy
  - Severe dry eye—injection into the medial part of upper and lower lids causes punctal eversion and decreases tear drainage
  - Spastic lower lid entropion
  - Apraxia of eyelid
  - *Crocodile tears*—hyper lacrimation following seventh nerve injury or Bell's palsy.

Preparation

Botulinum toxin is commercially available in sterile vials comprising of 50 units, 100 units or 200 units vacuum-dried powder, which is reconstituted with sterile, preservative-free 0.9% sodium chloride injection. Depending on the indication, a concentration of 1.25–5 IU/0.1 mL is formulated.

The first noticeable effect is visible after 3 days of the injection, while it reaches a peak around 1–2 weeks. The effect lasts for duration of 3–6 months after which repetition of the injection is required (Figs. 2 and 3).

Complications

Patients can develop the following complications after injection:

- Extraocular muscle weakness
- Diplopia
- Ptosis
- Swelling of eyelid
- Corneal exposure and ulceration
- Blurred vision

- Dysphonia, dysarthria, dyspnea, and dysphagia
- Allergic reaction or anaphylaxis
- Exacerbation of the preexisting neuromuscular disorder
- Death.

Precautions

Cosmetic use of botulinum toxin is not recommended for use in children younger than 18 years of age, while therapeutic use is limited to more than 12 years of age. It is contraindicated in following situations:

- Previous allergic reaction
- Infection at the injection site
- Lactating mother or pregnancy
- Neuromuscular disorder such as myasthenia gravis or Lambert Eaton syndrome
- Urinary tract infection or urinary retention.

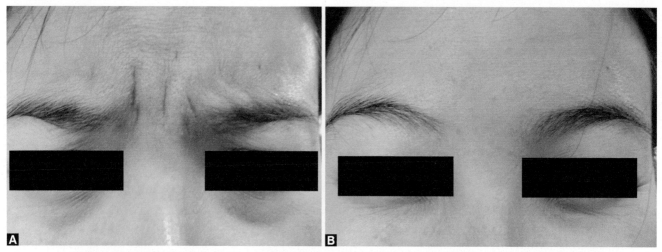

Figs. 2A and B: (A) Glabellar Furrows; (B) Disappearance of furrows after injection of botulinum toxin.

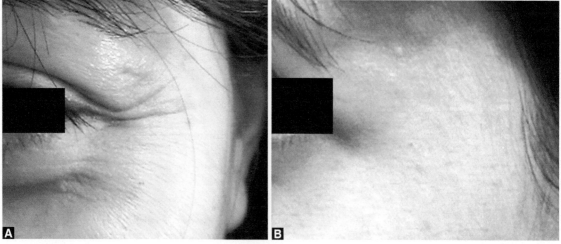

Figs. 3A and B: (A) Crow's feet; (B) Disappearance of Crow's feet after injection of botulinum toxin.

Dermal Fillers

Since the introduction of injectable dermal fillers in 1981, its usage has grown rapidly in the esthetic field. It is used for facial rejuvenation in patients looking for nonsurgical means of correcting age-related changes. The introduction of the newer hyaluronic acid (HA) based agents has revived the interest in dermal fillers as they promise better outcomes with a lesser side effect profile.

Dermal fillers, based on the duration of the effect, can be divided into mainly three groups:

1. *Temporary agents: (2–12 months)*
   Collagen compounds:
   - Bovine collagen (Zyderm 1 and Zyderm 2)
   - Human collagen (Cosmo Derm)
   Hyaluronic acid compounds:
   HA-based fillers can be divided into:
   - *Lighter HA*—mainly used for superficial and periorbital rhytides
   - *Denser HA*—mainly useful for deeper rhytides and mid to lower face.
   Some of the commercially available preparations are:
   - Restylane and perlane
   - Hylaform/hylaform plus
   - Juvéderm ultra
   - Juvéderm ultra plus
   - Juvéderm voluma
   - Juvéderm volbella.
2. Semipermanent compounds (1–2 years)
   - Calcium hydroxyapatite (radiesse, radiance)
   - PLLA (Sculptra).
3. Permanent compounds (>2 years)
   - Silicone (SILIKON 1000)
   - PMMA spheres (ArteFill)
   - Autologous fat.

Hyaluronic Acid Derivatives

Hyaluronic acid is one of the most commonly used agents for dermal fillers in recent times. This nonanimal, noncadaveric biomaterial has a set of properties, which makes it a desirable agent for injection. It is naturally found in various tissues including the spaces between the collagen fibers of the skin. HA has hydrophilic property and the ability to imbibe water, thereby acting as a natural filler. With increasing age, the production of hyaluronic acid goes down along with its ability to draw water, thereby playing an important role in facial soft tissue atrophy.

Properties of HA
♦ Glycosaminoglycan, a major component of the connective tissue
♦ Ground substance of the dermis
♦ Immunologically inactive
♦ No species or tissue specificity
♦ Binds to water molecules
♦ Expands many times in volume

For commercial filler injection, it needs to be converted into a polymerized form. HA is naturally unstable in its noncross-linked form, and is rapidly degraded in the body. Once it is cross-linked, it becomes more stabilized and resilient. A cross-linked polymer is added for this purpose, which converts its liquid form into a gel-like form. The consistency of the injection HA gel is based on the amount of cross-linked polymers that is present in the preparation.

Advantages of HA based fillers:
♦ Nonanimal product
♦ Noninfectious material
♦ Longer lasting esthetic effect
♦ Minimal morbidity
♦ Very few side effects

Each HA filler product has different sized particles, thus, each type of product has different indications which are used to address specific problems in various layers of the skin. Small gel particle size containing fillers are used in superficial wrinkles in the perioral area, while larger gel size particle containing fillers should be used in the deeper skin layer for correction of deeper folds (e.g. nasolabial and melolabial folds) and for lip/chin augmentation.

Use of HA based fillers
- Fine superficial wrinkles
- Temporal brow lift
- Glabellar furrows
- Nasojugal folds or tear trough deformity
- Chin augmentation (Fig. 4A)
- Mid face lift (Figs. 4B and C)
- Traumatic liner scars

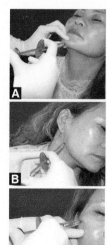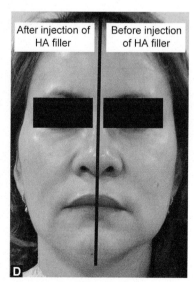

Figs. 4A to D: (A) Chin augmentation using injection HA filler; (B and C) Points of injection for a midface lift using injection HA filler; (D) Comparison between the right half of the face showing a desired lift (postinjection) vs. the left half of the face showing mid face ptosis (preinjection).

- Nasolabial lines
- Lip augmentation (Fig. 5)
- Marionette lines
- Peri-mental hollows
- Non invasive facelift
- Nose augmentation (Figs. 6A and B).

Adverse Reaction

Transient adverse effects: Pain, intermittent swelling, edema, lumpiness, itching, erythema, bruising, and discoloration.

These are temporary and resolve within few days of the injection.

Other adverse reaction can be:
- *Hypersensitivity-related:*
  - Urticaria
  - Granuloma formation
  - Scar formation.
- *Non-hypersensitivity related:*
  - Bruising, infection at injection site, and reactivation of herpes

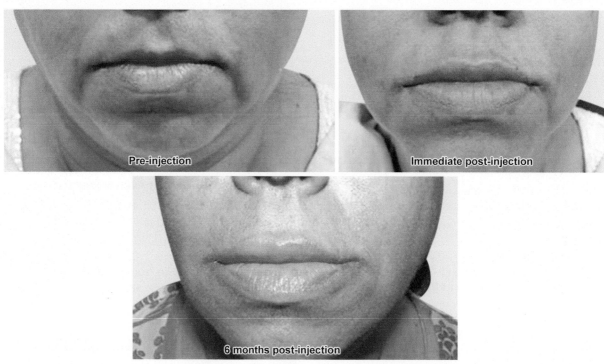

Fig. 5: Lip augmentation using injection HA filler.

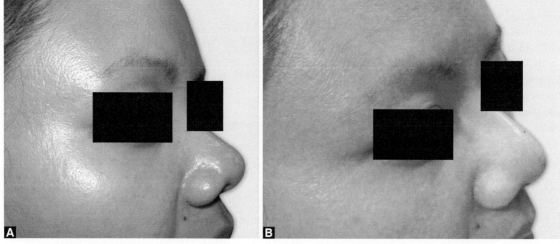

Figs. 6A and B: (A) Nose augmentation pre-HA filler; (B) Nose augmentation post-HA filler.

– Bluish discoloration of the skin, known as the Tyndall effect
– Tissue necrosis and intravascular injection.
  - Central retinal artery occlusion (CRAO) leading to blindness can occur in 1 in 10,000 cases.

Laser Skin Resurfacing

Laser skin resurfacing is used to reduce wrinkles and enrich the texture and appearance of the facial and periorbital skin.

Lasers Used

- Superpulsed and ultra-pulsed CO_2 lasers
  - Deliver small pulses of high energy light to the skin
  - Between the two pulses, a pause allows cooling of the soft tissue leading to decrease in the collateral damage in treated area.
- The Erbium: YAG laser
  - Has a primarily ablative effect on collagen and water-containing tissues
  - Less heat transfer and a lesser zone of ablation to the tissues than the CO_2 lasers.

Advantages

- Useful adjunct to lower eyelid blepharoplasty
- Has a skin-shrinking and collagen-tightening effect
- Skin tightening effect can be achieved without external incision and removing skin.

Contraindications

- Patients on isotretinoin therapy
- Collagen vascular disease
- Significant lower eyelid laxity
- Inappropriate, unrealistic expectations.

Complications

- Lower eyelid retraction
- Exposure keratitis
- Corneal injury
- Lagophthalmos
- Ectropion.

SURGICAL PROCEDURES

Upper Eyelid Blepharoplasty

- Introduction
- Indications
- Preoperative evaluation
- Surgical procedure
- Complications

Introduction

Blepharoplasty comes from the ancient Greek words "Blepharon" which means eyelids and "plastikos" which means to mold. It is a common surgical procedure performed for correction of the involutional changes in the periocular region in which the eyelid skin, orbicularis oculi muscle, and orbital fat are excised, molded, or sculpted to enhance the esthetic look of the patient while also correcting any functional abnormality that may coexist. The upper eyelid blepharoplasty has both esthetic and functional applications while the lower eyelid blepharoplasty is mainly useful for esthetic rationales. Karl Ferdinand Von Graefe (father of Albrecht von Graefe, Ophthalmologist) first coined the term blepharoplasty in 1818, while reporting an eyelid reconstruction. Thenceforth, blepharoplasty has been evolving and has now become the most commonly performed facial esthetic surgery.

Indications of Upper Eyelid Blepharoplasty

Indications of blepharoplasty are either for functional or for esthetic concerns. Some of the common indications are:
- *Functional:*
  - *Dermatochalasis:* Dermatochalasis, typically a bilateral condition, is a common aging change associated with sagging of excess and lax eyelid skin. Older individuals, after 50 years of age are most commonly affected. The eyelid skin being the thinnest, is more prone to develop early signs of aging such as skin redundancy and lid atrophy of the upper eyelids.

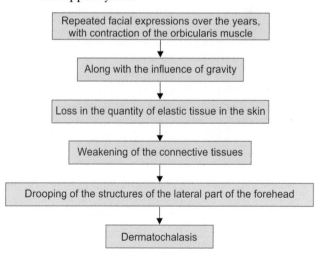

Clinical features: Patient presents with cosmetic concerns and complains of drooping of eyelids or swelling of the lids (Fig. 7). Other problems are a tired look or an appearance older than their age. Moreover, functional problems such as obstruction in

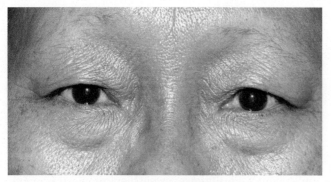

Fig. 7: Bilateral age related dermatochalasis along with lower lid fat prolapse in old female patient.

the outer and upper visual field, decreased quality of vision; and reduction in contrast sensitivity can occur. Blepharoplasty addresses all such problems along with the enhancement of the cosmetic look.

Changes in parameters after blepharoplasty:
♦ Improvement in the visual field
♦ Improvement in contrast sensitivity
♦ Reduction of ocular aberrations specifically the high order aberrations
♦ Significant corneal shape changes, correlated with topographical corneal changes

- *Upper eyelid epiblepharon*: Upper eyelid epiblepharon causing lash ptosis due to vertical configuration of the eyelashes can cause microtrauma to ocular surface provoking a cascade of inflammation and dry eyes. Correction of the lash ptosis by means of blepharoplasty may even revert such changes
- *Blepharochalasis:* Recurrent inflammatory swelling of the lid produces redundancy of the upper eyelid skin. It is characterized by relaxation and atrophy of the tissues of the upper lids following attacks of edema
- Inflammatory disorders such as Grave's ophthalmopathy
- *Others:* Trauma, large xanthelasma, mass or tumor, and developmental eyelid anomaly.
- **Esthetic**
Esthetic practice of upper eyelid blepharoplasty is on the rise. Main cosmetic concerns for blepharoplasty include:
  - Correction of asymmetrical lid folds
  - Double lid crease formation from Single lid fold
  - Creation of a higher lid crease
  - Typical Asian eyelid features.

Preoperative Evaluation

While evaluating patients for blepharoplasty, following points should be kept in mind for complete preoperative check-up:

- Complete medical and ocular history
- Thorough ophthalmologic examination
- Eyelid examination including palpebral fissure height, lid contour, lid crease, lid fold distance, tarsal plate show (TPS), brow fat span (BFS), eyebrow position, frontalis action, medial and lateral canthal laxity, Bell's phenomenon, marginal reflex distance, lagophthalmos
- Tear film and ocular surface evaluation
- Associated conditions such as thyroid disease, angioneurotic edema dry eye disease, seventh nerve function
- Written and informed consent
- Preoperative photographs in straight and lateral view (Figs. 8 to 11).

Surgical Technique (Figs. 8 and 9)

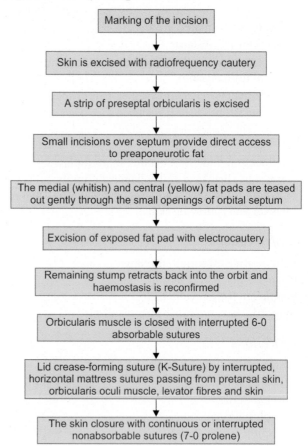

Complications

- Superficial hematoma/ecchymosis
- Asymmetry of lids
- Lagophthalmos
- Sunken eye appearance and superior sulcus deformity
- Ptosis
- Scaring
- Dry eye syndrome.

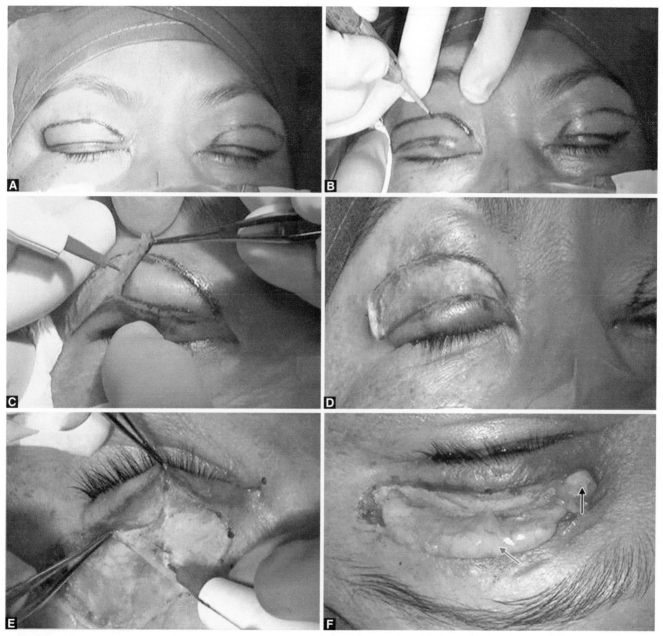

Figs. 8A to F: (A) Marking of the incision prior to surgery; (B) Skin incision using the radiofrequency tip; (C) Excision of the skin using electrocautery probe; (D) Exposure of the underlying orbicularis oculi muscle; (E) Excision of the orbicularis oculi muscle fibers using electrocautery; (F) Exposure of the central yellow fat pad (green arrow) and the whitish nasal fat pad (black arrow).

LOWER LID BLEPHAROPLASTY

Lower eyelid blepharoplasty aims to remove excess and prolapsed orbital fat in the lower lid, while a more recent approach is focused on repositioning the herniated fat into a subperiosteal pocket in cases of tear trough deformity.

Indications of Lower Lid Blepharoplasty
- Lower eyelid fat prolapse
- Sagging of lower eyelid skin
- Tear trough deformity
- Wrinkles or circles around the eye
- Displacement of the canthal position.

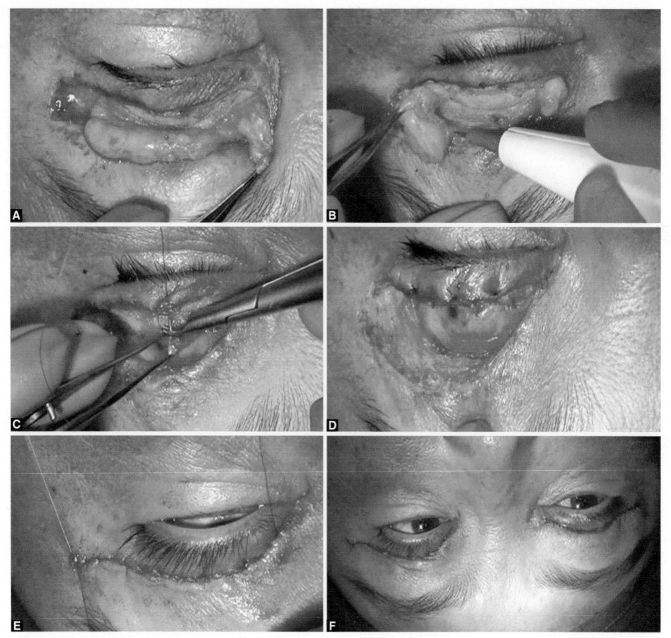

Figs. 9A to F: (A) Exposure of central and nasal fat pads; (B) Excision of the fat pads using electrocautery; (C) Placing of the lid crease forming sutures (K suture); (D) Showing all three cardinal lid crease sutures; (E) Skin closure using running 6-0 prolene; (F) Both eyes after completion of surgery.

Surgical Procedure

There are two surgical approaches:

1. *Transconjunctival approach:* This approach is preferred in patients with lower orbital fat prolapse without significant skin laxity. It leaves no external scar, making it the favored approach for young patients. After local infiltration with anesthetic agents, incision is marked 6–8 mm below the lower lid margin. Using the electrocautery, conjunctiva is incised and is tagged with two 6-0 polyglactin sutures. Blunt dissection is carried out to reach the orbital septum. A careful incision in the septum and further extension would lead to exposure of the all three fat pads. The inferior oblique muscle, which lies between the medial and central fat pads should not be damaged. Desired amount of fat is either excised or reposited into the subperiosteal pockets. Conjunctiva is closed with 6-0 polyglactin sutures.

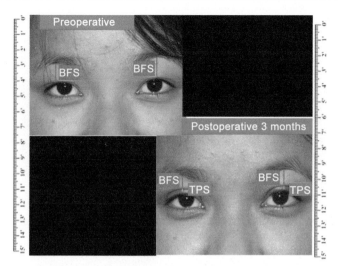

Fig. 10: Upper lid blepharoplasty postoperative 3 months, showing improvement in TPS and reduction in BFS.
(BFS: brow fat show; TPS: tarsal plate span

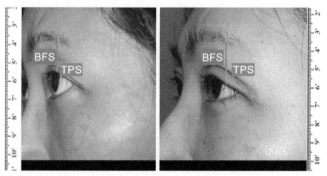

Fig. 11: Lateral view photo following upper lid blepharoplasty postoperative 3 months, showing improvement in TPS and reduction in BFS.
(BFS: brow fat show; TPS: tarsal plate span)

This approach provides scarless cosmetic correction but its disadvantage is that excessive skin laxity is not addressed (Fig. 12).

2. *Transcutaneous approach:* This approach provides an added advantage of dealing with excessive skin laxity. Preoperatively, using skin pinch test, marking is done. A subcilliary incision is given. The desired amount of the skin is resected along with the preseptal orbicularis flap. Orbital septum is identified and a small incision is made to expose the orbital fats. Excessive fat is removed and wound is closed with 6-0 prolene.

Complications

- Hematoma
- Ecchymosis
- Lower lid retraction
- Scleral show
- Excess fat removal
- Asymmetry of lid contour

- Corneal exposure
- Inferior orbicularis trauma
- Acquired strabismus.

Mid-Face Lift

Dropping or sagging of the mid face structures namely the cheeks, orbital fat, and the sub orbicularis oculi fat (SOOF), is evident by an increased prominence of the nasojugal folds and the double convex deformity around the eyes. For a mid-face rejuvenation, various approaches can be used to lift the ptotic SOOF and debulk the prolapsed orbital fats. The incision sites can vary and any of the following may be chosen:

- The lateral
- Superolateral
- Superotemporal coronal/temple incision
- Endoscopic corono-canthoplasty
- Extended infraciliary incision.

Thus, depending on the amount of lift required either a subperiosteal or a preperiosteal tissue lift can be done. For advanced cases associated with a lower lid retraction, a subperiosteal approach is preferred.

Other minimally invasive techniques available for the midface lift include endoscopic elevation of the soft tissues and fixing it to a higher point at the periosteum. To keep the tissues anchored to the underlying periosteum either the threading technique or the endotine technique may be used. Threading is a simple technique in which the ptotic mid facial tissues are held in its new position by "barbed threads" that provide the lift. The effects may not last very long with threading and there may be complications like "cheese-wiring" of the threads through the skin, whereas the endotine is a biodegradable suspension device that can be used endoscopically to anchor the facial soft tissues in the desired place till the healing takes place, after which the tissues remain fixed at the desired point of suspension for a longer duration. Thus, this technique provides effective minimally invasive mid face lift lasting for a longer duration.

Liposculpture: A technique in which the autologous fat is injected into the volume deficit areas of the mid face can also be done. As it addresses the volume deficiency associated with the aging face, this technique can also be used.

BROW PTOSIS CORRECTION

- Introduction
- Etiopathogenesis
- Preoperative assessment
- Treatment
  - Medical
  - Surgical
- Complications

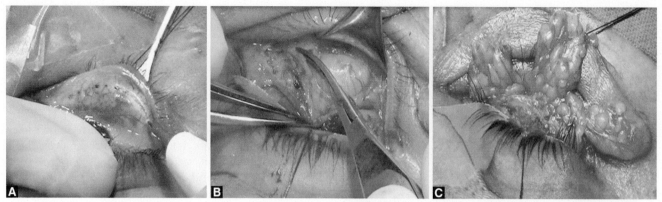

Figs. 12A to C: Steps of lower lid blepharoplasty: (A) Incision over the conjunctiva; (B) Incision over the orbital septum to expose underlying fat pads; (C) Exposure of the medial, central, and lateral fat pads.

Introduction

Eyebrows are situated in a strategic part of upper third of the face with a prominent role in facial expression and cosmetic appearance. The position of the eyebrows provides a glimpse of mood and emotion of the person.

The ideal brow position has been described by many authors and is a matter of debate. Although, the simplest concept provided by Westmore[1] is as follows:

- The medial and lateral ends of the brow should be at approximately the same horizontal level
- The medial end of the ideal brow is club shaped and it gradually tapers laterally
- The apex of the brow curve should lie directly above the lateral limbus
- The medial brow should be on the same vertical plane as the lateral extent of the nasal ala and the inner canthus
- The lateral end should be at an oblique line from the most lateral point of the nasal ala and the outer canthus.

Beside this, Ellenbogen added that in women the brow should arch above the supraorbital rim, whereas in men it should arch along the rim. So any age related changes that disturbs this anatomical relationship would lead to cosmetic alterations in the brow region, which would warrant a correction. The correction of brow ptosis can lead to a dramatic cosmetic improvement.

Etiopathogenesis

- Age-related changes of periorbital and facial soft tissues
  - The eyebrow position becomes lower due to involutional changes due to gravity, deflation of tissues and action of the depressors of the eyebrow (corrugator supercilii, the depressor supercilii, the procerus, and the orbicularis oculi muscles), along with the resorption of the underlying bone.

- Paralysis or weakness of the frontalis muscle
  - The frontal branch of the facial nerve innervates the frontalis muscle. This muscle is responsible for elevating the medial two-thirds of the brow. Therefore, any paralysis of the facial nerve will lead to brow ptosis mainly in the medial and central brow region.
- Involuntary contraction of the orbicularis oculi:
  - Blepharospasm
  - Facial dystonia.
- Mechanical causes:
  - Basal cell carcinoma
  - Squamous cell carcinoma
  - Keratoacanthoma
  - Melanoma.
- Miscellaneous:
  - Facial nerve palsy—Bell's palsy, acoustic neuroma, surgical trauma, birth trauma
  - Myasthenia gravis
  - Myotonic dystrophy
  - Oculopharyngeal dystrophy.

Preoperative Evaluation

History: The patient may complain of one or more of the following due to brow ptosis:
- Drooping of the upper eyelids
- Heaviness in the eye
- Foreign body sensation
- Restriction of upper-outer visual field
- Headache
- Tired appearance.

These complaints may be due to brow ptosis or associated upper eyelid dermatochalasis. Sometimes, severe dermatochalasis may mask the lateral brow ptosis;

so true eyelid and eyebrow position should be evaluated and noted. In such patients, combined approach of upper eyelid blepharoplasty with browlift or browpexy is useful. A complete and thorough ophthalmic examination is necessary along with extra notes on the following points:
- Position of eyebrow
- Mobility of eyebrow
- Frontalis overaction
- Position of hairline and prominence of frontal bone
- Position of the upper eyelid
- Degree of upper eyelid laxity
- Degree of excess upper eyelid skin
- Eyelid crease
- Palpebral apparatus
- Tear film assessment.

Management

After careful assessment and diagnosis, based on associated conditions and patient's choice, medical or surgical treatment can be planned.
- *Non-surgical treatment:*
  Botulinum toxin is a useful nonsurgical approach to correct the brow ptosis. It is injected into brow depressor muscles, leading to a chemical brow lift. This is particularly more convenient and effective in dysthyroid patients with medial brow ptosis and deep glabellar frown lines, which create an aggressive appearance. The botulinum injection can also be combined with dermal fillers in selected cases.
- *Surgical correction:*
  The surgical approaches for management of brow ptosis are:
  – Internal browpexy
  – External browplasty
  A browpexy is a suture suspension of the brow to the underlying frontal bone. It can be performed from within the eyelid (internal browpexy) or from a small incision above the brow (external browpexy).
  Various surgical approaches to browlift surgery have been described.
- *Direct Browlift*
  – This simple technique is more suitable for older patients who have severe drooping of the brow or facial nerve palsy. It provides a long lasting result with excellent correction
  – The temporal direct brow lift poses no risk to the supraorbital and supratrochlear nerves
  – The only disadvantage is a resultant scar, especially in younger patients. Although, this is usually not a

problem in old age as the scar is well hidden within the natural crease.

Surgical procedure:

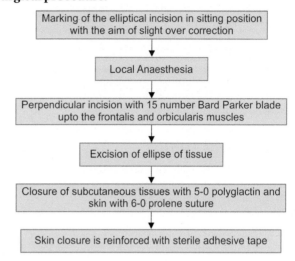

- *Transblepharoplasty browpexy:*
  – In this procedure, browpexy is combined with blepharoplasty. A browpexy is a suspension of the retro orbicularis fat and brow tissue to the underlying periosteum of the supraorbital frontal bone
  – It can be performed from within the eyelid (internal browpexy) or from a small incision above the brow (external browpexy)
  – It mainly prevents or stabilizes the brow rather than providing a significant lift.

Other techniques are:
- Gull-wing direct brow lift
- Mid forehead brow lift
- Temporal brow lift
- Transblepharoplasty brow lift
- Pretrichial brow lift
- Coronal brow lift
- Endoscopic brow lift.

Endoscopy brow lift: Endoscopic brow lift has become widely accepted as a procedure for restoring a youthful brow, as only three, hardly noticeable incisions of the scalp are needed for this subperiosteal dissection and final repositioning of the brow.

Complications

- Facial nerve trauma
- Sensory nerve trauma
- Hematoma
- Scarring
- Alopecia.

ACKNOWLEDGMENT

The authors would like to acknowledge and thank Dr. Harsha Bhattacharjee Medical director and Trustee Sri Sankaradeva Nethralaya, Guwahati, for being a constant source of inspiration and support throughout.

REFERENCE

1. Westmore M. Facial cosmetics in conjunction with surgery. In: Proceedings of the Aesthetic Plastic Surgical Society Meeting. Vancouver, British Columbia; 1974.

SUGGESTED READING

1. Basic and Clinical Science Course, Section 7: Orbit, eyelids, and lacrimal system. San Francisco, CA: American Academy of Ophthalmology; 2014. pp. 230-4.
2. Bhattacharjee K, Misra DK, Deori N. Updates on upper eyelid blepharoplasty. Indian J Ophthalmol. 2017;65(7):551.
3. Booth AJ, Murray A, Tyers AG. The direct brow lift: Efficacy, complications, and patient satisfaction. Br J Ophthalmol. 2004;88(5):688-91.
4. Cohen BD, Reiffel AJ, Spinelli HM. Browpexy through the upper lid (BUL): A new technique of lifting the brow with a standard blepharoplasty incision. Aesthet Surg J. 2011;31(2):163-9.
5. Czyz C, Burns JA, Petrie TP, et al. Long-term botulinum toxin treatment of benign essential blepharospasm, hemifacial spasm, and meige syndrome. Am J Ophthalmol. 2013;156(1):173-7.e2.
6. Dutton JJ, Fowler AM. Botulinum toxin in ophthalmology. Surv Ophthalmol. 2007;52(1):13-31.
7. Lipham W, Melicher J. Cosmetic and clinical applications of botox and dermal fillers.
8. Park J, Yun S, Son D. Changes in eyebrow position and movement with aging. Arch Plast Surg. 2017;44(1):65-71.
9. Pascali M, Bocchini I, Avantaggiato A, et al. Our experience with brow ptosis correction: A comparison of 4 techniques. Plast Reconstr Surg Glob Open. 2015;3(3):e337.

Lacrimal System

- Embryology, Anatomy and Physiology of Lacrimal Secretory and Drainage System
- Evaluation and Abnormalities of Lacrimal Secretory and Drainage System
- Lacrimal Surgeries
- Recent Advances in Dacryology

Embryology, Anatomy and Physiology of Lacrimal Secretory and Drainage System

Mohit Chhabra, Ruchi Goel

INTRODUCTION

The lacrimal apparatus comprises of structures involved in secretion and transport of tears from the lacrimal gland in the orbit to the end of the nasolacrimal duct.

- The secretory system comprises of the main and accessory lacrimal glands, conjunctival goblet cells and crypts of Henle
- The excretory system comprises of osseous and soft tissue components from the lacrimal punctum to the nasolacrimal duct.

EMBRYOLOGY

The lacrimal gland as well as the epithelial lining of the lacrimal apparatus is derived from the surface ectoderm. The development begins at 22–25 mm stage of the embryo.

- The ectodermal epithelium of the superolateral conjunctival fornix proliferates and gives rise to a series of tubular buds at around 2nd month of fetal life. The buds are arranged into:
  - Lacrimal gland proper
  - Palpebral processes of the lacrimal gland
- The lacrimal sac, nasolacrimal duct and canaliculi develop from the ectoderm of the nasomaxillary groove extending from the lateral nasal process to the maxillary process of the developing face
  - *5 weeks of gestation:* An ectodermal invagination forms between lateral nasal process and maxillary process, that becomes pinched off from the surface (Fig. 1A)
  - *6 weeks of gestation:* A solid cord is formed between primitive medial canthus and nose (Fig. 1B)
  - *12 weeks of gestation:* Latero-inferior proliferation of cord (Fig. 1C)

- *3–4 months of gestation:* Cavities appear within the solid cord
- *7th month of gestation:* Canalization nearly complete (Fig. 1D)
- The upper part of the developing ectoderm forms the lacrimal sac.
- Ectodermal buds arising from the medial margins of the eyelids are canalized to form the canaliculi
- During the 5th month of life developing tendon of the levator palpebrae superioris (LPS) cuts the gland into two parts—early buds forming the orbital portion and secondary buds forming the palpebral portion.

ANATOMY

Secretory System

The secretory system is responsible for tear production, both basal and reflex.

A. Basal tear production:
  - *Meibomian glands, glands of Zeiss and Moll:* Lipid layer
  - *Accessory lacrimal glands of Krause and Wolfring:* Aqueous layer
  - *Conjunctival goblet cells and crypts of Henle:* Mucoid layer
B. Reflex tear production:
  - Main lacrimal gland.

Meibomian Glands

- Modified sebaceous glands
- *Location:* Present in the posterior part of the stroma of the tarsal plates

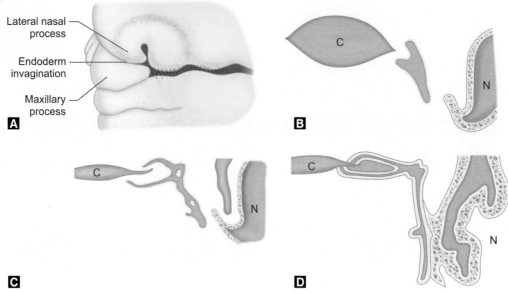

Figs. 1A to D: Development of lacrimal excretory system. N—nasal cavity; C—conjunctival fornix.

- Arranged vertically in a single row, parallel to each other
- Openings are located along the lid margins between the gray line and posterior border of the lid
- Approximately 20–30 in the upper lid, 10 in the lower lid.
- *Histology:* Branched acinar glands with 10–15 acini opening into a long central duct
  - Acini are lined by glandular epithelium
  - Ducts are lined by keratinized squamous epithelium.

Glands of Zeiss

- Modified sebaceous glands
- *Location:* Directly attached to eyelid follicles, usually 2 per cilium
- *Histology:* Acini lined by actively dividing cuboidal cells on a basement membrane.

Glands of Moll

- Modified sweat glands
- 2 mm long, unbranched, spiral glands which lie between the eyelashes
- More in lower lid than in upper lid
- *Parts:* Fundus, body, ampulla, neck
- *Histology:* Glands and their ducts are lined by myoepithelial cells. The secretory portion is lined by columnar cells containing secretory granules.

Accessory Lacrimal Glands (Fig. 2)

- *Glands of Krause:* Subconjunctival microscopic glands in the fornices (40–42 in upper lid and 6–8 in lower lid)

- *Glands of Wolfring:* Microscopic glands located along the upper border and lower border of the upper and lower tarsus, respectively (2–4 in each lid)
- Other accessory glands include infra-orbital glands and glands of the plica and caruncle.

Conjunctival Goblet Cells

- Present in the entire conjunctiva except at the grey line and limbus
- Holocrine glands
- Maximum in inferonasal fornix and bulbar conjunctiva
- Decrease in number with age and increase in inflammation
- Loss of these cells leads to xerosis
- *Crypts of Henle:* Folds of palpebral conjunctiva between the tarsus and the fornix
- *Glands of Manz:* Existence in humans is controversial, present in limbal conjunctiva in animals.

Main Lacrimal Gland

- *Location:* Fossa glandulae lacrimalis of the frontal bone (superotemporal orbit)
- *Parts:* Gland is divided into orbital and palpebral lobes by the lateral horn of the LPS.
Both lobes are continuous posteriorly.
- *Histology:* Modified mucous gland, covered by simple fascia and no true capsule
- *Orbital Part:*
  - 20 mm × 12 mm × 5 mm almond shaped part conforming to the space between orbital wall and the globe. Two surfaces, two borders and two extremities

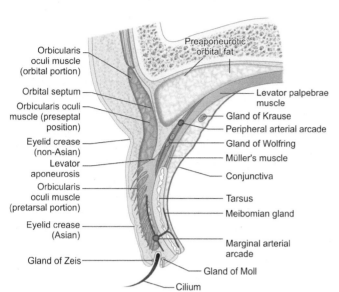

Fig. 2: Section of lid showing accessory lacrimal glands.

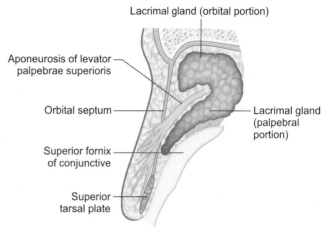

Fig. 3: Lacrimal gland is divided into orbital and palperbral lobes by the lateral horn of the levator palpebrae superioris.

– Superior surface is attached (via fine trabeculae) to the periorbita lining the fossa for the lacrimal gland in the frontal bone
– Inferior surface lies on the LPS and lateral horn of levator aponeurosis
– Anterior border runs parallel to the orbital margin and is bound in front by the orbital septum, preaponeurotic fat, orbicularis and skin
– Posterior border is in contact with orbital fat and is continuous with the palpebral part of the lacrimal gland
– Lateral extremity is in contact with the lateral rectus
– Medial extremity is related to the LPS and intermuscular septum between superior rectus (SR) and lateral rectus (LR) (Fig. 3).
- *Palpebral part:*
  – Smaller, flatter, lying underneath the levator aponeurosis in the sub-aponeurotic space of Jones
  – Related to the superior fornix inferiorly and continuous with the orbital part posteriorly
  – It is secured by the conjunctiva and inter-muscular membranes below, lacrimal fascia linking it to the Whitnall's ligament and by the surrounding LPS horn
  – Disruption of the Whitnall's ligament during LPS surgery may lead to lacrimal gland prolapse.
- *Lacrimal gland ducts:*
  – 10–12 ducts pass from the main gland into the superotemporal conjunctival fornix. Few ducts also drain inferotemporally
  – Ducts from the orbital part pass via the palpebral part. Hence palpebral dacryoadenectomy interrupts the drainage of the orbital part as well.

- *Fascial supports:*
  – Sommering's ligament—superior surface to the periosteum
  – LPS and lateral levator aponeurosis
  – Whitnall's ligament/superior transverse ligament—main support, pass through the orbital part and insert on the roof of the orbit
  – Inferior ligament of Schwalbe—associated with the lacrimal artery and nerve and passes under the posterior lip of the gland.
- *Histopathology:*
  – Branched tubulo-alveolar gland containing acini draining into ducts and divided into lobules by septa
  – Acini are serous and lined by myoepithelial cells and secretory columnar cells
  – Ducts are lined by inner cylindrical cells and outer flat cells
  – Stroma is mesodermal with connective tissue, blood vessels, nerve terminals, and lymphatics.
- *Arterial supply:*

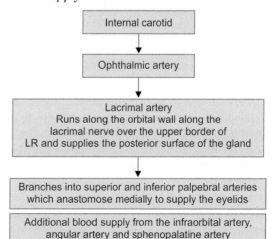

The autonomic innervation of the lacrimal gland.

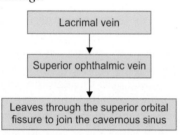

Fig. 4: Autonomic innervation of lacrimal gland.

- *Venous drainage:*

```
Lacrimal vein
     ↓
Superior ophthalmic vein
     ↓
Leaves through the superior orbital
fissure to join the cavernous sinus
```

- *Lymphatic drainage:* Preauricular LN.
- *Nerve Supply (Fig. 4):*
  - *Sensory:* Lacrimal branch of the ophthalmic division of the trigeminal nerve
  - *Sympathetic:* Sympathetic plexus from superior cervical ganglion responsible for basal secretion
  - *Parasympathetic:* Secretomotor fibers from the lacrimatory nucleus (pons).

Excretory System (Fig. 5)

Osteology

- Lower part of medial orbital margin contains the "lacrimal fossa" (different from fossa for the lacrimal gland). 16 mm × 8 mm × 2 mm (H × W × D)
  Formed by: Anteriorly—anterior lacrimal crest (frontal process of maxillary bone) and posteriorly—posterior lacrimal crest (lacrimal bone).
- A *maxillary lacrimal suture* runs between the crests and its position varies depending upon which bone is dominant in forming the fossa floor. This knowledge of anatomical variation carries significance during dacryocystorhinostomy (DCR) surgery
- The *anterior lacrimal crest* continues as the inferior orbital rim inferiorly, attaches to the medial canthal

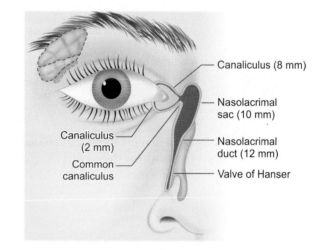

Fig. 5: Lacrimal excretory system.

tendon superiorly and gives rise to the lacrimal fascia posteriorly
- The *posterior lacrimal crest* terminates at the start of the nasolacrimal duct (NLD) inferiorly, gives attachment to Horner's muscle (pretarsal deep head of the orbicularis) superiorly and insertion to the orbital septum posteriorly
- The lacrimal fossa continues inferiorly into the osseous part of the *nasolacrimal canal*. It comprises of the maxillary bone anterolaterally and lacrimal bone posteromedially
- Since the maxillary bone develops before the lacrimal bone in the embryonal stages, it may sometimes have a greater contribution to the medial nasolacrimal canal, leading to a *physiologically narrow NLD*. Females also have a relatively narrower NLD compared to males, leading to greater incidence of chronic dacryocystitis in females.

Lacrimal Puncta

- Small oval opening at medial end of each lid, at the junction of ciliary and lacrimal portion of the lid margin
- Located atop the lacrimal papilla of Arruga
- Upper puncta lies 6 mm lateral to inner canthus and lower puncta lies 6.5 mm lateral to the inner canthus. Thus, the puncta does not overlap when the eyes close
- The posterior pull of the Horner's muscle causes posteriorly directed puncta, hence requiring lid eversion to examine them
- Surrounding rim of fibrous tissue keeps the puncta patent to diameter up to 0.4 mm.

Lacrimal Canaliculi

- Join the upper and lower puncta to the lacrimal sac.
- Usually buried within the orbicularis muscle
- 0.5–1.0 mm in diameter but highly variable due to elasticity
- 2 mm vertical part followed by 8 mm horizontal part at right angles, with an ampulla at the junction
- Horizontal parts converge and join after piercing the lacrimal fascia to form the common canaliculus (4 mm long) which opens into the lacrimal sinus of Maier, which is a small diverticulum of the lacrimal sac. At this opening, the valve of Rosenmuller prevents reflux from sac to puncta
- *Anatomical variation:* 10% of the population has separate openings for the canaliculi into the sac.

Lacrimal Sac

- *Three parts:*
  - *Fundus:* 3–5 mm above the opening of the canaliculi
  - *Body:* 10–12 mm
  - *Neck:* Lower narrow part which continues into the NLD.
- *Relations:*
  - *Medially:* Periorbita and bone, anterior ethmoidal cells and middle meatus of the nose
  - *Anterolaterally:* (from deep to superficial) Lacrimal fascia, Horner's muscle, medial palpebral ligament (MPL), orbicularis fibers, angular vein and skin
    - Sac distention always occurs inferiorly as the MPL covering the superior part prevents distention. Hence lacrimal abscess and fistulae open below the MPL owing to lesser resistance
    - Angular vein crosses MPL 8 mm medial to the medial canthus with the occasional tributary between the vein and canthus. Hence DCR incision should be made in the 3–8 mm zone from the medial canthus

  - *Posteriorly:* (from anterior to posterior) Lacrimal fascia, orbicularis fibers, orbital septum and check ligaments of MR muscle. Hence the sac is a preseptal structure.

Nasolacrimal Duct

- 15–24 mm long, 3–7 mm in diameter. Two parts—bony (12.5 mm); intrameatal (2–5 mm)
- Opens into the inferior meatus of the nose 30–40 mm from the anterior nares
- Upper end is the narrowest and not adherent to the bone unlike the lower parts
- NLD travels downward, backward and laterally, represented externally by a line joining the inner canthus with the ala of the nose
- Numerous mucosal folds known as valves are present (Fig. 6)
- Histology shows a transition from the stratified squamous epithelium of the canaliculi to the fibrous coat and columnar epithelium of the sac to the fibrous wall and erectile venous plexus of the NLD. Engorgement of these plexus may lead to blockage.

Vascular Supply of the Lacrimal Passage

- *Arterial supply:* Superior and inferior palpebral branches of the ophthalmic artery, angular artery, infraorbital artery and nasal branches of the sphenopalatine artery
- *Venous drainage:* Angular and infraorbital vein from above, nasal vein from below
- *Lymphatics:* Submandibular and deep cervical lymph nodes.

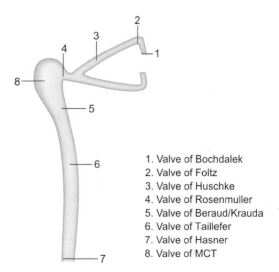

1. Valve of Bochdalek
2. Valve of Foltz
3. Valve of Huschke
4. Valve of Rosenmuller
5. Valve of Beraud/Krauda
6. Valve of Taillefer
7. Valve of Hasner
8. Valve of MCT

Fig. 6: Valves in lacrimal excretory system.

Nerve Supply of the Lacrimal Passage

- *Sensory:* Infratrochlear branch of the nasociliary nerve (V1) and anterior superior alveolar branch of the maxillary nerve (V2)
- Reflex relation between the sac and the gland is responsible for reduced tear production after sac removal and may play a role in decreased symptoms after DCT surgery.

PHYSIOLOGY

The Tear Film

Structure

- Wolff in 1946 coined the term precorneal film and assumed that it consists of three layers which still holds good (Fig. 7)
- A six-layered model was suggested by Tiffany who included three layers and three interfaces
- *Lipid layer:*
  - Outermost layer
  - Derived from meibomian, Zeiss and Moll glands
  - Thickness is 0.1–0.2 μm, varies on palpebral fissure width
  - Chemically contains both polar and nonpolar lipids. Polar lipids face the aqueous layer and the nonpolar lipids face the air

- Secretion of lipid layer is controlled by androgen sex hormones and neurotransmitters surrounding the glands
- Main function is to retard evaporation of tears and prevent their overflow
- Provides a smooth surface for uniform optical function
- It also acts as a surfactant, lubricant and barrier for preventing contamination.

- *Aqueous layer:*
  - Middle layer, 60% of the tear film
  - Derived from main and accessory lacrimal glands.
  - Thickness is 7–8 μm
  - Chemically comprises of an aqueous solution of low viscosity containing salts, glucose, enzymes, proteins, immunoglobulins, lysozyme and tear-specific prealbumin
  - Presence of both bicarbonate ions and proteins provides buffering capacity
  - Tonicity varies with tear flow rate, i.e. hypertonic at low flow rates and isotonic at high flow rates
  - Main functions include providing oxygen to cornea, washing away debris and noxious molecules
  - Also functions as an antibacterial layer due to immunoglobulins, lysozymes and betalysin.

- *Mucous layer:*
  - Innermost layer

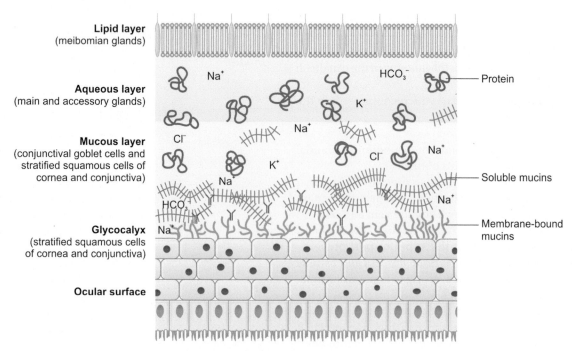

Fig. 7: Structure of tear film.

- Derived from conjunctival goblet cells and crypts of Henle
- Thickness is 0.02–0.05 um
- Contains two types of mucin—aqueous soluble and membrane adherent
- Current concept of the tear film eliminates the need of three layers and simply divides the tear film into a lipid layer and an aqueous-mucinous phase
- Mucin converts the hydrophobic corneal surface into a hydrophilic one that allows complete wetting of the cornea
- Also acts as a lubricating layer and a protective barrier against the ill effects of foreign bodies by providing them with a slippery coating to minimize abrasive effects (Table 1).

Tear Film Dynamics

The primary role of the tear film is to establish a high quality and protective refractive surface over the ocular surface.

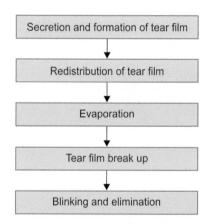

- *Tear secretion:* 95% of all full-term infants achieve normal tear secretion by the age of 1 week. However, low innervation of the cornea results in lower reflex stimulation. Various layers of the tear film are secreted by different glands (discussed before)

TABLE 1: Tear film properties.

Thickness	7–8 μm
Volume	4–13 μL
Rate of secretion	1.2 μL/min
Refractive index	1.357
pH	7.3–7.7
Na⁺/K⁺	140/25 mEq/L
Glucose	3–10 mg/100 mL

- *Formation of the precorneal tear film:* The lids surface the cornea with the mucus layer while blinking. The aqueous component spreads spontaneously over the film and finally the lipid layer spreads over to increase stability and reduce evaporation
- *Tear film retention:* Due to its structure, the tear film is retained despite its vertical configuration and downward gravitational pull. A marginal strip of tear fluid helps in constant flow and redistribution of tears
- *Tear film evaporation:* Lipid layer retards evaporation. It is estimated to be 10% of the secretion rate
- *Tear film break up:* When blinking is prevented, the tear film ruptures after around 15 seconds followed by dry spots on the cornea. Thinning of the aqueous layer causes lipid molecules to be attracted to the mucin layer, making it hydrophobic and causing the tear film to rupture (Fig. 8)
- *Tear elimination:* 25% of the tears are lost by evaporation and rest are drained via lacrimal apparatus (Figs. 9A to D)
  - *On eyelid closure:* Contraction of pretarsal orbicularis compresses the ampulla and shortens the canaliculi. This propels the tear present in the ampulla toward the lacrimal sac. The preseptal fibers also contract to pull the lacrimal sac laterally and produce a negative pressure in it to draw tears from the canaliculi
  - *On eyelid opening:* Relaxation of pretarsal orbicularis allows canaliculi to expand and open, drawing the lacrimal fluid through the puncti from the lacus lacrimalis. The preseptal fibers also relax, causing the lacrimal sac to collapse, expelling the lacrimal fluid downward into the NLD and finally into the nasal cavity. Flow of tears along the NLD is influenced by:
    - Gravity
    - Air current within the nasal cavity
    - Hasner's valve.

Lacrimal Pump Theory

Old theory (Jones):
- *Contraction phase:* Nasal shift of canaliculi and compression of Horner's muscle causing lacrimal sac to be pulled laterally, pulling tears from the shortened canaliculus
- *Relaxation phase:* Opening up of the canaliculi and collapse of the lacrimal sac.

New theory (Doanes):
- *Contraction phase:* Closure of the eye causes the puncta to meet and occlude, causing the canaliculi and sac to empty into NLD
- *Relaxation phase:* Puncta and passages open causing tears to flow into the sac.

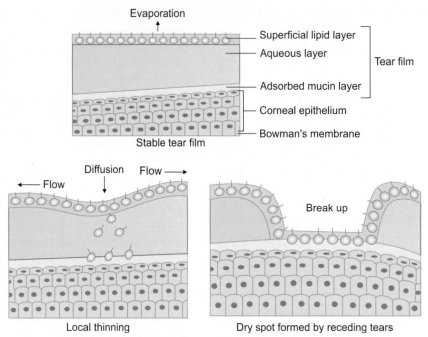

Fig. 8: Tear film break up on blinking.

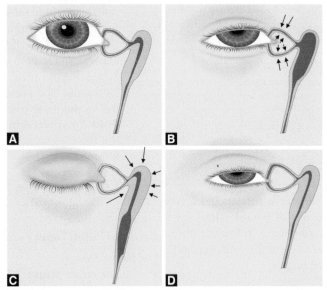

Figs. 9A to D: Schematic of the lacrimal pump: (A) In between the blinks, the lids are open and the lacrimal canaliculi are filled with tears; (B) *Lid closure:* In the early phase of the blink, the pretarsal orbicularis muscle and Riolan muscle contract causing canalicular shortening and pushing the tears into the lacrimal sac; (C) During the late phase of the blink deep pretarsal orbicularis muscle (Horner–Duverney muscle) and preseptal orbicularis contract leading to compression of lacrimal sac pushing the tears into the NLD; (D) The lid reopening phase marks the end of the blink. The orbicularis compression ceases, negative pressure is created inside the ampulla and canaliculi, and tears enter the canaliculi.

SUMMARY

To conclude, lacrimal apparatus consists of excretory and secretory system. It develops from surface ectoderm. The aqueous layer of the tear film is secreted by the lacrimal and the accessory lacrimal gland. The tears are eliminated by evaporation and drainage through the lacrimal excretory system.

Evaluation and Abnormalities of Lacrimal Secretory and Drainage System

Sumit Kumar, Ruchi Goel

INTRODUCTION

Watering is the commonest presentation of disorders of lacrimal drainage system.

Patients with complain of tearing can be grossly divided into two groups (Table 1).

Those with:
1. Hypersecretion of tears (lacrimation)
2. Impairment of drainage (epiphora).

A detailed history and examination is performed to decide the further course of management.

CLINICAL HISTORY

History of Present Illness

- *Duration*—congenital/acquired
- Does the eye feel wet, or does the patient need to wipe their cheek as the tears spill on to it?

TABLE 1: Causes of tearing.

Causes of tearing		
Lacrimation (hypersecretion)	Epiphora (decreased tear elimination)	
	Anatomic factors	Physiologic factors
Corneal foreign bodies	Strictures	Orbicularis muscle weakness (lacrimal pump failure)
Refractive errors	Obstruction	
Corneal irritation with dry spots	Foreign bodies	
Thyroid dysfunction	Tumors	Punctal and eyelid malpositions
Ocular surface inflammation		Nasal obstruction with normal lacrimal pathway
Nasal irritation and inflammation		

- Is there irritation on wiping?
- How often do they need to wipe their eyes?
- Is the vision blurred?
- Unilateral/bilateral
- Aggravating/alleviating factors
- Constant versus intermittent tearing
- Seasonal/environmental allergy
  Allergic rhinitis → edema of the nasal mucosa → obstruction of the outflow pathway → epiphora
- *Associated symptoms*—pain, redness, discharge, glare, photophobia, itchiness, foreign body sensation, and burning
  - Pain:
    - *Pain at the site of lacrimal sac:* Rule out acute dacryocystitis
    - Pain in the eye may be due to foreign body, keratitits, recurrent corneal erosions, iritis, or glaucoma
  - Itching is suggestive of allergic phenomenon
  - Grittiness and burning may be due to tear film instability (keratitis sicca/thyroid eye disease)
- History of bloody tears could be due to malignancy.

History of Past Illness

- History of probing during childhood
- Prior surgical history:
  - Lid/lacrimal surgery
  - Sinus surgery
- Lid/facial trauma
- History of Bell's palsy → aberrant regeneration of facial nerve can result in tearing while chewing

- Systemic diseases:
  - *Immunologic disorders:* Thyroid disease, rheumatic arthritis
  - *Inflammatory disorders:* Sarcoid, Wegeners
- History of medication which can cause punctal and/or canalicular obstruction
  - Topical antivirals
  - Echothiophate iodide (phospholine iodide), pilocarpine, epinephrine
  - Antiglaucoma therapy
  - *Systemic chemotherapy:* Docetaxel (commonly used in treating breast cancer and can result in epiphora by causing canalicular stenosis)
- History of orbital irradiation, treatment with radioactive iodine (I^{131}) for thyroid carcinoma.

PHYSICAL EXAMINATION

- *Lid examination:*
  - *Lid tone:* Poor orbicularis tone (either due to aging or seventh nerve dysfunction) leads to:
    - Lacrimal pump dysfunction
    - Rapid tear breakup, corneal irritation, and reflex tearing due to incomplete blinking.
  - Orbicularis oculi function should be assessed by examining strength of forced voluntary closure of the lids and lid tone, and snap-back test
  - Poor orbicularis muscle tone may be presumed if the lid can be pulled more than 6 mm away from the globe, decreased snap back
  - *Lid position:*
    - *Ectropion* Leads to abnormality in drainage of tears
      Entropion Leads to reflex tearing due to irritation of ocular surface.
    - *Lid retraction* Increases exposure and tear evaporation may lead to reflex tearing.
- *Lacrimal passages:* Medial canthal area is examined for any mass—
  - *Dacryocystitis:* Visible or palpable fullness of the lacrimal sac, erythema of the overlying skin, and/or reflux of mucus, or exudate from the lacrimal punctum on palpation
  - *Lacrimal sac tumors and mucoceles* may also present as palpable masses in the region of the medial canthus. Unlike dacryocystitis, these entities may extend above the medial canthal tendon.
- *Nasal examination:*
  Proper nasal examination using high powered light source and nasal speculum is an essential part of every lacrimal evaluation to rule out any mucosal

inflammation, nasal mass, hypertrophy of turbinates, and adhesions between septum and lateral wall of nose.

Slit-Lamp Examination

- *Tear film*
  - *Tear volume:* Very low tear volumes with watering raises the possibility of reflex tearing in the setting of dry eye
  - *Tear break up time:* Normal tear breakup time is 15–30 seconds
    Tear breakup time of less than 10 seconds indicates dry eye syndrome resulting reflex hypersecretion.
  - *Tear meniscus level:* Normal tear meniscus height is ~0.2 mm which may increase up to ~0.6 mm in patients with nasolacrimal duct obstruction
  - Presence of debris/exudates
- *Punctum*
  - Size
  - Position in relation to tear lake
  - Discharge
  - Inflammation
  - Kissing puncta—condition in which upper and lower puncta come in contact with each other preventing tear outflow
- *Caruncle*—megalo-caruncle can cause epiphora by occluding the opening to the punctum or by displacing the punctum away from globe
- *Conjunctiva*:
  - Signs of inflammation:
    - Chemosis and/or injection
    - Follicles
    - Papillae
  - Conjunctivochalasis—a condition of unknown etiology in which redundant conjunctiva may drape over and cover the punctum, preventing tear outflow
  - Foreign body
- *Cornea*—look for any subtle surface abnormalities
- *Anterior chamber*—rule out uveitis.

CLINICAL DIAGNOSTIC TESTS

Secretory Tests

Schirmer's Test

Schirmer testing is essential in evaluating the tearing patient to establish whether severe dry eye is the cause of tearing.

The Schirmer I test: To evaluate gross tear production (basic and reflex tear production):
- Performed without topical anesthetic
- The tear lake is wiped from the conjunctiva before inserting the paper strips, to prevent excessive degree of wetting

- A strip of #41 Whatman filter paper, 50 mm long and 5 mm wide, is folded 5 mm from one end, and the small folded end is placed into the inferior conjunctival fornix at the junction of the lateral and middle thirds of the lower eyelid
- The amount of wetting on the filter paper is measured at 5 minutes
- The test should be performed in subdued lighting, and both eyes must be tested simultaneously
- *Disadvantage:* The paper itself may stimulate reflex lacrimation
  Normal value: 10–30 mm at 5 minutes, with values more than 15 mm typical of patients younger than age 40 and at least 10 mm or less in those older than age 40.
- If the Schirmer I test is abnormal, the test may be modified to separate the reflex component from basic secretion.
  Basic secretion test: A drop of topical anesthetic is instilled into the eye and the test is repeated. This test must be performed in the dark, because light can stimulate reflex tearing.
  Normal values: Basal secretion is expected to be 10 mm in a normal patient younger than 40 years and at least 5 mm in a patient older than 40 years.

Schirmer II test: For stressed reflex capability
- When Schirmer I test results are below normal
- Topical anesthetic is used in the eye, and the nasal mucosa is stimulated mechanically with a cotton swab or chemically with ammonium chloride
- The amount by which the Schirmer II test exceeds basic production represents stressed reflex secretion.

Excretory Tests

Dye Disappearance Test

The dye disappearance test is usually performed as part of the primary Jones dye test (Jones I test). It is a rudimentary measurement of the rate of tear flow out of the conjunctival sac.
- One drop of 2% sodium fluorescein is instilled in the lower conjunctival fornix
- The volume of the tear lake is then noted with a cobalt blue-filtered light
- The amount remaining at 5 minutes is graded on a 0 to 4+ scale, with 0 representing no dye remaining and 4+ representing all the dye remaining
- Both sides are compared simultaneously.

Interpretation of result:
- *Positive test:* Little or no fluorescein remaining in the conjunctival sac indicating probable normal drainage outflow

- *Negative test:* Most or all of the dye remaining indicates partial or complete obstruction or pump failure.

Disadvantage: Site of lacrimal drainage obstruction cannot be determined.

Primary Jones Dye Test

This test differentiates partial obstruction of the lacrimal passages and lacrimal pump failure from primary hypersecretion of tears.

Steps:
1. The patient should be in an upright position and should blink normally.
2. A drop of 2% fluorescein is instilled into the conjunctival sac.
3. A fine cotton-tipped applicator moistened in local anesthetic is passed beneath the inferior turbinate to the level of the nasolacrimal ostium after 2 minutes and again after 5 minutes.

Interpretation of results (Figs. 1A and B):
- *Positive test:* Retrieval of dye is a "positive" test, and establishes that neither an anatomic nor functional blockage is present within the lacrimal drainage system
- *Negative test:* This indicates either a partial obstruction or failure of lacrimal pump mechanism.

Disadvantage: High false-negative rate, i.e. dye is commonly not recovered even in presence of a functionally patent drainage system.

Modifications:
- *Flach modification* of the primary Jones dye test:
  - It is designed to avoid the difficulty and variability involved in recovering dye from the inferior meatus
  - 2% fluorescein is placed in the conjunctival sac and the oropharynx is examined with ultraviolet light, beginning at 5 minutes and continuing up to 1 hour if necessary
  - With this technique, 90% of normal individuals are said to show oropharyngeal fluorescence within 30 minutes and 100% within 60 minutes
  - This procedure is best used as a supplement to a negative primary Jones test and can be performed 20–30 minutes later
- *Hornblass* variation of the primary Jones dye test:
  - 0.4 mL of 1% sterile solution of sodium saccharin is instilled into the conjunctival sac and the patient is asked to report when he or she tastes the solution
  - Hornblass found a mean transit time to the nose of 3.5 minutes, with 65% of normal individuals reporting a positive test within 6 minutes and 90% reporting positive results within 15 minutes

– Transit times in excess of 15 minutes suggest partial nasolacrimal duct obstruction.

Secondary Jones Dye Test

This test indicates in patients with negative primary Jones dye test to differentiate anatomic patency of the system or lacrimal pump failure.

- Topical anesthetic is instilled and any residual fluorescein is flushed out from the conjunctival sac.
- The drainage system is then irrigated with a cotton bud under the inferior turbinate.

Interpretation of results (Figs. 1C and D):

- *Positive:* Recovery of dye-stained saline demonstrates normal punctal and canalicular anatomy because the dye must have passed freely into the sac during the previous Jones I test. Partial obstruction distal of nasolacrimal duct distal to sac is inferred
- *Negative:* Recovery of clear saline without fluorescein suggests upper lacrimal (punctal or canalicular) dysfunction, which may be due to partial physical occlusion and/or pump failure.

Lacrimal Irrigation

Probing and irrigation help in detection and localization of obstruction in the lacrimal drainage outflow tract (canalicular, common canalicular, and nasolacrimal duct obstruction)

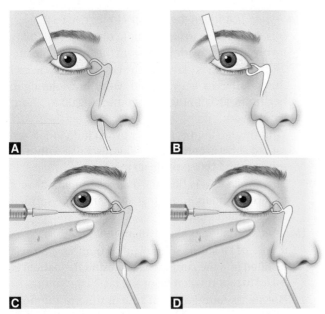

Figs. 1A to D: (A) Jones dye test 1 positive; (B) Jones dye test 1 negative; (C) Jones dye test 2 positive; (D) Jones dye test 2 negative.

Steps:
1. Topical anesthesia is instilled.
2. The punctum is gently dilated with a punctal dilator by advancing the tip vertically into the punctum with a gentle twisting motion for 2 mm.
3. The dilator is then rotated to a horizontal position (consistent with the course of the canaliculus) and the dilator is advanced slightly.
   Important: Lateral traction should always be applied to the eyelid during this maneuver to reduce the risk of creating a false passage.
4. The dilator is withdrawn and a lacrimal cannula on a syringe containing saline is advanced into the mid to distal canaliculus while maintaining lateral traction on the lid.
5. *Remaining too proximal in the canaliculus while irrigating may result in reflux during irrigation creating a false impression of obstruction.*
6. Irrigation then proceeds into the lacrimal drainage system
   Important: Irrigation should be performed gently.
   - As any forceful irrigation into the canaliculus may result in reflux from the opposite punctum causing the false impression that an obstruction is present
   - If a partial obstruction is present in the lacrimal drainage pathway, forceful irrigation may be able to overcome the partial blockage and lead the examiner to conclude that no obstruction is present.

Interpretation of results:
- Reflux from the same punctum in which the cannula is placed indicates canalicular obstruction
- Reflux from the opposite punctum indicates obstruction at the level of either the common canaliculus, the lacrimal sac, or the nasolacrimal duct
- Saline entering the nasopharynx documents anatomic patency of the lacrimal drainage system
- When partial obstruction exists, some of the saline will enter the nose while some will reflux from the opposite punctum
- Presence of mucus suggests nasolacrimal duct obstruction whereas clear fluid indicates common canalicular obstruction.

Probing: Probing helps to determine the site of obstruction.
Steps*:*
1. After punctal anesthesia and dilatation as described previously, a No. 00 Bowman probe is advanced into the canaliculus.
2. If an obstruction is encountered, the probe is grasped with forceps at its entrance to the punctum and then withdrawn.
   i. The distance from the forceps to the end of the probe gives the location of the canalicular obstruction.

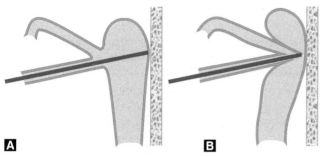

Figs. 2A and B: Probing: (A) Hard stop; (B) Soft stop.

Important: This is essential in guiding surgery to address the obstruction. For example, distal canalicular or common canalicular obstructions may be addressed by modifying standard dacryocystorhinostomy (DCR) surgical techniques. However, proximal or mid-canalicular obstruction typically requires placement of a Jones tube.

ii. Consistency of stop will also tell about nature of obstruction (Fig. 2).

   a. Nasolacrimal duct obstruction—"hard stop" when the probe encounters the medial wall of the lacrimal sac in the lacrimal sac fossa.

   b. Common canalicular obstruction—distal soft stop to passage of the probe.

3. Probing the nasolacrimal duct is painful and has no value in adults as either a diagnostic test or a therapeutic modality.

DIAGNOSTIC IMAGING

Diagnostic Ultrasonography

It is a simple, noninvasive method of evaluating gross anatomic abnormalities of the lacrimal drainage system. In the B-scan mode probe is oriented vertically, placed on the medial canthus, and aimed toward the lacrimal sac fossa, an oblique longitudinal cross-section of the lacrimal sac and upper duct is obtained.

Advantages:
- Helpful in differentiating the contents of lacrimal sac:
  - *Sac filled with air*—echolucent defect bound by sharply defined vertical anterior and posterior sac walls
  - *Mucus*—uniform, homogeneous, low-density internal echoes
  - *Inflammatory exudates and membranes*—stronger, more irregular echoes
  - *Tumors:* Multiple high-density, irregular echoes with infiltration of the sac walls suggest a sac tumor

- The diameter of the sac and upper duct may be evaluated and the thickness of the walls can often be appreciated.

Disadvantages: The canaliculi cannot usually be visualized unless they are dilated.

Contrast Dacryocystography

Gold standard for imaging of the nasolacrimal system, but it does not allow for imaging of the soft tissue or bony structures surrounding the nasolacrimal sac or duct. It is combined with CT and MRI to give complete picture of the nasolacrimal system and the surrounding anatomy.

Contrast material used:
- *Digital subtraction DCG*—aqueous contrast media such as sinografin and angiografin
- *Conventional DCG*—low-viscosity iodized oils such as Pantopaque, ethiodol, and ultrafluid lipiodol.

Steps of standard DCG:
1. Canaliculi are intubated with intravenous catheters and contrast material is injected into the lower canaliculus on each side, and films are taken immediately in Caldwell's posteroanterior frontal projection and in both lateral projections.
2. Repeat films are obtained at 5 and 15 minutes and upright films may be taken to evaluate the effects of gravity on lacrimal drainage.

Normal dacryocystogram:
- The dacryocystogram of a normal lacrimal drainage system will usually show the canaliculi when less viscous aqueous contrast media are used
- The sac appears as a smooth, straight, or gently curved passage with the concavity facing laterally
- The anteroposterior dimension is wider than the transverse. There is usually a constriction at the sac–duct junction caused by the split fascia of the orbicularis muscle as it passes around the system
- The duct widens at the level of the bony rim and its inner surface becomes more irregular because of the presence of mucosal folds, well developed in younger children
- Further constrictions are seen in the duct's midportion in the region of Hytle's and Taillefers' valves
- Finally, in its lower third, the duct widens again.

Interpretation of result:
- Imaging of the canaliculi with dye failing to pass into the sac or duct implies obstruction at the common canaliculus
- Obstruction at the sac–duct junction usually results in a dilated sac with no dye reaching the duct or nose, even on late films

- Obstruction at the level of the nasolacrimal duct will show dilatation of the sac, with dye in the duct, but not reaching the nose
- A patent dacryocystorhinostomy ostium is easily demonstrated by passage of contrast into the nose at the level of the middle meatus.

Computed Tomography

High resolution CT in the axial and coronal plane is a useful technique to assess the patients with disease in the structures adjacent to the nasolacrimal drainage pathways. When combined with DCG, CT scan is excellent at identifying bony structures around the nasolacrimal system.

Disadvantages:
- Inferior for evaluating soft tissue masses of the nasolacrimal system
- In standard CT, the images are presented as a series of axial images and make identification of small obstructions difficult
- Longitudinal and oblique images can be created, but this reconstruction results in decreased spatial resolution in the reformatted images
- The exposure to ionizing radiation is also more than for standard DCG.

Advantages:
- Relatively cheaper
- Good for study of bony details.

Magnetic Resonance Imaging

It as an adjunctive diagnostic test in the evaluation of lacrimal system pathology that allows for excellent resolution of the nasolacrimal system, especially when combined with a contrast agent, MRI offers several advantages over other imaging studies.

- Topical solution of gadolinium (Magnevist) diluted in 1:10 to 1:100 ratio with normal saline, is instilled one drop in each eye per minute for 5 minutes
- The patient is instructed to be in upright position until just before image acquisition.

Advantages:
- It gives a picture of the functional status of the nasolacrimal system
- No ocular complications from the administration of topical gadolinium
- No risk of exposure to ionizing radiation
- MRI allows very fine resolution of soft tissue structures within and surrounding the nasolacrimal system compared with dacryoscintigraphy, DCG, and even CT

- The superficial location of the nasolacrimal system facilitates imaging with small surface coils which can give a spatial resolution of 0.3 × 0.3 × 3 mm or better
- Allows for differentiation of mucous or blood from solid neoplasms
- Because of volumetric acquisition, magnetic resonance images can be viewed in any plane without degradation of the quality of images, compared to CT-DCG which requires reformatting of images that are out of plane and results in degradation of image resolution
- Coronal images are superior for determining the distal extent of contrast transit and axial images are excellent for examining the lumen of the nasolacrimal duct and intraductal pathology.

Disadvantages:
- Expensive
- Poor ability to image bony structures
- MRI is also susceptible to movement of artifacts because of the relatively long acquisition times required.

Radionuclide Dacryoscintigraphy (Lacrimal Scintillography)

Scintigraphy assesses tear drainage under more physiological conditions than DCG.

Rossomondo et al. introduced the first modern nuclear imaging technique for the lacrimal drainage system.

Steps:
1. A drop of saline with (99mTc) sodium pertechnetate is instilled into conjunctival sac, and a pinhole collimator of a gamma camera is used to record its transit to the nose.
2. The patient is advised to blink normally and the nasolacrimal system is imaged every 10 seconds for the first 2–3 minutes, and then late images are taken every 5 minutes for a total of 20 minutes.
3. The sac and duct are usually well-outlined.

Disadvantages:
- Proximal canalicular system is usually poorly imaged unless it is dilated
- Complete blocks in the sac or duct can be detected, but the precise localization of the obstruction may be difficult
- It is more sensitive to incomplete blocks than DCG especially in the upper system, but it does not provide the detailed anatomic visualization available with contrast DCG
- This technique is most accurate and reproducible for the upper lacrimal system, but at times becomes quite variable for the lower system, with 25–32% of asymptomatic individuals showing no tracer in the nose after 12 minutes.

Other Diagnostic Techniques

Percutaneous Contrast Dacryocystography

Routine DCG is not possible with complete common canalicular block, hence the concomitant presence of lower sac or duct pathology cannot be easily demonstrated unless echography is used to detect a dilated sac.

Putterman described a technique of percutaneous injection of aqueous contrast material directly into the lacrimal sac to bypass the occluded common canaliculus.

Chemiluminescence

It is a nonradiologic technique using luminescent agents such as *dimethylphthalate* and *tertiary butyl alcohol* activated by *dibutylphthalate*, which produce an intense cold light.

- When these agents are injected into the lacrimal system, the glow is visible through the skin and clearly outlines the upper system
- The lower duct is not readily demonstrated
- The compounds are safe and nontoxic, if confined within the lacrimal system, but extravasation into tissues or onto the globe can produce severe complications of corneal scarring and vascularization, purulent infection, granuloma formation, and fibrosis.

Lacrimal Thermography

The canaliculi and lacrimal sac have been visualized by thermography, using an infrared scanner and color monitor with a resolution of 0.5°C.

- The lacrimal system can be differentiated from surrounding tissues by irrigation with cold water
  - Decreased temperature in the nose demonstrates patency
  - A large dilated sac can be visualized, and persistent inflammation will produce increased temperature within the sac
  - The duct is not demonstrated with this method
- In a related technique, a mini-thermocouple probe has been used to detect temperature differences with the lacrimal sac
- Increased temperatures are seen with vascularity and inflammation, and decreased temperatures with hemorrhage and mucocele formation.

Nasolacrimal Endoscopy

Nasal endoscopy using rigid or flexible endoscope is useful to observe the anatomy of the opening of the nasal lacrimal duct in inferior meatus and to diagnose any nasal condition. Also helpful following lacrimal surgery to view the size and location of dacrycystorhinostomy opening and to determine the cause of ostium obstruction if present (fibrous tissue, polyp, granuloma, or foreign bodies).

ACQUIRED LACRIMAL DISORDERS

Acquired lacrimal drainage obstruction may be classified into primary or secondary.

- *Primary acquired nasolacrimal duct obstruction* results from inflammation of unknown cause that eventually leads to occlusive fibrosis
  - Female > male
  - The majority of acquired obstructions occuring in adulthood experience the onset of epiphora, typically after the age of 40, and subsequently develop signs and symptoms of chronic or acute dacryocystitis
- *Secondary acquired lacrimal drainage obstruction* is a term used to define all the secondary causes of lacrimal obstruction.

Bartley GB, et al. described five categories of secondary obstructions, namely:
1. Infectious
2. Inflammatory
3. Traumatic
4. Mechanical
5. Neoplastic.

Punctal Obstruction

- *Primary punctal stenosis:* It occurs in absence of punctal eversion

  It may be idiopathic, drug induced (idoxuridine, pilocarpine, and chemotherapeutic agents), following irradiation, lid infections like herpes simplex or trachoma.

  Treatment: Please refer to chapter 25 for details.
- *Secondary punctal stenosis:* It is seen commonly secondary to punctal eversion.

Treatment: Medial ectropion repair by resection of a diamond-shaped piece of tarsoconjunctiva below the punctum with reapposition of the edges turns the punctum inward. A lacrimal probe during surgery prevents damage to the canaliculus.

Canaliculus Obstruction

Canalicular obstructions may involve:
- *The proximal segment*—the first 2–3 mm
- *The midcanalicular segment*—3–8 mm from the puncta, and/or
- *The distal segment*—at the opening of the common canaliculus into the lacrimal sac.

Obstruction may occur in the upper or lower canaliculus or in the common canaliculus.

Membranous stenosis at the internal common canaliculus is one of the most common locations for canalicular stenosis.

Canalicular obstruction can be secondary to trauma, infection, drugs or repeated probing.

Syringing, probing, and radiographic contrast studies help in determining the location and extent of obstruction.

Treatment

Obstruction in the medial part is treated by canaliculo-dacryocystorhinostomy while in the lateral part is treated by conjunctivodacryocystorhinostomy.

Canaliculitis

This may be caused by a variety of organisms. Most commonly it is caused by a Gram positive bacillus, *Actinomyces*. Other organisms like *Propionibacterium propionicum*, *Fusobacterium* and *Bacteroides* have also been cultured from canaliculitis.

Patient often presents with features of chronic conjunctivitis and epiphora.

Treatment:
It consists of warm compresses, topical antibiotics (ciprofloxacin, penicillin).

Canaliculotomy along with curettage is recommended to remove the concretions and to allow better penetration of drugs.

Canalicular Laceration

It occurs due to penetrating or avulsion injury. Syringing and probing help to diagnose the condition.

Management:
- *Identification:* First and most important step in management is to identify the cut ends of the canaliculus. The lateral end is easily identified by passing a lacrimal probe
  Exploration and direct visualization of the medial cut end of the canaliculus is attempted under a microscope.
  In difficult situations techniques like irrigation of air, viscoelastic, fluorescein, or pigtail probe may be used.
- *Silicone intubation:* A monocanalicular Monoka stent passed through the punctum is ideal if both the cut ends of the canaliculus can be visualized.
  Direct anastomosis of the cut ends can be carried out over the stent, which is left *in situ* for 6 weeks.

Nasolacrimal Duct

Nasolacrimal Duct Obstruction

Primary acquired nasolacrimal duct (NLD) obstruction (idiopathic) is the cause in nearly 80% of patients. Other causes include trauma, chronic sinus disease like Wegeners granulomatosis, granulomatous diseases like tuberculosis and tumors.

Treatment:
- *Complete obstruction:* It is managed by dacryocysto-rhinostomy
- *Incomplete obstruction or partial NLD obstruction:* It may be managed by stenting of the lacrimal system with silicone intubation. If symptoms are significant, a standard DCR surgery may be required.

Dacryocystitis

It is usually secondary to obstruction of NLD.

Adult dacryocystitis: It may present in chronic or acute form.

Chronic dacryocystitis: This is more common than the acute form. Stasis and mild infection of long duration results in dacryocystitis.

Predisposing factors: Females are predominantly affected due to the narrow lumen of the bony canal. It affects mainly the 40–60 years age group. Negros are affected less often due to their wide and short NLD. It is seen commonly in patients from low socio-economic strata with poor personal hygiene.

Factors responsible for stasis of tears: A narrow bony canal, partial obstruction of NLD, foreign body in the sac, excessive lacrimation, recurrent conjunctivitis, and obstruction of lower end of NLD by polyps, hypertrophied inferior concha, marked degree of deviated nasal septum, tumors, etc. contribute to stasis of tears. Lacrimal sac may get infected from conjunctiva, nasal cavity, or paranasal sinuses.

Causative organisms: The common organisms are staphylococci, pneumococci, streptococci, *Pseudomonas pyocyanea*, etc. Rarely tuberculosis, syphilis, leprosy, or rhinosporidiosis may cause dacryocystitis.

Stages of chronic dacryocystitis:
- *Stage of chronic catarrhal dacryocystitis:*
  - *Presentation:* Watering and mild redness in the inner canthus
  - *Syringing:* Clear fluid or few fibrinous mucoid flakes regurgitate
  - *Dacryocystography:* Block in NLD, normal sized lacrimal sac with healthy mucosa.
- *Stage of lacrimal mucocele:*
  - *Presentation:* Constant epiphora associated with swelling just below the inner canthus

- On pressing the swelling, milky or gelatinous fluid regurgitates from the punctum. On chronic infection the opening of both the canaliculi into the sac may get blocked resulting in an encysted mucocele with negative regurgitation
- Dacryocystography: Distended lacrimal sac with NLD obstruction
- *Stage of chronic suppurative dacryocystitis:*
  - *Presentation:* Epiphora, recurrent conjunctivitis, swelling at the inner canthus with mild erythema of the overlying skin
  - Regurgitation results in frank purulent discharge from the punctum. If canalicular openings get blocked it results in encysted pyocoele
- *Stage of chronic fibrotic sac:*

Presentation: Persistent epiphora and discharge. Low grade repeated infections result in fibrotic sac with mucosal thickening.

Dacryocystography shows small sac with irregular folds.

Complications of dacryocystitis:
- Chronic conjunctivitis, acute on chronic conjunctivitis
- Maceration and edema of lower lid skin due to prolonged watering
- Infection of trivial corneal abrasion
- Occurrence of endophthalmitis following intraocular surgery.

Acute dacryocystitis: Acute suppurative inflammation of the lacrimal sac results in painful swelling in the region of the lacrimal sac. It may develop as a result of exacerbation of chronic dacryocystitis or due to direct involvement of neighboring infected structures such as paranasal sinuses, dental abscess, etc. The frequently involved causative organisms are *Streptococcus haemolyticus, Pneumococcus,* and *Staphylococcus.*

Stages of acute dacryocystitis:
- *Stage of cellulitis:* There is painful swelling in the region of lacrimal sac, epiphora, fever, and malaise. The swelling is red, hot, and tender
- *Stage of lacrimal abscess:* Continued inflammation leads to canalicular blockage with distension of sac with pus. The swelling later points below and to the outer side of the sac (Fig. 3)
- *Stage of fistula formation:* A neglected lacrimal abscess may lead to external fistula formation below the medial canthal ligament or sometimes it may burst open into the nasal cavity forming internal fistula (Fig. 4).

Complications: Acute conjunctivitis, corneal ulceration following corneal abrasion, lid abcess, orbital cellulitis, osteomyelitis of lacrimal bone, and rarely cavernous sinus thrombosis.

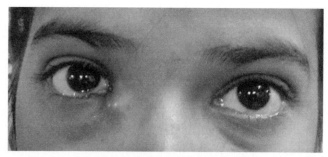
Fig. 3: Right-sided lacrimal abscess.

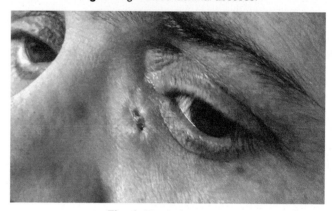
Fig. 4: Fistula formation.

Treatment of acute dacryocystitis: Systemic and local antibiotics, systemic anti-inflammatory, and hot fermentation relieve pain and swelling during the cellulitis stage. Once the lacrimal abscess forms and pus starts pointing, it is drained with a small incision. DCR is performed after 7–10 days. External fistula if present is dealt with fistulectomy at the time of DCR.

Nowadays, lacrimal surgeons prefer to perform endoscopic DCR in acute dacryocystitis under cover of antibiotics at an early stage. The passage created helps in early drainage of pus and rehabilitation of the patient.

Atonic Sac

This is another cause of lacrimal pump failure. Diagnosed when the syringing through lacrimal passages is patent but fluid regurgitates on pressure on lacrimal sac area.

Dacryolithiasis

Dacryoliths, or cast formation, within the lacrimal sac can also produce obstruction of the NLD. Dacryoliths consist of shed epithelial cells, lipids, and amorphous debris with or without calcium.

It can occur due to infection with *Actinomyces israelii* or *Candida.* Long-term administration of topical medications such as epinephrine can also lead to the formation of such a cast.

Patient may present with intermittent epiphora, pain due to acute impaction of dacryolith in the NLD leading to lacrimal sac distension.

Treatment is with mechanical removal of stones along with DCR.

Lacrimal Sac Tumors

- Primary tumors are predominantly epithelial. They are more commonly malignant than benign
- Squamous cell carcinoma is the most common lacrimal sac tumor followed by lymphoma, malignant melanoma, and adenocarcinoma.

Presentation: This is with chronic dacryocystitis, nonpalpable nontender mass with a bloody discharge from punctum.

Treatment: Dacryocystectomy is indicated in cases without bone erosion. It prevents extension of tumor into the nose.

Lateral rhinotomy, subtotal maxillectomy if tumor extends beyond the sac.

CONGENITAL ETIOLOGY OF LACRIMAL SYSTEM OBSTRUCTIONS

Congenital NLD obstruction can grossly be grouped into:
- *Upper system blockage:* Obstruction before the canalicular-lacrimal sac junction (punctae, canaliculi, and common canaliculus)
- *Lower system blockage:* Obstruction after this junction (lacrimal sac and nasolacrimal duct)

Upper System Obstructions

As there is no connection between upper system with the mucus-secreting goblet cells located in the nasolacrimal sac. These obstructions generally present with epiphora without any mucus discharge or mucus mattering of the lashes.

Punctal Abnormalities

During embryogenesis, canalization of the solid ectodermal cord, progresses laterally terminating at the superior and inferior punctum, any disruption in this process can lead to punctal atresia or punctal agenesis.

Congenital punctal atresia: It commonly presents as a thin membranous veil over the punctum that may appear as a small depression in the lid margin around 6 mm lateral to the medial canthus.

Theory:
- Failure of the epithelial bud to open at the punctum results in an imperforate punctum

- *Mesenchymal origin:* During development of the canaliculi and punctum, the orbicularis muscle is also developing from local mesenchyme. The orbicularis covers the surface of the lids while the lids are fused. The membranous veil found overlying the punctum may have its origin from the orbicularis muscle or
- May be secondary to failure of the conjunctiva to perforate properly.

Presentation:
Inferior punctal atresia is more common than upper punctal atresia, and typically, only one punctum demonstrates atresia.

During embryogenesis, the frontal nasal process gives rise to the upper lid bud, while the lower lid bud originates from the maxillary process. The distinct embryologic origin of the upper lid and lower lid may be the reason for only one punctum being affected more often than both.

Management:
- This veil may be lysed with a pin or with a sharp punctal dilator
- Temporary intubation or placement of a silicone plug may help prevent recurrence.

Congenital punctal agenesis: Congenital absence of the punctum is less common than atresia; however, it can also be attributed to abnormal canalization of the ectodermal cord during embryogenesis.

It can be associated with canalicular agenesis.

Management:
- Retrograde probing through an open lacrimal sac with direct visualization of the common canalicular opening (common internal punctum) or
- Surgeon may cut down through the eyelid margin in the expected area of the lateral canaliculus
- Conjunctivodacryocystorhinostomy (CDCR): When the patient is old enough to allow manipulation of, and to care for, the Jones tube.

Canalicular Abnormalities
Canalicular atresia and agenesis:
If the surface ectoderm cord migration during embryogenesis is retarded before reaching the eyelid margin or if incomplete canalization of the cord occurs, canalicular atresia or agenesis will occur.

The atresia can be classified as proximal, mid-canalicular, or distal, depending on the extent and location of canalicular abnormality.

Management:
- Retropassage of silicone tubes from the lacrimal sac
- Canaliculodacryocystorhinostomy—if no canalicular tissue identified.

Accessory canaliculi and accessory canalicular channels:
If more than two cords of surface ectoderm from the canalicular system are directed toward the lid margin, accessory canaliculi may develop.

If these cords terminate below the lid margin on the cutaneous surface of the lid, accessory channels can form.

Lower System Obstructions

Congenital Dacryocystocele (Amniotocele, Lacrimal Sac Mucocele)

A mucocele is an unusual presentation of a nonpatent nasolacrimal sac that is obstructed both proximally and distally.

Pathophysiology:
- Distal NLD obstruction
- Obstruction to reflux through common canaliculus—functional block as the expansion of the lacrimal sac collapses common canaliculus at junction with the sac. Mucous glands lining the lacrimal sac continue to secrete mucus and further distend the sac.

Clinical presentation:
- Mucoceles can be seen at birth or shortly after birth as a bluish subcutaneous mass just below the medial palpebral ligament
- Epiphora
- Slowly progressive
- Female preponderance
- Sterile fluid.

Differential diagnosis:
- Encephalocele
- Hemangioma
- Dermoid cyst.

Complications:
- Dacryocystitis is common (unsterile fluid)
- Astigmatism and amblyopia
- Permanent canthal deformity
- Airway obstruction.

Management:
- Short-term observation may be appropriate (weeks) as it may resolve spontaneously
- Warm compress and lacrimal sac massage
- Close watch to be kept for dacryocystitis (hospitalize)—intravenous antibiotics
- Watch for respiratory distress.

Surgical treatment:
- Early intervention often needed
- Simple probing ineffective
- Endoscopy and resection of nasal cyst is most definitive approach, combined with silicone stent.

Lacrimal Diverticulum

It refers to an outpouching from the lacrimal apparatus. Lacrimal diverticulum appears as a soft reducible swelling at the medial canthus.

Congenital Lacrimal Fistula

Congenital lacrimal fistulae are rare developmental conditions. They are accessory or anlage ducts that connect the lacrimal drainage system (lacrimal sac, the common canaliculus or nasolacrimal duct) to the skin.

It is usually situated *inferonasally* from the medial canthus though it may occur anywhere along the skin surface of the eyelids, around the medial canthal angle and even on the conjunctival surface (Fig. 5).

Epidemiology:
- Most cases are unilateral, though familial and syndromal cases reported to date have demonstrated an increased incidence of bilaterality
- *Prevalence:* 1 in 2,000 live births
- *Age:* Variable, ranging from the immediate postnatal period to the fifth decade
- *Sex:* M = F
- No racial or ethnic predilection.

Etiopathogenesis of congenital lacrimal fistula:

Duke-Elderhad theory: This theory proposed that the fistula originates due to one of the following factors:
- Overgrowth of the outer wall of the nasolacrimal duct, amniotic bands, dysfunctional closure of the embryonic fissure or
- Resultant inflammation from purulent dacrocystitis.
  Jones and Wobig referred to the cord of cells extending inward as the lacrimal anlage. They suggested that the failure of involution of the lacrimal anlage and subsequent canalization of this cord of cells results in congenital lacrimal fistulae.

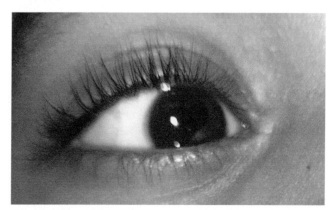

Fig. 5: Congenital fistula located inferonasal to medial canthus.

Levine proposed that the fistula occurs secondary to dysfunctional fusion of surface ectoderm after invagination. The hypotheses converge on the idea that anlage ducts occur when lacrimal cells proliferate and canalize instead of involuting.

Histopathology:
- Similar to normal canaliculus
- Stratified squamous epithelium in the external part
- Cuboidal epithelium near connection to sac.

Clinical presentation:
Congenital lacrimal fistulae are frequently asymptomatic. Symptomatic cases may present with:
- *Epiphora:* Most patients with epiphora have symptoms since birth, yet others experience late-onset epiphora from underlying intermittent functional nasolacrimal duct obstruction
  Precipitating factors:
  - Valsalva maneuver can be used to accentuate the extrusion of discharge from the fistula orifice
  - They may also be noticed to have clear discharge from the fistula site when coughing or blowing the nose
  - Constant tearing from the fistula orifice may be observed when the child cries
- May present with redness of the medial canthal angle with mucus or pus oozing from the fistula opening
- *Blepharitis:* It may develop subsequently and presents with redness and swelling of the eyelid
- *Persistent suppurative dacryocystitis* (rare cases): However, typically, patients have patent nasolacrimal ducts and do not suffer from dacryocystitis.

Management:
Investigations: Standard methods of diagnostic investigations include:
- Probing
- Irrigation
- Radiological methods such as a dacryocystography or nuclear scintigraphy.
  Several studies suggest various alternatives to visualize the anatomy of the nasolacrimal duct in the detection of congenital lacrimal fistulae:
- Dacryoendoscopy
- Computerized tomography (CT)
- Polyvinyl siloxane cast.

Conservative: Conservative treatment is generally reserved for uncomplicated and asymptomatic congenital lacrimal fistulae especially when not associated with NLDO.

Surgical: Treatment modalities for symptomatic fistula include—
- Nasolacrimal duct probing

- Cauterization of the external ostium
- Fistulectomy with or without dacryocystorhinostomy.

Complications:
- Recurrence of the fistula tract (~11%)
- Persistent symptoms of epiphora and discharge postoperatively
- Infection (e.g. dacryocystitis)
- Poor cosmesis
- Bleeding and damage to lid or nasal structures.

CONGENITAL NASOLACRIMAL DUCT OBSTRUCTION

Congenital obstruction of the lacrimal drainage system, which is usually caused by a membranous blockage of the valve of Hasner covering the nasal end of the NLD, is the most common cause of childhood epiphora.

Epidemiology

- Nasolacrimal duct obstruction may be present in roughly 50% of newborn infants
- Most obstructions open spontaneously within 4–6 weeks after birth, it becomes clinically evident in only 2–6% of full-term infants at 3–4 weeks of age
- Of these, one-third have bilateral involvement
- Approximately 90% of all symptomatic congenital NLD obstructions resolve in the first year of life.

Symptoms

- Epiphora
- Mucous discharge
- Periocular skin soreness and excoriation
- Dacryocystitis—acute /chronic.

Medical Therapy

- *Crigler massage:* First described by Crigler in 1923.
  Technique:
  - The index finger is placed medial to the medial canthus; massage should be performed only in the medial canthal area
  - A common mistake is to continue the maneuver down the nasal bone. At this point the duct is interosseus and the pressure on nose would exert no influence on duct itself
  - Initially motion should be to milk any discharge from the sac by applying gentle pressure to it and stroking upward
  - Following this, firm downward pressure should be applied to the nasolacrimal sac, this pressure allows

residual fluid in the sac to be forced against the thin obstructing membrane in an effort to perforate it and relieve the obstruction
- The complete maneuver should be repeated twice or thrice a day when the sac is inflated
- Topical broad-spectrum antibiotics are given only if significant mucoid discharge is present
- Systemic antibiotics are prescribed if dacryocystitis is present
- Probing is deferred until 9 months of age.

Probing

Prerequisites:
- Familiarity with lacrimal and nasal anatomy and developmental variations
- Under restraint/sedation/general anesthesia
- General anesthesia
  - Cuffed endotracheal tube
  - Laryngeal mask—preferred
- Confirmation of the clinical diagnosis.

Preparation:
- Decongestant nasal spray and packing.

Instruments:
- Punctal dilator—sharp and blunt tipped
- Standard lacrimal probes size No. 0000 to No. 2
  - No. 0000: 0.70 mm
  - No. 000: 0.80 mm
  - No. 00: 0.90 mm
  - No. 0: 1.00 mm
  - No. 1: 1.10 mm
- Lacrimal cannula: 22–24 gauge
- Syringe: 2–5 cc
- Caliper
- Nasal speculum
- Light source
- Straight artery forceps
- Cotton swabs
- Suction.

Procedure:
1. The upper eyelid is stabilized.
2. Upper punctum is dilated with a punctal dilator.
3. The initial position is vertical in the coronal plane with slight medial angulation.
4. The probe is then turned 90° (horizontal in the coronal plane) to enter the proximal canaliculus for 2–3 mm.
5. Probe size depends on age of the child.
   - Probe No. 000: Neonates
   - Probe No. 00: Younger than 3 months
   - Probe No. 0: 3 months to <1 year
   - Probe No. 1: 1 year and beyond

- Probe No. 2: Rarely used for children aged >3 years or for "reaming" tight bony obstructions.
6. The lateral canthus is stretched to straighten the canaliculus while gently turning the probe to a horizontal plane.
7. The probe is advanced toward the root of the nose until a hard stop is encountered.
8. While releasing the stretch over the lateral canthus, the probe is gently turned vertically down and advance in a downward, posterior, and lateral direction.
9. The upper end of the probe in a right anatomical plane should be-
   - Flat on the child's forehead
   - Aligned with the trochlea
   - Able to "spring-back" into position.
10. The pressure is increased if resistance is felt.
11. The probe is advanced till a hard stop of the floor of the nose is encountered or the probe is advanced for 45 mm.
12. The presence of probe in the nose is confirmed by-
    - Metal to metal contact with an instrument passed into the inferior meatus
    - Nasal endoscopy.
13. The patency of the lacrimal system is confirmed using syringing coupled with nasal suction.

Difficult probing:
- Incorrect diagnosis
- False passage
- Tight bony obstruction
  - Within the NLD
    "Graduated" or "step-wise" probing
    "Reaming" maneuver
- Beyond the NLD
  - Infracture inferior turbinate

Post-operative measures:
- Nasal decongestant drops
- Topical antibiotics
- Continue lacrimal sac massage for 1–2 weeks
- Office evaluation at 2 weeks.

Repeat probing:
- Any time after 6 weeks if the child remains symptomatic
- Consider other therapeutic measures if 2–3 probing attempts fail.

Intubation

Intubation is usually performed with a silicone stent.

Indications:
- Recurrent epiphora following nasolacrimal system probing

- For older children when initial probing reveals significant stenosis or scarring
- For upper system abnormalities such as canalicular stenosis and agenesis of the puncta.
  Intubation after failed probing has a reported success rate greater than 70%.

Balloon Dacryoplasty (Fig. 6)

- This is a useful adjunctive procedure in cases with incomplete NLD obstructions, where probing has failed especially in children older than 13 months of age
- The balloon is introduced until it is in the NLD
- The balloon is then inflated to a pressure of 8 atmospheres for 90 seconds and deflated for 10 seconds
- The balloon is retracted 5 mm, to lie at the junction of sac and the NLD and two more inflations are performed.

Pediatric Dacryocystorhinostomy

Dacryocystorhinostomy is usually reserved for children who have persistent epiphora following intubation and balloon dacryoplasty and for patients with extensive developmental abnormalities of the nasolacrimal drainage system that prevent probing and intubation.

- *Indications for pediatric DCR:*
  - In soft tissue obstruction, failed silicone stenting and/or balloon dacryoplasty
  - In bony obstruction
- *Anatomic/physiological differences:*
  - Flatter anterior and posterior lacrimal crests
  - Shallower lacrimal sac fossa
  - Anterior ethmoidal air cells
  - Rapidly growing facial bones
  - Exuberant wound healing response
- *Preoperative considerations:*
  - In cases of dacryocystitis systemic antibiotics should be used to quieten the inflammation and infection prior to surgery

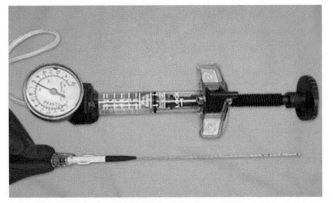

Fig. 6: Instrument for balloon dacryoplasty.

- In cases with epiphora with minimal discharge, surgery deferred until preschool years
- *Operative considerations:*
  - Ostium size at least 1 cm in size to account for bony growth and exaggerated wound-healing response
  - Anterior and posterior flaps to be sutured if possible
  - Use of silicone stents with nasal anchor (suture)
  - Blood loss in infants is tolerated much less well than in adults. Circulating blood volume is much less and blood loss greater than 50 cc's should raise the possibility of transfusion
  - Success rates for pediatric DCR is approximately 83%
  - Most failures occur due to anatomic obstruction caused by granulation at the osteotomy site.

SWELLINGS OF THE LACRIMAL GLAND

Dacryoadenitis

Acute dacryoadenitis may occur as a primary inflammation of the gland or secondary to some local or systemic infection. Local infection may develop following trauma, erysipelas of face, conjunctivitis, or orbital cellulitis. Systemic causes can be mumps, infectious mononucleosis, and measles.

The patient presents with a painful swelling in the lateral part of the upper lid. The lid may become red, edematous and may develop an "S"-shaped curve. The eye may be pushed down and medially. Suppurative dacryoadenitis may result in fistula formation.

The patient is managed with systemic antibiotic, analgesic, and anti-inflammatory drugs along with hot formentation. Incision and drainage may be required if pus forms.

Chronic dacryoadenitis may develop as sequelae to acute inflammation, in association with chronic conjunctivitis or systemic diseases like tuberculosis, syphilis, and sarcoidosis. Recently IgG-4 related diseases are recognized to cause dacryoadenitis.

The patient presents with a painless swelling in upper and outer part of lid associated with ptosis. The eyeball may be displaced down and in and diplopia may occur in up and out gaze.

Treatment depends on the cause and biopsy may be required to come to a conclusion.

Mikulicz Syndrome

The syndrome is characterized with bilateral and symmetrical enlargement of lacrimal glands and salivary glands along with systemic diseases like leukemia, lymphosarcomas, benign lymphoid hyperplasia, Hodgkin's disease, sarcoidosis, and tuberculosis.

Dacryops

Dacryops is a benign condition characterized by a fluid-filled cyst in association with normal lacrimal tissue that occurs most commonly in lacrimal gland but also in accessory lacrimal gland and ectopic lacrimal tissue. The proposed causation due to retention of lacrimal secretions following blockage of lacrimal ducts has given way to other theories. Hypersecretion of IgA into the cyst lumen with resultant osmotic retention of fluid and expansion of the cyst and damage to the walls of lacrimal ducts, perhaps secondary to trauma or inflammatory conditions are other proposed mechanisms. It presents as a cystic swelling and is usually diagnosed clinically. It is managed by simple excision.

Epithelial Tumors of the Lacrimal Gland (*See* tumors of the orbit in Chapter 27)

Approximately 50% of epithelial tumors are benign mixed tumors (pleomorphic adenoma) and about 50% are carcinomas. About 50% of the carcinomas are adenoid cystic carcinomas and the remainders are malignant mixed tumor primary adenocarcinoma, mucoepidermoid carcinoma, and squamous carcinoma.

CONCLUSION

The lacrimal system consists of secretory and the excretory apparatus. The excretory system is responsible for tear drainage into the nose. Blockage in the drainage pathway results in epiphora. Watering due to blockage needs to be differentiated from hyperlacrimation. Tests are performed to ascertain the level of block and manage accordingly.

Lacrimal Surgeries

Swati Singh, Saurabh Kamal, Akshay Gopinathan Nair, Ruchi Goel

INTRODUCTION

Lacrimal surgeries have been constantly evolving over the years with the introduction of newer diagnostic and treatment modalities. With ophthalmic surgeries becoming less invasive, lacrimal surgeries have also followed the trend. This chapter focuses upon the basics of some of the routinely performed lacrimal surgeries.

LACRIMAL PROBING

This procedure, known by many names—"lacrimal probing", "syringing and probing", and "probing and irrigation"—is the primary modality to treat congenital nasolacrimal duct obstruction (CNLDO). Probing is indicated when symptoms of CNLDO persist even after lacrimal sac compressions, and in complex CNLDO. The age at which probing should be performed as per available literature, is debatable.[1-3] PEDIG studies advocate late probing versus early probing (<6 months of age).[4] Early probing in less than 6 months of age is indicated in congenital dacryocele with respiratory distress while feeding.[5] Given the high rates of spontaneous resolution in CNLDO by 1 year of age (95%), early probing would lead to intervention in cases which otherwise would have resolved with sac compressions alone.[1,3] Therefore 9–12 months age is considered appropriate in case of persistent symptoms.[1-3] It is advisable to employ general anesthesia so as to avoid creating false passage in an uncooperative crying child.

TECHNIQUE

Nasal cavity is decongested with cotton buds soaked in 0.25% xylometazoline placed along inferior meatus. Punctal dilator is used to dilate the upper punctum and proximal canaliculus. Upper punctum lies more in line with NLDO; hence, chances of creating false passages become low. A Bowman probe no. 1 (for age 1 year or more) is advanced into upper punctum first perpendicularly and then turned very gently at junction of vertical and horizontal canaliculus. The lid is stretched laterally, and probe is advanced further toward common canaliculus till hard stop is reached. Probe should be placed parallel to lid margin in order to avoid false passage. No undue force should be used to navigate through. After reaching hard stop, probe is tilted against supraorbital notch and directed backward, outward, and downward. NLD makes an angle of 15° with sagittal plane. Soft stop at lower end of NLD is overcome by probe. Syringing is then performed with fluorescein stained distilled water/normal saline. Sequential dilation with larger number probe is needed in cases with stenosis at sac-duct junction/common canaliculus. Ideal way of confirming it is endoscopic visualization of inferior meatus. Inferior turbinate may be lifted off with the blunt end of periosteal elevator to visualize lower end of NLD. If endoscopic assessment is not available, then metal-to-metal touch or presence of fluorescein stained fluid in throat aspirations are indirect signs of patency. Careful assessment of sac-duct junction should be performed where narrowing can be expected.

Nasal decongestants along with topical antibiotic-steroid drops are administered for 2 weeks. Periodic follow-ups are done at 4 weeks, 12 weeks, and 1 year. Monocanalicular intubation with Monoka-crawford or bicanalicular intubation with 27G Crawford tubes is advisable wherever needed.

Indications for intubation in CNLDO:[6]
- Persistent CNLDO after probing

- Diffuse NLD stenosis
- Canalicular stenosis with persistent CNLDO
- Complex CNLDO.

CANALICULAR LACERATION REPAIR

Lacrimal trauma most commonly involves canaliculi (lower, upper, and bicanalicular) followed by nasolacrimal duct, lacrimal sac/naso-orbit-ethmoid (NOE) fractures (Fig. 1A).[7] Any eyelid laceration located medial to punctum should be considered as eyelid laceration involving canaliculus until proven otherwise. It is important to address and repair canaliculus irrespective of whether lower or upper, as both are important for drainage of tears.

- Surgery can be performed under general or local anesthesia depending upon age, extent of injury, and associated orbital trauma. Repair should be performed under high magnification using an operating microscope
- Thorough wound toileting is performed with 5% betadine followed by syringing via intact system. Cut end of canaliculus can be identified—
  - Canalicular mucosa appears smooth, whitish elevated typically resembling the ring of a "Calamari" and hence is known as *calamari sign* (Fig. 1B)
  - Medial end of canaliculus gets pulled away posteriorly and inward (toward posterior lacrimal crest). Gentle retraction of tissues will expose the medial end
  - *Using pigtail probe*—A blunt nontraumatic instrument with curved ends can be introduced via other canaliculus and navigated through common canaliculus, lacrimal sac to emerge via injured medial end.

Although this instrument is blunt, even in experienced hands manipulation via normal canaliculus has led to iatrogenic injury to normal canaliculus.

  - Injecting fluorescein stained viscoelastic, methylene blue has been mentioned in literature but diffuse egress of material does not help in exact location of cut ends most of the times
- After identifying cut ends, punctum is dilated and probe is passed through identified medial cut end of canaliculus to assess hard stop. Syringing can be done through the medial cut end of canaliculus to confirm the patency. Once confirmed, monocanalicular stent (Mini-Monoka/Aurostent/20G) silicone rod (Fig. 1C) is introduced with nontraumatic forceps.[8] The available length of these stents is 40 mm, so half of the length is trimmed off. In situations where self-retaining stents are unavailable, annular stent in the form of 20G silicone rod threaded over 6-0 prolene passed across both canaliculi can be used
- Pericanalicular tissue is approximated with 6-0 vicryl in horizontal mattress manner (Fig. 1D). Medial canthal tendon is repaired thereafter with 5-0 prolene followed by orbicularis and skin closure (Fig. 1E).

Postoperative Care

Stent is removed at 4–6 weeks. Syringing is performed thereafter, which indicates anatomical success. Functional success is documented with negative fluorescein dye disappearance (FDDT).

PUNCTOPLASTY

Management of punctal stenosis is traditionally performed with one-, two- or three-snip punctoplasty.[9] Punctoplasty is performed under local anesthesia with vannas scissors. One-snip involves placing a vertical incision along ampulla whereas two-snip involves two vertical incisions along medial and lateral wall of punctum and then excising flap at its base. Three-snip punctoplasty involves incising horizontal canaliculus and punctal ampulla to create a triangular flap, which is then excised (Fig. 2). Rectangular four-snip punctoplasty involves excising a posterior canalicular lining of vertical canaliculus in the shape of a rectangle. Other alternative to snip procedures is a simple punctal dilation with monocanalicular stent which has shown promising success in 90% cases by Caesar and McNabb.[10] It has advantage of preserving punctal ampulla, which has a functional role in tear drainage. Perforated punctal plugs are also used and have the advantage of being an OPD procedure (Fig. 3).

DACRYOCYSTORHINOSTOMY

Dacryocystorhinostomy (DCR) is among the common oculoplastics surgeries performed for managing epiphora due to nasolacrimal duct obstruction. The goal of DCR procedure is to make a large bony ostium into the nose with mucosa lined anastomosis.[11]

History

Addeo Toti in 1904 introduced the technique of excising medial sac and nasal walls to form anastomosis between sac and nasal cavity. Later on modifications were introduced by Dupuy-Dutens in 1920 to create epithelial lined tract with flaps formation.

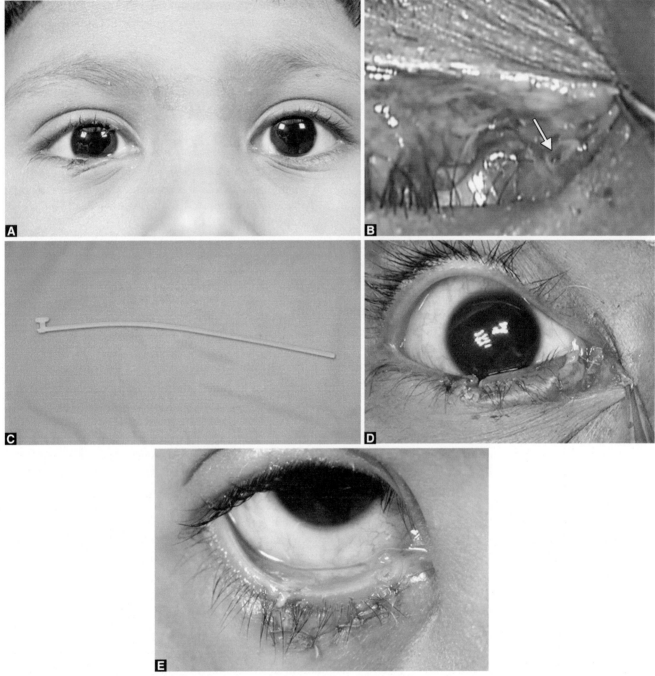

Figs. 1A to E: (A) Right lower eyelid laceration involving canaliculus; (B) Calamari's sign: Smooth, whitish elevated canalicular mucosa; (C) Minimonoka stent; (D) Pericanalicular tissue is approximated with 6-0 vicryl in horizontal mattress manner; (E) Skin closed with vicryl suture.

Indications

- Persistent congenital nasolacrimal duct obstructions unresponsive to previous therapies
- Bony congenital nasolacrimal duct obstruction

- Primary acquired nasolacrimal duct obstructions (PANDO)
- Acute dacryocystitis (Endoscopic surgical/laser and nonendoscopic nonlaser DCR)

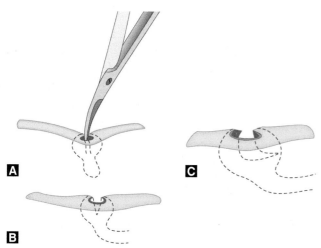

Figs. 2A to C: (A) One snip involves placing a vertical incision along ampulla; (B) Two-snip involves two vertical incisions along medial and lateral wall of punctum and then excising flap at its base; (C) Three-snip punctoplasty involves incising horizontal canaliculus and punctal ampulla to create a triangular flap, which is then excised.

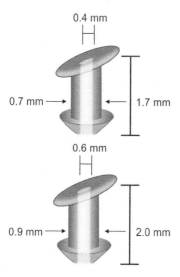

Fig. 3: Perforated punctal plug.

- Secondary acquired nasolacrimal duct obstructions (SALDO) posttrauma
- Functional nasolacrimal duct obstruction.

Contraindications
- Bleeding diathesis
- Suspected malignancy of lacrimal sac
- Suspected tuberculosis of lacrimal sac.

Preoperative Work-up
- Hemoglobin and complete blood count
- Blood sugar and blood pressure

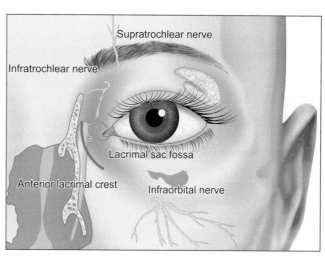

Fig. 4: All the nerves to be blocked in dacryocystorhinostomy and surface anatomy landmarks.

- Bleeding time, clotting time (prothrombin time if on anti-coagulants)
- ECG in elderly population, associated cardiac morbidity
- General anesthesia related investigations if planned.

Anesthesia

The surgery can be done under general anesthesia or local anesthesia. The latter is the most commonly employed modality. Local anesthesia is given by both infiltration as well as topical application. For infiltration 2% lignocaine with 0.5% bupivacaine with or without adrenaline is used. Infraorbital nerve block is first given at about a centimeter below the inferior orbital rim. Infratrochlear nerve is then blocked by inserting needle medial to supraorbital notch (Fig. 4). The nondominant hand marks the supraorbital notch and the needle is inserted into the lateral edge of the medial third of the eyebrow and advanced to just medial to medial canthus, and 2 cc of the drug is injected. The tissues along the anterior lacrimal crest are infiltrated subcutaneously and the needle enters deeper at about 3 mm medial to medial canthus, and without withdrawing the needle the drug is injected deep upto periosteum superiorly and inferiorly for anterior ethmoidal block. Nasal mucosa is sprayed with 10% lignocaine 1–2 puffs followed by packing with 4% lignocaine and 0.5% xylometazoline.

Surgical Technique of External DCR

Incision

A curvilinear incision of about 10–12 mm in length, 3–4 mm from the medial canthus along the anterior lacrimal crest in line with relaxed skin tension lines is given with No. 15 blade Bard-parker knife. Blunt dissection of orbicularis is carried to reach the periosteum. This can be done by tenotomy scissors but radiofrequency knife which cuts and coagulates, reduces blood loss, and keep field relatively blood less.

Lacrimal Fossa Exposure

Periosteal incision is given with radiofrequency knife. A Freer's elevator is used to separate the periosteum from the bone and reflect it laterally along with the lacrimal sac to expose the lacrimal fossa (Fig. 5).

Creating Bony Ostium

Once the lacrimal fossa is exposed, bone punching should be started at the junction of thick frontal process of maxillary bone and thin lacrimal bone. The differences in anatomy of lacrimal fossa are quite commonly seen, with variable contribution of maxillary and lacrimal bone. The Kerrison bone punch should be gently inserted between the bone and the nasal mucosa, taking care to avoid damaging nasal mucosa. Bone punching is started with 1.5 mm and progressively increased to larger diameters. Ostium is sequentially enlarged to achieve adequate size.

Boundaries of Ostium

Anteriorly osteotomy is carried out till the punch cannot be inserted further between the frontal process of maxilla and nasal mucosa. Posterior boundary involves posterior lacrimal crest and anterior ethmoid bone (anterior lamina papyracea). Superiorly extension is about 3–5 mm above the level of medial canthus to expose the fundus of sac completely. Inferiorly osteotomy is carried up to the lacrimal sac and nasolacrimal duct junction along with partial de-roofing of superior most nasolacrimal duct.

Flaps Formation

Sac flaps are created in a way to have a large anterior and small posterior flap. For beginners, fluorescein stained viscoelastic can be injected from the upper punctum to dilate the sac, to help in creation of flaps. Using the probe as guide, an "H"-shaped incision is made with the help of a number 11 or 15 blade right across the sac from the fundus to the nasolacrimal duct. Flaps are raised and posterior flap can either be retained or cut. Nasal mucosal flaps are fashioned with the help of number 11 blade initially and then by Stevens scissors. Incisions are made in the nasal mucosa along the bony ostium except anteriorly to have a hinged flap. It is important to avoid injury to nasal septum, as it can lead to the formation of ostio-septal synechiae with possibility of failure.

Flap Anastomosis

Anterior nasal and sac flaps are sutured with 6-0 vicryl in intermittent manner. If posterior flaps are preserved, then they are sutured as well. Flaps might require trimming and/ or anchoring to preperiosteal tissue if found to be lax.

Adjunctive Measures

Mitomycin C in a concentration of 0.04% for 3–5 minutes is used if there are intrasac synechiae, soft tissue scarring like in failed DCR, episodes of acute dacryocystitis, and in a complicated surgery. Intubation is advisable for similar indications or in cases with canalicular stenosis.

Wound Closure

Once flaps are secured, the orbicularis is sutured with interrupted 6-0 vicryl and skin with interrupted 6-0 vicryl

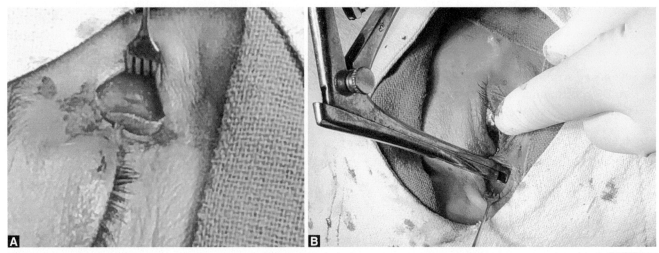

Figs. 5A and B: (A) External dacryocystorhinostomy (DCR): Exposure of lacrimal fossa; (B) Creation on bony osteotomy in external DCR.

or silk. Nasal packing is performed to ensure hemostasis postoperatively.

Postoperative Care

Analgesics and oral antibiotics are given for 5–7 days. At first postoperative day, the nasal pack is gently removed and hemostasis is assessed. The wound hygiene is maintained with 5% betadine and application of antibiotic ointment. Nasal decongestants with or without steroid nasal sprays are advised. Rose maneuver should be taught in case small amount of bleeding happens postoperatively. Both the nostrils are pinched with head bent forward and maintained in same position for 20 minutes. If excessive epistaxis is noted, patient should be asked to contact hospital or visit nearest medical care. Sutures are removed at one week postoperatively. Syringing is performed at 1 week to check patency. The patient is reviewed at 6 weeks and 12 weeks. Tube removal is usually done at 4 weeks whenever used. Success rate in the range of 85–99% has been reported in published literature.[12] Causes of failure include inadequate osteotomy, inaccurate positioning of ostium, stenosis of internal canalicular opening, incomplete marsupialization of lacrimal sac, intranasal adhesions (ostio-septal), and cicatricial closure of ostium. Sump syndrome is a cause of failed DCR where inferior remnant of lacrimal sac retains secretions and interferes with tear drainage.

Complications

- Early (1–4 weeks):
  - Bleeding, epistaxis
  - Wound dehiscence, infection
  - Tube prolapse
- Intermediate (4–12 weeks)
  - Intranasal synechiae
  - Ostial granulomas
  - Cicatricial closure of ostium
  - Punctal cheese-wiring, if intubated
  - Webbed skin scar (incision extends above medial canthus)
  - Failure of DCR
- Late (>12 weeks):
  - Failure of DCR.

Endoscopic DCR

Endoscopic endonasal DCR was first introduced by Caldwell in 1893 and then popularized by McDonogh and Meiring in 1989.[13] Endoscopic DCR can be surgical or laser. The commonly used laser is 980 nm diode laser through transcanalicular route. Other lasers that have been used are argon, CO_2, potassium titanyl phosphate, Holmium: Yag and Erbium laser.

Ultrasonic endoscopic DCR is where piezoelectric waves are used for osteotomy without risk of damage to soft tissues in vicinity, if touched inadvertently. Powered endoscopic DCR is used when superior thick bone removal is achieved with a powered drill/burr.

Surgical Technique

Endoscopic DCR can be performed under general anesthesia or local anesthesia. For local anesthesia, similar block as for external DCR and local infiltration near external nares is given. Nasal cavity is packed with ribbon gauze/gel foam soaked in 2% lignocaine + adrenaline (1:70,000). Area of intended osteotomy is infiltrated with 1.5–2 cc of 2% lignocaine + adrenaline (1:70,000) for endoscopic surgical DCR.

Identification of landmarks: The most important landmark to identify is the axilla of middle turbinate (Fig. 6A). Axilla of middle turbinate is the area where middle turbinate attaches on lateral nasal wall. Maxillary line is another important landmark, which can be visualized as a curvilinear ridge running from axilla of middle turbinate to the root of inferior turbinate (Fig. 6B).

Nasal mucosal flaps: Nasal mucosal incision is placed just anterior to maxillary line in a C-shape with the sickle knife/15 no. blade. It starts above and 10 mm anterior to the axilla of middle turbinate and extends downward up to the point corresponding to two-thirds of length of middle turbinate. Mucoperiosteal flap is elevated with Freer's elevator and reflected onto middle turbinate (Fig. 6C). Lacrimal fossa is exposed and osteotomy is started.

Osteotomy: Thin lacrimal bone is differentiated from thick frontal process of maxilla. A kerisson rongeur/forward-biting Hajek Koeffler punch is used to start osteotomy at the lower end of maxillary line. Frontal process of maxilla is removed, which exposes lower half of lacrimal sac and lower end of NLD. Thin lacrimal bone can be removed with Blakesley's ethmoid forceps. Superiorly, bone becomes too thick which might need assistance of a drill/ultrasonic burr for removal. Fundus of sac should be deroofed of all bone (Fig. 6D). Boundaries for ostium—superiorly, exposed fundus of sac (2 mm above common canalicular opening); anteriorly, orbicularis muscle should be just exposed; inferiorly, sac-duct junction and posteriorly agger nasi air cells/anterior ethmoid should be exposed.

Lacrimal sac flaps: After exposing lacrimal sac in toto, Bowman probe is inserted via upper canaliculus oriented horizontally to tent lacrimal sac. Good idea of an adequate

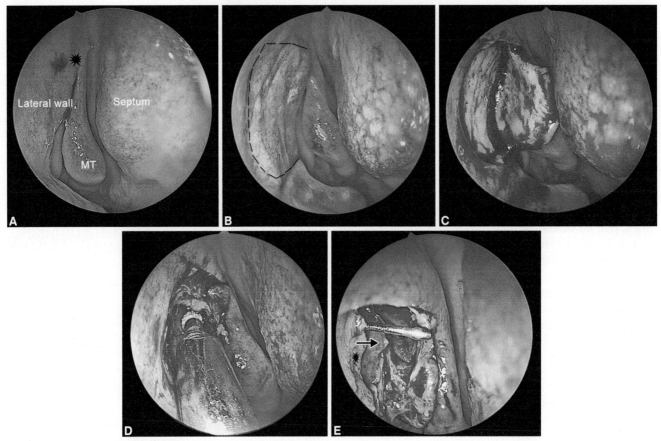

Figs. 6A to E: (A) Endoscopic landmarks; (B) Maxillary line is another important landmark, which can be visualized as a curvilinear ridge running from axilla of middle turbinate to the root of inferior turbinate; (C) Mucoperiosteal flap is elevated with Freer's elevator and reflected onto middle turbinate; (D) Fundus of sac should be deroofed of all bone; (E) Anterior and posterior sac flaps are reflected upon lateral nasal wall. Reflected nasal mucosa flap is apposed to the posterior sac flap with fibrin glue/suture.

osteotomy can be obtained by verifying bone-free area 2 mm above the probe. Flaps are fashioned with crescent knife placed vertically over lacrimal sac. Relaxing cuts are given superiorly and inferiorly with crescent knife in order to completely marsupialise the lacrimal sac. Anterior and posterior sac flaps are reflected upon lateral nasal wall. No bone or mucosal remnant should be lying against/falling onto lacrimal sac. Reflected nasal mucosa flap is apposed to the posterior sac flap with fibrin glue/suture (Fig. 6E).

Adjunctive measures like use of mitomycin C in a concentration of 0.04% for 3 minutes are used if there are intrasac synechiae, soft tissue scarring like in failed DCR and in a complicated surgery. Circumostial 0.04% MMC can be injected into sac flaps and along osteotomy superiorly and inferiorly in difficult cases. Intubation is also advisable for similar indications.

Laser Conjunctivo-DCR[14]

The puncta are dilated with a punctum dilator and a lacrimal probe is passed till a hard stop is felt. The nasal cavity is visualized with a 0° 4-mm nasal endoscope. The laser fiber-optic cable of the 980 nm diode laser via the canaliculus, to reach the sac (Fig. 7A). The aiming beam of the laser fiber is pinpointed to the lowermost part of the sac and visualized with help of the nasal endoscope. Laser energy is delivered at 8 W to vaporize the mucosa, and a 4 × 4 mm ostium is created (Fig. 7B). The ostium is further enlarged surgically to 8 × 8 mm using Blakesley's forceps. Nasal packing is performed at the end of the procedure.

Postoperative Care

Similar to external DCR except wound care is not needed, however, a dedicated follow up with syringing is required.

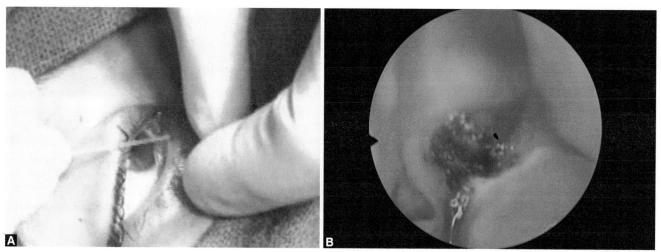

Figs. 7A and B: (A) Laser fiberoptic passed through the canaliculus; (B) Osteotomy is created by 980 nm diode laser.

Outcomes

Success rates across published studies vary from 90% to 95% with external or endoscopic DCR.[15,16] Advantages of endoscopic DCR over external are preservation of lacrimal pump, lack of cutaneous scar, faster recovery, and no contraindication in acute dacryocystitis.

Conjunctivo-DCR

Epiphora due to the absence or secondary proximal canalicular obstruction (<8 mm from the punctum) is treated by conjunctivodacryocystorhinostomy (CDCR) with the insertion of bypass tube. It can be performed both by external route as well as using 980 nm diode laser. The original bypass tube made up of pyrex was introduced by Jones. Since then various modifications have come up to prevent its extrusion such as Putterman–Gladstone tube that has an extra intranasal dilatation of the glass tube, frosted tubes with extra lightly textured outer surface, extended angled tubes, Medpor-coated tubes that promote fibrovascular ingrowth, and the StopLoss tube with an intranasal silicone flange. Also, numerous fixation techniques have also been described.

Laser Conjunctivo-DCR

The caruncle is partly excised and a tract is created from the caruncle to lacrimal fossa with Von Grafe knife. The fiberoptic cable is introduced and aiming beam is turned on. The nasal pack is removed and a 0° 4-mm nasal endoscope is passed into the nasal cavity and the middle turbinate is identified. The endoscope light is turned off to visualize the aiming beam at the medial wall of the sac. An osteotomy 6 mm × 6 mm is created at the root of the middle turbinate under direct visualization using 980 nm diode laser with a power of 8 W in continuous mode. Any overhanging tissue is removed and a smooth opening created using a Weil Blakesley nasal forceps.

External Conjunctivo-DCR

An incision is made with a No. 11 blade 10 mm from medial canthal angle starting slightly above the medial palpebral ligament and extending downward for an inch and a half. Dissection is carried down to the level of periosteum. The sac is separated from the underlying bone for 5 mm from anterior to the posterior lacrimal crest. The thin lacrimal bone is fractured. An osteotomy of 6 mm × 6 mm is created using Citelli bone punch. The lacrimal sac is opened and an anterior based nasal mucosal flap is created. The caruncle is partly excised and a Von Graefe's knife is passed through the medial angle through the lacrimal sac and into the middle meatus of the nose.

After this step the procedure of the tube placement was similar in both the laser and external groups. A lacrimal probe is passed through the caruncle into the tract created till it hits the nasal septum. The length of this segment is measured against a scale. Tube sized 2 mm less than this length is placed and the proximal end sutured with 6-0 prolene to the adjacent episclera and conjunctiva using "mirror tuck technique" (Fig. 8).[17] The tube is placed as vertically as possible with the lateral end in the tear lake and medial end exposed in the nasal cavity. Syringing is done to confirm patency of the tract. Postoperatively nasal packing is done using a solution of 2% lignocaine with adrenaline 1:80,000.

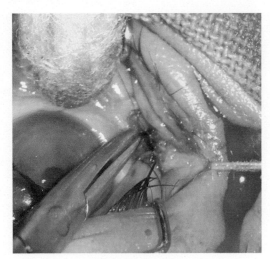

Fig. 8: Jones tube fixation using mirror-tuck technique in conjunctivo-dacryocystorhinostomy.

Canaliculodacryocystorhinostomy

For total obstruction at the common canaliculus, the common canaliculus is removed and the remaining canalicular system is directly anastomosed to the lacrimal sac mucosa over the silicone stent.

DACRYOCYSTECTOMY

Dacryocystectomy (DCT) was first described by Thomas Woolhouse in 1724 and popularized by Rudolph Berlin in nineteenth century. DCT refers to complete extirpation of lacrimal sac with proximal nasolacrimal duct. Extended DCT refers to complete removal of lacrimal sac along with any of the surrounding structures such as nasolacrimal duct, overlying lacrimal fossa bone, adjacent soft tissues, and bony structures like maxilla, lateral nasal wall depending upon the extent of disease.[18]

Indications

- Malignant lacrimal sac tumors
- Dacryocystitis in patients with severe dry eyes like Steven Johnson syndrome, Sjögren syndrome
- Recurrent dacryocystitis in multiple times failed DCR
- Dacryocystitis in patient with systemic co-morbidities like frail elderly population with neurologic or cardiac co-morbidities, bleeding diathesis, and high cardiac risk
- Dacryocystitis in patients with nasal morbidities like atrophic rhinitis, Wegener granulomatosis, cicatricial pemphigoid, etc.
- Relative indication in elderly patients with ocular morbidities, which require immediate intervention

like advanced cataract, microbial keratitis, and endophthalmitis.

Surgical Technique

Surgery can be performed under local or general anesthesia. Local infiltration is given subcutaneously along anterior lacrimal crest and infraorbital block. For block, 2% lignocaine and 0.5% bupivacaine with adrenaline (1:200,000) is used. A curvilinear incision of about 10–12 mm in length, 3–4 mm from the medial canthus along the anterior lacrimal crest is given. Blunt dissection is performed to separate the subcutaneous tissues and orbicularis muscle and expose the periosteum. A Freer elevator is used to lift off the periosteum from the bone and reflect it laterally. Anterior limb of medial canthal tendon is cut to expose fundus of the sac. The lateral wall of lacrimal sac is separated with the help of Westcott scissors from the orbicularis oculi. One should be careful to avoid perforating lacrimal sac. Further, superior wall and posterior walls are separated from the fascia with a Westcott scissor till nasolacrimal duct. After exposing the sac in toto, it is severed at its junction with the nasolacrimal duct. In cases of lacrimal sac tumors, the amputation is carried at a point as far as possible toward the distal nasolacrimal duct. After the sac removal, the common internal canaliculus, canaliculi, nasolacrimal duct stump, and any remnant sac lining, if any should be cauterized. Once hemostasis is achieved, the orbicularis is sutured back with 6-0 vicryl followed by skin closure with 6-0 prolene, vicryl, or silk based on the surgeon's preference.

Postoperative Care

Oral analgesics and topical antibiotics are given on the day of surgery. After patch removal, local wound care in the form of antibiotic ointment and betadine cleaning is advised. Sutures are removed at 1 week. Histopathology should be followed up for ensuring if lacrimal sac is removed completely.

Complications

Profuse bleeding due to inadvert injury to angular vein, wound related like infection, dehiscence, and recurrent dacryocystitis due to incomplete sac removal are among few rarely seen complications of this procedure.

REFERENCES

1. Paediatric Eye Disease Investigator Group. Resolution of congenital nasolacrimal duct obstruction with nonsurgical management. Arch Ophthalmol. 2012;130(6):730-4.

2. Ali MJ, Kamal S, Gupta A, et al. Simple vs complex congenital nasolacrimal duct obstructions: Etiology, management and outcomes. Int Forum Allergy Rhinol. 2015;5(2):174-7.

3. Paediatric Eye Disease Investigator Group. A randomized trial comparing the cost-effectiveness of 2 approaches for treating unilateral nasolacrimal duct obstruction. Arch Ophthalmol. 2012;130(12):1525-33.

4. Repka MX, Chandler DL, Beck RW, et al. Pediatric Eye Disease Investigator Group. Primary treatment of nasolacrimal duct obstruction with probing in children younger than 4 years. Ophthalmology. 2008;115(3):577-84.e3.

5. Ali MJ, Singh S, Naik MN. Long-term outcomes of cruciate marsupialization of intra-nasal cysts in patients with congenital dacryocele. Int J Pediatr Otorhinolaryngol. 2016;86:34-6.

6. Andalib D, Gharabaghi D, Nabai R, et al. Monocanalicular versus bicanalicular silicone intubation for congenital nasolacrimal duct obstruction. JAAPOS. 2010;14(5):421-4.

7. Naik MN, Kelapure A, Rath S, et al. Management of canalicular lacerations: Epidemiological aspects and experience with Mini-Monoka monocanalicular stent. Am J Ophthalmol. 2008;145(2):375-80.

8. Singh S, Ganguly A, Hardas A, et al. Canalicular lacerations: Factors predicting outcome at a tertiary eye care center. Orbit. 2017;36(1):13-8.

9. Kashkouli MB, Beigi B, Astbury N. Acquired external punctal stenosis: Surgical management and long-term follow-up. Orbit. 2005;24(2):73-8.

10. Caesar RH, McNab AA. A brief history of punctoplasty: The 3-snip revisited. Eye (Lond). 2005;19(1):16-8.

11. McNab A. Dacryocystorhinostomy. Manual of Orbital and Lacrimal Surgery, 2nd edition. Oxford: Butterworth-Hienemann; 1998.

12. Rosen N, Sharir M, Moverman DC, et al. Dacryocystorhinostomy with silicone tubes: Evaluation of 253 cases. Ophthalmic Surg. 1989;20(2):115-9.

13. McDonogh M, Meiring JH. Endoscopic transnasal dacryocystorhinostomy. J Laryngol Otol. 1989;103(6):585-7.

14. Goel R, Nagpal S, Kumar S, et al. Transcanalicular laser-assisted dacryocystorhinostomy with endonasal augmentation in primary nasolacrimal duct obstruction: Our experience. Ophthalmic Plast Reconstr Surg. 2017;33(6):408-12.

15. Wormald PJ, Kew J, Van Hasselt A. Intranasal anatomy of the nasolacrimal sac in endoscopic dacryocystorhinostomy. Otolaryngol Head Neck Surg. 2000;123(3):307-10.

16. Kamal S, Ali MJ, Naik MN. Circumostial injection of mitomycin C (COS MMC) in external and endoscopic dacryocystorhinostomy: Efficacy, safety profiles and outcomes. Ophthalmic Plast Reconstr Surg. 2014;30:187-90.

17. Goel R, Kishore D, Nagpal S, et al. Results of a new "mirror tuck technique" for fixation of lacrimal bypass tube in conjunctivodacryocystorhinostomy. Indian J Ophthalmol. 2017;65(4):282-7.

18. Ali MJ. Dacryocystectomy: Goals, indications, techniques and complications. Ophthalmic Plast Reconstr Surg. 2014;30(6):512-6.

Recent Advances in Dacryology

Swati Singh, Mohammad Javed Ali

INTRODUCTION

The science of dacryology is progressing at a rapid pace taking leaps and bounds in both clinical and basic sciences arena across the globe. There is an increasing interest in this subspecialty of ophthalmic plastic surgery and this augurs well for both the science and the patients it deals with. The advances in recent past are numerous and outside the purview of this chapter. The authors, however, discuss a few of them in brief, where they have been directly involved in the past 3 years.

ULTRASTRUCTURE OF LACRIMAL SYSTEM

Recently, ultrastructural anatomy of lacrimal system has been revisited with scanning electron microscopy (SEM) (Fig. 1). SEM study of normal adult lacrimal system revealed presence of distinct features of canalicular valves, specific orbicularis muscles arrangement in the periphery of the canalicular walls, and variably rugged external surfaces of the lacrimal system owing to criss-cross arrangement of collagen bundles in lacrimal sac and nasolacrimal ducts (NLD).[1] Presence of dense vascular plexus around lacrimal sac and NLD was noted similar to as shown by Paulsen et al.,[2] which facilitates tear outflow via "wrung out" mechanism. No valvular areas were seen in NLD. Reasonably well discernable thickened junctional areas between inner-punctal surface-vertical canaliculus and lacrimal sac–NLD, were noted, leading to a speculation about their possible functional roles. The exact role of these areas needs to be studied further, which might help in understanding the etiopathogenesis of NLD obstructions (NLDO).

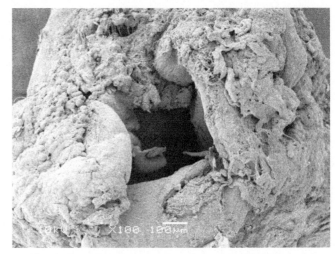

Fig. 1: Scanning electron microphotograph of the external surface of a punctum.

ETIOPATHOGENESIS OF PUNCTAL STENOSIS

Punctal stenosis is one of the commonly encountered etiologies of epiphora but its exact pathogenic mechanism is elusive as of yet. A step toward unraveling its etiopathogenesis was attempted where immuno-phenotyping and electron microscopy of punctae was performed (Fig. 2).[3] Infiltration of CD45+ and CD3+ T lymphocytes, focal B cell and plasma cell immunoreactivity along with numerous fibroblasts were the significant findings. Electron microscopy showed blunting of epithelial microvilli, abundant fibroblasts, disorderly arranged collagen bundles, and mononuclear infiltration in the vicinity of fibroblasts or in between collagen bundles. The presence of specific T-lymphocytes in the vicinity of fibroblasts had led to speculation about the possible role of immune cells rather than fibroblasts in triggering the events.

LACRIMAL SYSTEM OPTICAL COHERENCE TOMOGRAPHY

Proximal lacrimal system imaging using Fourier-domain optical coherence tomography (OCT) gave a throwback to the idea of 2 mm long vertical canaliculus (Fig. 3). Maximal visualized depth of vertical canaliculus across published literature on OCT was 1,400 microns, with an average of 890 microns.[4] Imaging with spectralis R using EDI technology has been found to be of prognostic value in punctal disorders like punctal stenosis, thereby helping in better preoperative counseling.[5] In addition, OCT features of numerous disorders of the proximal lacrimal system like incomplete punctal canalization,[6] punctal keratin cyst,[7] and canaliculops[8] have been explored recently.

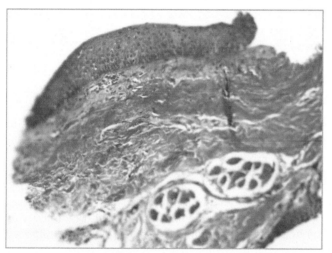

Fig. 2: Microphotograph showing pathological changes in punctal stenosis (Stain: Masson Trichrome).

MITOMYCIN C

Mitomycin C (MMC) has been used extensively in DCR surgery, however, the appropriate concentrations and duration has not been standardized. A concentration of 0.2 mg/mL for 3 minutes was noted to inhibit proliferation of human nasal mucosal fibroblasts without inducing apoptosis[9] and also correlated with in vitro collagen contractility and wound simulation[10] and hence was considered as an appropriate dose and duration in dacryocystorhinostomy surgeries (Fig. 4).[9] Clinically wound healing in the postoperative ostium is mediated by several cell types and occurs over a period of 6–8 weeks. Maintenance dose of MMC during healing period can be attained with injectable rather than topical application of MMC. Hence, a newer technique of using circumostial (COS) MMC injection in DCR at defined time-points have been proposed, which resulted in anatomical success of 89% in revision DCR (93% after one repeat surgery) and 97% in combined primary DCR and complex cases.[11] These effects were maintained in long-term assessments as well.[12] Transmission electron microscopic studies later confirmed the beneficial effects of both topical and circumostial MMC on the nasal mucosal healing, hence having implications in healing following dacryocystorhinostomy.[13]

LACRIMAL STENTS

The great debate for and against stent usage in DCR surgeries is still unsettled. However, many surgeons agree upon selective intubation for canalicular stenosis, revision DCR, prolong surgeries, poor flaps, and postacute dacryocystitis. Bio-films have recently been studied on the external and luminal surfaces of extubated stents (Fig. 5).[14-17] Biofilms were noted to be significant beyond 4 weeks of intubation. This combined with the data on postoperative ostium healing[18] suggests that stents, when used in lacrimal

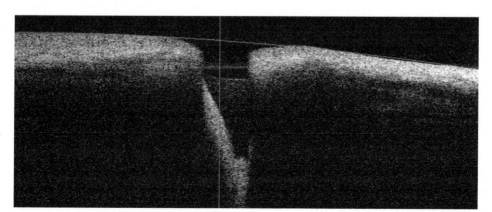

Fig. 3: Ocular coherence tomography image depicting the punctum and the vertical canaliculus.

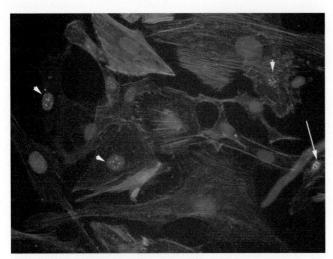

Fig. 4: Effect of mitomycin C on fibroblast. The image shows the phalloidin-DAPI merge image of cellular proliferation arrest with the use of mitomycin C.
(DAPI: 4′, 6-diamidino-2-phenylindole)

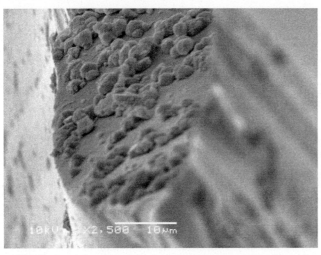

Fig. 5: Scanning electron microscopic image of a surface of lacrimal stent showing biofilms.

surgeries, should ideally not be kept beyond 4 weeks. In addition, extensive deposits and thick mixed biofilms constituted by fungal filaments and bacteria were found within the lumen and this led to a speculation about the possible use of nonluminal stents.

IMAGE-GUIDED LACRIMAL SURGERIES

Complex secondary acquired lacrimal drainage obstructions (SALDO) with distorted facial anatomy pose a difficult surgical challenge. Stereotactic navigation facilitates safe and precise dacryolocalization in such cases (Fig. 6).[19] Imaging data is acquired preoperatively in the form of 3D CT/MRI and built into the navigation system, which then can be used for radio-anatomic correlation during surgery. Successful outcomes have been demonstrated in all complex cases in one of the series using Stealth navigation system.[20,21] Newer introductions like telescopes enabled navigation, use of continuously variable viewing telescope (Endochameleon) have transformed the endoscopic lacrimal surgeries.[21,22]

I-131 AND NASOLACRIMAL DUCT OBSTRUCTION

The reported frequency of NLDO ranges from 3.4% to 11% following iodine therapy.[23] Radio-uptake studies showed a significant intranasal localization of I-131 in patients receiving dose more than 150 millicurie.[24] This could possibly reflect the underlying etiology for bilateral acquired NLDO observed in these cases. Screening of all patients (pre- and post-I-131 therapy), specifically those who receive a dose of more than 150 mCi should be performed. A screening protocol is now in place for patients receiving I-131 along with their risk stratification and clinical assessments.[23]

LACRIMAL PIEZOSURGERY

The advent of ultrasonic bone emulsification in neurosurgery helped multiple subspecialties to explore this option. Ultrasonic endoscopic DCR has been explored as an alternative modality of managing NLD obstructions.[25] It was found to be safe and effective in both adult and pediatric populations and surgical outcomes were comparable to that of regular powered endoscopic DCRs.[26] In addition it was also found that the time taken for superior osteotomy with the help of piezo techniques is not significantly different from mechanical drills.[27] There is also evidence to suggest that this may be a better modality to use for training in endoscopic DCR as compared to mechanical drills in view of its safety even in the hands of beginners.

THREE-DIMENSIONAL ENDOSCOPIC LACRIMAL SURGERIES

The recent development of a 3D enabled 4 mm rigid telescope for nasal surgeries has the potential to revolutionize the way we perform endoscopic lacrimal surgeries. Operating lacrimal surgeries like probing and DCR in 3D planes was found to enhance depth perception, dexterity, and precision as compared to the routine 2D intraoperative views.[28] The surgical observers noted enhanced anatomical and surgical understanding as compared to the 2D views.[28] Further detailed comparisons would help formulate guidelines for the routine use of 3D endoscopy in lacrimal surgeries.

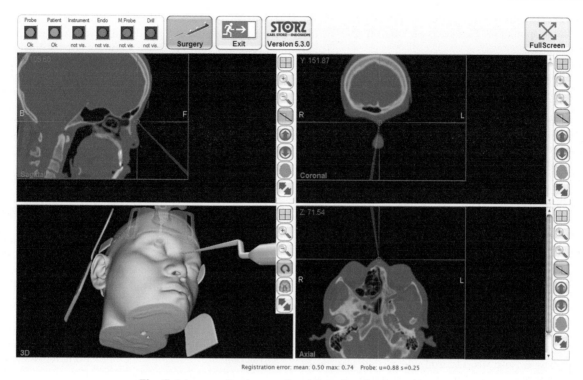

Fig. 6: Intraoperative image of an infrared navigation guidance.

QUALITY OF LIFE IN LACRIMAL DISORDERS

There is an increasing shift from surgeon-reported outcomes to patient reported outcomes in lacrimal disorders and quality of life (QOL) assessment is an essential outcome measure. Numerous QOL questionnaires like the Holmes, Glasgow benefit inventory, NLDO-symptom score (NLDO-SS), and lacrimal symptom scores (Lac-Q) are available. The use of Lac-Q is simple and reliable and has specific components addressing the lacrimal symptoms and social symptoms in brief.[29] The usefulness of Lac-Q has been studied in assessing the outcomes of powered endoscopic DCR and monoka stent dilatation for punctal stenosis.[30]

REFERENCES

1. Ali MJ, Baig F, Lakshman M, et al. Scanning electron microscopic features of the external and internal surfaces of normal adult lacrimal drainage system. Ophthalmic Plast Reconstr Surg. 2015;31(5):414-7.
2. Paulsen FP, Thale AB, Hallmann UJ, et al. The cavernous body of the human efferent tear ducts: Function in tear outflow mechanism. Invest Ophthalmol Vis Sci. 2000;41(5):965-70.
3. Ali MJ, Mishra DK, Baig F, et al. Punctal stenosis: Histopathology, immunology, and electron microscopic features-a step toward unraveling the mysterious etiopathogenesis. Ophthalmic Plast Reconstr Surg. 2015;31(2):98-102.
4. Kamal S, Ali MJ, Ali MH, et al. Fourier domain optical coherence tomography with 3D and En face imaging of the punctum and vertical canaliculus: A step towards establishing a normative database. Ophthalmic Plast Reconstr Surg. 2016;32(3):170-3.
5. Timlin HM, Keane PA, Rose GE, et al. Characterizing the occluded lacrimal punctum using anterior segment optical coherence tomography. Ophthalmic Plast Reconstr Surg. 2018;34(1):26-30.
6. Singh S, Ali MJ, Naik MN. Familial incomplete punctal canalization: Clinical and fourier domain optical coherence tomography features. Ophthalmic Plast Reconstr Surg. 2017;33(3):e66-e69.
7. Kamal S, Ali MJ, Naik MN. Punctal keratinizing cyst: report in a pediatric patient with Fourier domain optical coherence tomography features. Ophthalmic Plast Reconstr Surg. 2015;31:161-3.
8. Singh S, Ali MJ, Peguda HK, et al. Imaging the canaliculops with ultrasound biomicroscopy and anterior segment ocular coherence tomography. Ophthalmic Plast Reconstr Surg. 2017;33(6):e143-e144.
9. Ali MJ, Mariappan I, Maddileti S, et al. Mitomycin C in dacryocystorhinostomy: The search for the right concentration and duration—A fundamental study on human nasal mucosa fibroblasts. Ophthalmic Plast Reconstr Surg. 2013;29(6):469-74.
10. Kumar V, Ali MJ, Ramachandran C. Effect of Mitomycin-C on contraction and migration of human nasal mucosal fibroblasts: Implications in dacryocystorhinostomy. Br J Ophthalmol. 2015;99(9):1295-300.
11. Kamal S, Ali MJ, Naik MN. Circumostial injection of mitomycin C (COS-MMC) in external and endoscopic

dacryocystorhinostomy: Efficacy, safety profile, and outcomes. Ophthalmic Plast Reconstr Surg. 2014;30(2):187-90.

12. Singh M, Ali MJ, Naik MN. Long-term outcomes of circumostial injection of Mitomycin C (COS-MMC) in dacryocystorhinostomy. Ophthalmic Plast Reconstr Surg. 2015;31(5):423-4.

13. Ali MJ, Baig F, Lakshman M, et al. Electron microscopic features of nasal mucosa treated with topical and circumostial injection of Mitomycin C: Implications in dacryocystorhinostomy. Ophthalmic Plast Reconstr Surg. 2015;31(2):103-7.

14. Murphy J, Ali MJ, Psaltis AJ. Biofilm quantification on nasolacrimal silastic stents after dacryocystorhinostomy. Ophthalmic Plast Reconstr Surg. 2015;31(5):396-400.

15. Ali MJ, Baig F, Lakshman M, et al. Biofilms and physical deposits on nasolacrimal silastic stents following dacryocystorhinostomy: Is there a difference between ocular and nasal segments? Ophthalmic Plast Reconstr Surg. 2015;31(6):452-5.

16. Ali MJ, Baig F, Lakshman M, et al. Scanning electron microscopic features of nasolacrimal silastic stents retained for prolong durations following dacryocystorhinostomy. Ophthalmic Plast Reconstr Surg. 2016;32(1):20-3.

17. Ali MJ, Baig F, Naik MN. Electron microscopic features of intraluminal portion of nasolacrimal silastic stents following dacryocystorhinostomy: Is there a need for stents without a lumen? Ophthalmic Plast Reconstr Surg. 2016;32(4):252-6.

18. Ali MJ, Psaltis AJ, Ali MH, et al. Endoscopic assessment of the dacryocystorhinostomy ostium after powered endoscopic surgery: Behavior beyond 4 weeks. Clin Exp Ophthalmol. 2015;43(2):152-5.

19. Ali MJ, Naik MN. Image-guided dacryolocalization (IGDL) in traumatic secondary acquired lacrimal drainage obstructions (SALDO). Ophthalmic Plast Reconstr Surg. 2015;31(5):406-9.

20. Ali MJ, Singh S, Naik MN, et al. Interactive navigation-guided ophthalmic plastic surgery: The utility of 3D CT-DCG-guided dacryolocalization in secondary acquired lacrimal duct obstructions. Clin Ophthalmol. 2016;11:127-33.

21. Ali MJ, Singh S, Naik MN, et al. Interactive navigation-guided ophthalmic plastic surgery: Navigation enabling of telescopes and their use inendoscopic lacrimal surgeries. Clin Ophthalmol. 2016;10:2319-24.

22. Ali MJ, Singh S, Naik MN. The usefulness of continuously variable view rigid endoscope in lacrimal surgeries: First intraoperative experience. Ophthalmic Plast Reconstr Surg. 2016;32(6):477-80.

23. Ali MJ. Iodine-131 therapy and nasolacrimal duct obstructions: What we know and what we need to know. Ophthalmic Plast Reconstr Surg. 2016;32(4):243-8.

24. Ali MJ, Vyakaranam AR, Rao JE, et al. Iodine-131 therapy and lacrimal drainage system toxicity: Nasal localization studies using whole body nuclear scintigraphy and SPECT-CT. Ophthalmic Plast Reconstr Surg. 2017;33(1):13-6.

25. Ali MJ. Ultrasonic endoscopic dacryocystorhinostomy. In: Principles and Practice of Lacrimal Surgery. Ali MJ (Ed). New Delhi: Springer; 2015. pp. 203-12.

26. Ali MJ, Singh M, Chisty N, et al. Endoscopic ultrasonic dacryocystorhinostomy: Clinical profile and outcomes. Eur Arch Otorhinolaryngol. 2016;273(7):1789-93.

27. Ali MJ, Ganguly A, Ali MH, et al. Time taken for superior osteotomy in primary powered endoscopic dacryocystorhinostomy: Is there a difference between an ultrasonic aspirator and a mechanical burr? Int Forum Allergy Rhinol. 2015;5(8):764-7.

28. Ali MJ, Naik MN. First intraoperative experience with three-dimensional (3D) high-definition (HD) nasal endoscopy for lacrimal surgeries. Eur Arch Otorhinolaryngol. 2017;274(5):2161-4.

29. Ali MJ. Quality of life in lacrimal disorders and patient satisfaction following management. In: Principles and Practice of Lacrimal Surgery. Ali MJ (Ed). New Delhi: Springer; 2015. pp. 359-62.

30. Ali MJ, Iram S, Ali MH, et al. Assessing the outcomes of powered endoscopic Dacryocystorhinostomy in adults using the lacrimal symptom (Lac-Q) questionnaire. Ophthalmic Plast Reconstr Surg. 2017;33(1):65-8.

Tumors

Neoplasms and Malformations of the Orbit

Ruchi Goel, Bita Esmaeli

INTRODUCTION

Graves' disease constitutes 47% patients of orbital disease, and of the remaining 53% mass lesions, cystic and the inflammatory lesions are the commonest (Fig. 1).
The orbital tumors can be classified as follows:

- Vascular anomalies
- Neural tumors
- Mesenchymal tumors
- Lymphoproliferative disorders
- Histiocytic disorders
- Lacrimal gland tumors
- Secondary orbital tumors
- Metastatic tumors
- Orbital cysts

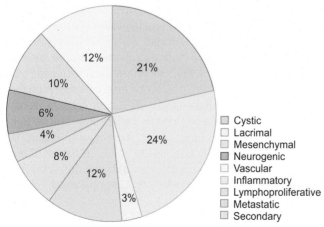

Fig. 1: Non-Graves orbital mass lesions.

- Retinoblastoma
- Secondary epithelial neoplasms
- Miscellaneous tumors.

VASCULAR ANOMALIES

The classification of vascular anomalies has been continuously evolving. Hemangiomas have been cited to proliferate by new vessel growth, with increased mitoses seen in vascular endothelium whereas, malformations expand by ectasia.

Conceptually, the vascular anomalies have been classified as follows:

- Malformation:
    - Lymphatic:
        - Microcystic
        - Macrocystic
    - Venous:
        - Encapsulated
        - Infiltrative
            Low flow
            High flow
- Hemangioma:
    - Focal
    - Segmental
- Rare vascular tumors.

Classification proposed by the International Society for the Study of Vascular Anomalies

- Malformations:
    - Arteriovenous
    - Venous (includes varices)

- Venular (includes port wine stain)
- Capillary
- Lymphatic
- Mixed (lymphaticovenous; cavernous hemangioma)
- Vascular tumors:
  - Infantile hemangiomas
  - Hemangiopericytoma
  - Kaposiform hemangioendothelioma
  - Noninvoluting congenital hemangioma
  - Rapidly involuting congenital hemangioma
  - Tufted angioma
  - Angiosarcoma
  - Hemangioblastoma
- Shunts and fistulas:
  - High flow (carotid artery-cavernous sinus)
  - Low flow (dural shunts).

Capillary Hemangiomas (Synonym: Infantile Hemangioma, Juvenile Hemangioma, Hemangioblastoma, Benign Hemangioendothelioma, Hypertrophic Hemangioma)

- It is the most common childhood tumor of eyelids and orbit
- It may present as small isolated lesion or a large mass causing visual impairment, systemic effects or may exist as part of a syndrome. The lesions are noticed in the initial months of life with 33–55% being present at birth (Figs. 2A and B)
- Predominance in females, premature infants, and Caucasians.

Haik's classification:[1]
- Classic superficial strawberry nevus; subcutaneous hemangiomas that appear bluish or purple through the overlying, unaffected skin
- Deep orbital tumors that present with proptosis without observable skin discoloration.[1]

Rootman's classification:[2]
- Strawberry nevus confined to the superficial dermis
- Superficial hemangiomas combined with subcutaneous involvement
- Combined subcutaneous and deep orbital involvement.

Cycle:
- Initial appearance
- Proliferative phase (within 3–6 months)
- Stabilization
- Involution (by age four to seven years, but may continue until 10 years of age).

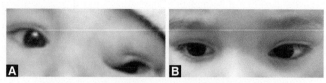

Figs. 2A and B: Capillary hemangioma left eye (A) Pretreatment; (B) One year after oral propranolol.

60% of the orbital capillary hemangiomas were found in the superior orbit, 16% in the inferior orbit, and 2% involving both upper and lower eyelids.

Large periocular lesions frequently cause functional defects such as amblyopia, strabismus, and optic atrophy.

Kasabach-Merrit syndrome, a critical thrombocytopenia occurs from platelet sequestration within the tumor's vascular channels.

Usually diagnosed on clinical examination. MRI may be required at times.

Management

Observation, refractive correction, and amblyopia therapy are the first-line of management.

Treatment Modalities

- Intralesional or systemic corticosteroids (most common)
- Interferon alpha
- Vincristine
- Laser therapy
- Surgical excision.

Oral propranolol, a nonselective beta-blocker, inhibits vascular proliferation of capillary hemangioma. Increased apoptosis and downregulation of vascular endothelial growth factor occurs due to vasoconstriction. It is given as 1–1.5 mg/kg/day orally. It is administered for a minimum of 2 months, with careful clinical monitoring of side effects.

Bradycardia, hypotension, hypoglycemia, rash, gastrointestinal discomfort/reflux, fatigue, and bronchospasm have been reported. Lethargy and hypothermia may require termination of therapy. Infants with PHACE syndrome (posterior fossa anomalies, hemangioma, arterial anomalies, cardiac anomalies, and eye anomalies) with tortuous, aneurysmal, or stenotic intracranial arteries are at high risk of stroke if treated with propranolol. A complete cardiovascular workup is required prior to initiation of propranolol therapy. Infants with large facial hemangioma should be evaluated for a PHACE association before initiation of oral propranolol. Intralesional propranolol injection 1 mg/mL has also been found effective.[3] Topical application further reduces the side effects.[4]

Intralesional steroid injection of triamcinolone 40 mg/mL has also been described. Kushner recommended a combination of 40 mg of triamcinolone acetate and 6 mg preparation of betamethasone acetate and betamethasone phosphate, with a total injection volume of 1–2 mL. The reported adverse effects of intralesional steroids are:

- Skin changes: Atrophy, depigmentation, and fat atrophy
- Adrenal-related changes: Reversible cushingoid facies, adrenal suppression that may require replacement therapy
- Central retinal artery occlusion.

Cavernous Venous Malformation of the Orbit (Previously Known as Cavernous Hemangioma of the Orbit)

Cavernous venous malformation (CVM) is the most common benign orbital lesion of adults. It usually presents in fourth and the fifth decade with female preponderance. It occurs as a solitary, unilateral lesion mostly (Fig. 3).

The classification in the malformation group is attributed to the immunohistochemical characterization. CD31 stains the endothelial layer and perivascular areas with microcapillary networks. It is immunonegative for glucose transporter type 1 protein (unique to infantile hemangiomas), similar to lymphatic malformations. Vascular stasis leads to intraluminal thrombosis resulting in neovascular activity and proliferation of CVM.

Middle third of the orbit is the most common site and it frequently occurs in the intraconal space leading to progressive axial proptosis.

Visual deterioration, motility deficits, and manifest strabismus, choroidal folds (retinal striae), optic disk changes may also be seen. Other infrequent manifestations are mechanical ptosis and corneal exposure. The symptoms tend to reverse on removal of the mass except in cases where permanent axial length modification ensues or there is a compromise of optic nerve function.

Differential diagnosis includes solitary fibrous tumor, lymphatic malformation, orbital lymphoma, and schwannoma.

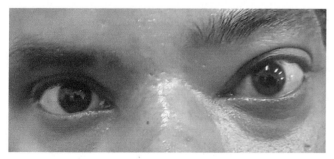

Fig. 3: Left axial proptosis due to cavernous venous malformation.

Imaging Characteristics[5]

On ultrasonography, A-scan shows high reflectivity, regular structure, and moderate attenuation of echoes. On B-scan, the mass is capsulated with medium-high reflectivity, and no signs of internal vascularization. On CT scan the well-circumscribed mass has homogeneous soft tissue density with bone remodeling. It enhances with contrast injection. It is isointense to muscle and gray matter but hypotense to fat on T1 weighted MRI. T2 weighted image shows hyperintensity to fat and brain.

Histopathology: Large vascular channels are present that are filled with blood and have regions of intralesional thrombosis indicating vascular stasis/extremely slow flow.

Treatment: Surgical excision is the main stay of management and is performed if there is a visual compromise or cosmetic disfigurement. The orbitotomy approach depends on the location of the lesion.

Nonsurgical treatment is used for lesions that are difficult to resect or patients unwilling for surgery. Pingyangmycin (bleomycin A5) is injected intralesionally. It induces vascular endothelial cell apoptosis with resulting sclerostenosis of the lumen resulting in marked decrease in the volume of the lesion leading to reduction in proptosis, swelling, and pain.

Hemangiopericytoma

Hemangiopericytomas are rare tumors that develop due to the proliferation of pericytes. They are encapsulated, hypervascular lesions that appear in midlife (can also occur in children). Symptoms usually include slowly progressive unilateral proptosis, mild pain, and decreased visual acuity. Resembles cavernous hemangiomas on imaging and the diagnosis is confirmed by histopathologic examination, complemented by immunohistochemistry. It has an uncertain malignant potential and high chance of relapse. Treatment involves complete excision with wide margins.

Lymphatic Malformation (LM; Earlier Called Lymphangiomas)

These occur from disruption of initially pluripotent vascular anlage that leads to aberrant development and congenital malformation. Orbital LM becomes apparent in first decade of life. Though typically stable or slowly progressive it may enlarge during upper respiratory infections and present as sudden proptosis caused by spontaneous intralesional hemorrhage (Figs. 4A to C).

The patients with acute manifestations may demonstrate compressive signs such as decreased visual acuity and afferent pupillary defects.

There can be pure lymphatic malformations or combined lymphaticovenous malformations. Pure

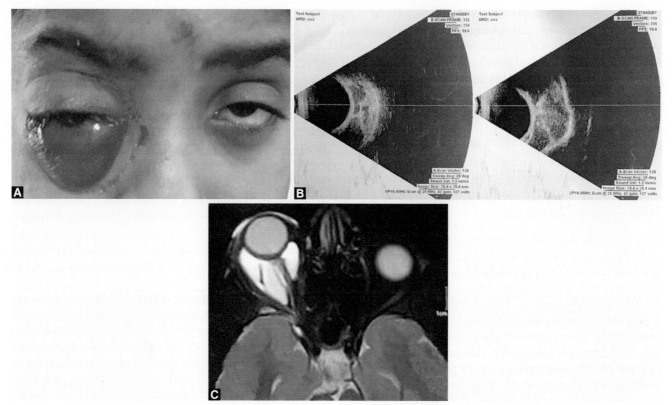

Figs. 4A to C: (A) Lymphatic malformation though typically slowly progressive may enlarge during upper respiratory infections and present as sudden proptosis caused by spontaneous intralesional hemorrhage; (B) B scan and (C) MRI showing large cystic spaces.

lymphatic malformations are classified as macrocystic, microcystic/diffuse, and mixed macrocystic/microcystic, all of which may have solid stromal components.

The Orbital Society classified orbital vascular malformations based on their internal flow into type 1 (no flow), type 2 (venous flow), and type 3 (arterial flow) lesions.[6]

Majority of these comprise of combined lymphaticovenous malformations that include venous dominant and lymphatic dominant types.

The venous dominant types are distensible on Valsalva and during dynamic investigations.

The lymphatic-dominant malformations are nondistensible lesions. The pure lymphatic malformations of the orbit are mostly located anteriorly and are seen as isolated, often irregular masses. Occasionally, they appear as single or sometimes septated macrocysts.

Histologically, they consist of multiple dilated sacs and lobules, lined with a single layer of endothelium, containing a proteinaceous or serosanguineous fluid and in some, neovascular tufts.

Treatment:
Asymptomatic lesions are kept under observation. Lesions that threaten vision will require more urgent treatment. Complete surgical resection is usually not possible.

If there is a *functional compromise* from bleeding, the cyst should be evacuated and a sclerosing agent is placed within the body of the cyst to collapse it.

Dual-drug chemoablation is performed with intracystic infusions of sodium tetradecyl sulfate 3%, followed by aspiration and then infusion of ethanol 98% solution, which is also removed. These work synergistically to destroy the cysts' linings.

Intralesional bleomycin has also been used successfully. Bleomycin is available as a freeze-dried powder in vials containing 15 international units (IU). The recommended dose is 0.25–0.5 IU/kg body weight. Bleomycin is reconstituted in sterile water and equal volume of 2% lignocaine is added in 1:1 ratio. The maximum allowed cumulative dose (including repeat injections) of bleomycin is 5 IU/kg body weight. The volume injected is about 20% of the aspirate not to exceed 5 mL at a time as too large a volume may lead to compressive effects and extravasation of the drug.

Oral sildenafil has recently shown favorable results in the dose of 1 mg/kg per day increased to 3 mg/kg per day over about a month and continued for about 5 months.

For microcystic lesions, multiple injections of ultrasound-guided intralesional sclerosing foam are given.

For a lymphoproliferative response, with upper respiratory tract infections and significant proptosis from proliferation of intraorbital lymphatic tissues, systemic steroids are administered.

Venous Malformation

Venous malformation or orbital varices are low flow vascular lesions that result from vascular dysgenesis. There may be enophthalmos at rest but on Valsalva's maneuver or on dependent position of head, the proptosis increases. The enlargement of the engorged veins are visualized on contrast enhanced CT scan during Valsalva's maneuver. Phleboliths may be seen.

Treatment is usually conservative and biopsy is avoided because of risk of hemorrhage. Surgery is indicated for relief of significant pain or when the malformation causes vision threatening compressive optic neuropathy. Surgical excision is difficult due to proximity of orbital structures and direct communication with cavernous sinus. Intraoperative embolization of the lesion may aid surgical removal. Excision following intralesional injection of cyanoacrylate has been described. Embolization with coils inserted through distal venous cut down has been found effective.

Arteriovenous malformations: These are high flow, developmental anomalies resulting from vascular dysgenesis and composed of abnormally formed anastomosing arteries and veins without intervening capillary bed (Figs. 5A and B). There may be dilated, episcleral corkscrew vessels. The lesions are studied by arteriography followed by selective occlusion of the feeding vessels and then surgical excision.

Arteriovenous fistula (AV fistula): These are acquired lesions that may be caused by trauma or degeneration and result in abnormal direct communication between an artery and vein. The blood flows directly from artery to vein without passing through the capillary bed.

The two forms of AV fistula are:

1. Carotid cavernous fistula: This typically occurs after a basal skull fracture. The high blood flow produces characteristic tortuous epibulbar vessels, bruit and pulsatile proptosis. Diversion of arterialized blood into the venous system may cause venous outflow obstruction and ischemic ocular damage. There may be elevated intraocular pressure (IOP), choroidal effusion, blood in Schlemm canal, and nongranulomatous iritis. There may be compression of cranial III, IV and VI nerve resulting in extraocular muscle palsy (Figs. 6A to C). Evaluation requires contrast angiography and treatment is required if the vision is threatened. Detachable balloon technique through endoarterial route where the balloon enters the fistula and is inflated till the fistula closes is the optimal treatment.

   Embolization, electrothrombosis, and direct surgery are other treatment modalities that are used.

2. Dural cavernous fistula: This usually occurs as a result of degenerative process in older patients with systemic hypertension and atherosclerosis. The small meningeal branches communicate with the venous drainage. The onset is insidious with only mild orbital congestion, proptosis, and pain. Arterialization of conjunctival veins may lead to chronic red eye. Asymmetric elevation of IOP may develop due to raised episcleral venous pressure. CT shows enlargement of all extraocular muscles due to venous engorgement and characteristically enlarged superior ophthalmic vein. Balloon occlusion is not possible in all cases due to small branches. For external carotid feeder vessels, embolization is possible with detachable balloons, isobutyl cyanoacrylate, and

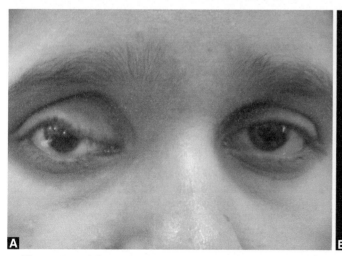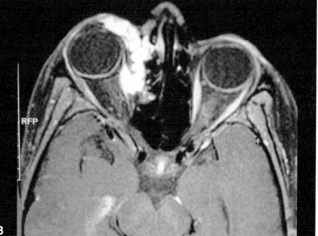

Figs. 5A and B: (A) Right upper lid A-V malformation; (B) MRI showing hyperintense lesion extending from lid to the extraconal compartment medially.

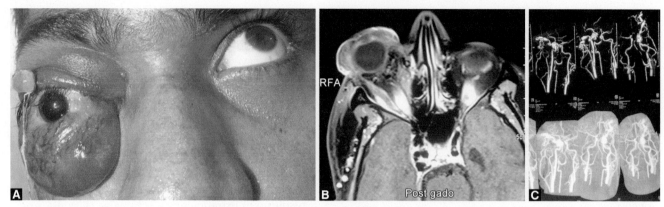

Figs. 6A to C: (A) Clinical picture with right proptosis and chemosis; (B) MRI of orbit showing enlargement of extraocular muscles and soft tissue edema; (C) Angiography showing A-V fistula.

polyvinyl alcohol particles. Electrothrombosis and direct surgery are associated with failure and morbidity.

NEURAL TUMORS

The optic nerve and the orbital peripheral nerves have major anatomic and cellular differences.

The meningeal tissues around the optic nerve are responsible for primary optic nerve meningiomas through the proliferation of meningoendothelial cells.

The intra-axial parenchymal portion of the optic nerve contains axons of the retinal ganglion cells that are enveloped in the myelin produced by oligodendroglial cells. The other type of cells, astrocytes, when transformed are responsible for optic nerve gliomas.

The peripheral orbital nerves include sensory branches of trigeminal nerve; 3rd, 4th, and 6th cranial nerves supplying the extraocular muscles; sympathetic and parasympathetic fibers. Most benign and malignant orbital peripheral nerve sheath tumors (PSNT) originate from divisions of trigeminal nerve. The peripheral nerves have an outer fibrous sheath called epineurium. Schwann cells serve as both astrocyte and oligodendrocyte in peripheral nerves. Each Schwann cell myelinates only one peripheral nerve. The nasociliary nerve is the only division of ophthalmic nerve that passes through the annular tendon. A PSNT arising from the nasociliary often causes compressive optic neuropathy which may be reversible on its removal.

Optic Nerve Gliomas

These are uncommon, usually benign tumors that present in the first decade of life. About half are confined to the orbit and rest may have intracranial extension. About 29% optic nerve gliomas are associated with neurofibromatosis 1 (NF1). Usual presentation is proptosis, decrease in visual acuity (NF1 patients have little if any visual acuity or visual field defect), and an afferent pupillary defect (Fig. 7).

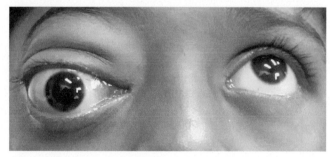

Fig. 7: Right optic nerve glioma with axial proptosis and RAPD.

Other findings may be optic atrophy, optic disk swelling, nystagmus, and strabismus.

MRI is the preferred imaging modality. It shows fusiform enlargement of the optic nerve. The two morphological patterns seen are:
1. Kinking as the nerve has an undulating appearance
2. Double intensity tubular thickening of the nerve.

Histologically, it is characterized as juvenile pilocytic astrocytoma consisting of cells with prominent eosinophilic processes called Rosenthal's fibers. The tumor may infiltrate the optic nerve substance or remain confined to the subarachnoid space.

Biopsy is rarely indicated. Close follow-up is required. Indications for surgical excision are:
- Disfiguring proptosis
- Continued deterioration of visual function
- Tumor extension documented on MRI

Chemotherapy is indicated for tumors affecting chiasma. Radiation therapy can be given for unresectable tumors. Stereotactic fractionated radiotherapy has shown to have good results.

Meningioma

Optic nerve sheath meningioma (ONSM)

Primary: Arises from cap cells of intraorbital or intracanalicular optic nerve sheath

Secondary: Arises intracranially from the region of sphenoid wing, tuberculum sella or olfactory groove.

Primary Optic Nerve Sheath Meningioma

Average age of onset is 5th decade and is more common in women.

Frequently associated with NF2 and may be bilateral.

Presentation: Blurred vision with little if any proptosis, opticociliary vein collaterals in presence of vision loss, and optic disk pallor suggest the diagnosis of ONSM. There is central or paracentral scotoma.

Radiological features:
- Fusiform enlargement of optic nerve sheath complex
- Flattening of posterior globe due tumor encroachment
- Enlargement of optic canal
- Circumferential calcification: Axial CT shows tram track sign; Coronal CT shows double ring sign.

Histopathological characteristic features:
Whorls and psammoma bodies are the characteristic features. Whorls are spindle-shaped cells, concentrically packed, producing onion skin appearance in cross section. Psammoma bodies are concentric lamellae of calcium deposits seen in the degenerative center of whorls.

Treatment:
Biopsy is rarely required for diagnosis and is indicated in patients with breast carcinoma to rule out metastasis.

Close follow-up is indicated due to slow growth. Three-dimensional conformal radiation therapy (3D-CRT) or stereotactic fractionated radiotherapy have been reported to have good results. Surgery is indicated in eyes that are already blind or to prevent extension to adjacent critical structures.

Secondary Optic Nerve Sheath Meningioma

- Associated with painless progressive vision loss with or without diplopia
- Sphenoid wing meningioma may present with proptosis
- Opticociliary shunts are absent but optic atrophy or papilledema may be present if there is direct tumor compression of the optic nerve or increased intracranial pressure
- Neuroimaging helps in diagnosis
- Close follow-up is indicated till symptoms worsen as the tumor shows a slow growth pattern. Surgical resection with or without radiation therapy is the definitive treatment.

Peripheral Nerve Sheath Tumors

Schwannoma (Neurilemoma)
- These arise from Schwann cells and account for 1% of all orbital tumors

- Associated with NF1
- Age group affected: Young to middle age adults
- Presents as slowly progressive proptosis
- Usually extraconal (especially superior orbit) but can be intraconal (Figs. 8A and B)
- Histopathology: Well encapsulated tumors with smooth surface, fish flesh to tan coloration on cut surface
- Microscopically, solid areas (Antoni A) alternate with myxoid areas (Antoni B). Spindle cell population oriented as fascicles is seen in a background of fibrillar material. Lateral palisading of nuclei and Verocay's bodies are other characteristic features
- Can undergo cystic degeneration
- The deposition of collagen is less than in neurofibromas, and is responsible for the friability of these tumors. It is vimentin and S-100 positive
- Encapsulated tumor that does not involve the axons and surgical resection leaves an intact nerve
- Malignant transformation is rare but recurrent tumors are aggressive.

Neurofibromas
- In contrast to Schwanomas, that are pure proliferations of Schwann cells, neurofibromas are composed of

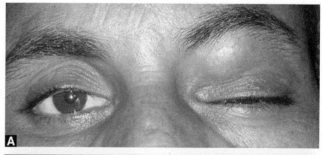
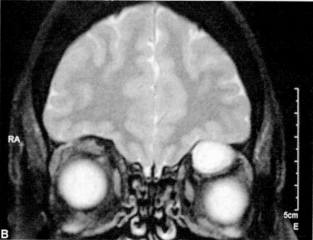

Figs. 8A and B: (A) Schwannoma presenting as left superior orbital mass pushing the globe downwards; (B) MRI of orbit showing well circumscribed mass in the superior orbit.

peripheral nerve axons, endoneural fibroblasts, and perineural cells
- Associated with NF1
- Non-encapsulated
- Types of orbital neurofibromas: Localized, plexiform, and diffuse
- Though benign can undergo malignant transformation.

Localized neurofibroma:
- Can occur singly or in multiples
- Non-encapsulated but circumscribed
- Insidious in onset
- Presents as localized orbital soft tissue mass, causing painless or mildly painful proptosis in young- to middle-aged adults. If located posteriorly, it may cause optic neuropathy
- It resembles schwannoma but is nonencapsulated, lacks friability due to greater deposition of collagen and does not show yellow discoloration or cystification
- Treatment involves excision.

Plexiform and diffuse neurofibromas:
- Present in first decade of life
- There is massive overgrowth of lids, infiltration of orbit and facial tissues (elephantiasis neuromatosa). On

palpation, the lids may feel like bag of worms; lacrimal gland involvement results in S shaped deformity (Figs. 9A and B)
- Other features of NF1 that may be present include café-au-lait spots, skin neurofibromas (fibroma molluscum), Lisch's iris nodules, axillary freckles, ectropion uveae, pigmented fundus lesions, uveal melanocytic, and ganglioneuromatous diffuse thickening, glaucoma, thickened corneal nerves, and pulsatile proptosis (caused by transmission of arterial pulsation of cerebrospinal fluid to the globe via bone defect usually greater wing of sphenoid). It may be associated with pilocytic astrocytoma or primary nerve sheath meningioma
- Management is unsatisfactory and complete excision is an exception. As the tumor is richly vascularized, robust bleeding may occur. There is 10% probability of malignant transformation.

MESENCHYMAL TUMORS

Rhabdomyosarcoma

Rhabdomyosarcoma is the most common primary malignancy of the orbit in children. The average age of

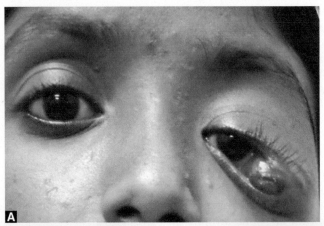

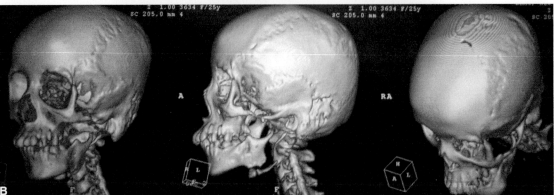

Figs. 9A and B: (A) Left plexiform neurofibroma; (B) 3D reconstruction showing sphenoid wing dysplasia.

patients affected by rhabdomyosarcoma is 7–8 years but it can also occur in adults.

Cause has been implicated to preexistent radiotherapy and germline mutation of p53 suppressor gene as in the rare cluster of families referred to as Li-Fraumeni syndrome.

Sudden onset, rapidly progressive unilateral proptosis developing in days to weeks is the classical picture (A less dramatic course is seen in teenagers.). There is marked edema and discoloration of lids that may be accompanied with ptosis and strabismus. The tumor may involve any quadrant, however, a palpable mass be felt usually in the superonasal quadrant.

A baseline CT scan and MRI for primary and metastatic sites, i.e. lung, liver, brain are required for preoperative evaluation. It also serves as a base line for adequacy of treatment. On CT scan, tumor appears isointense to muscle and shows homogeneous enhancement of soft tissue mass. Paranasal sinuses are usually clear of disease and helps in differentiating it from orbital cellulitis. On MRI, it is hyperintense to brain in T2 weighted images and enhance on gadolinium. Orbital biopsy helps in confirmation of diagnosis. The approach is to remove as much tumor as possible without risking the globe and optic nerve. Bone marrow aspirate and lumbar puncture helps in staging of the tumor and is performed under anesthesia at the time of initial biopsy.

Rhabdomyosarcoma arises from undifferentiated pluripotential mesenchymal elements in orbital soft tissues and not from extraocular muscles. Grossly, the fresh tumors are red to tan yellow and have a fish flesh appearance. The tumors are grouped as in Table 1.

Current treatment regimens avoid enucleation and exenteration. Local radiation and systemic chemotherapy are the main stay of treatment. Adverse effects of radiation are common in children and include cataract, radiation dermatitis, bony hypoplasia, etc. According to recent recommendation by Intergroup Rhabdomyosarcoma study group (IRS) the total amount of radiation is reduced to bring down the treatment induced side effects. So standard dose of vincristine is combined with 45 Gy of radiation in low-risk cases. The complications associated with chemotherapy are infertility after exposure to alkylating agents and cardiotoxicity after anthracycline exposure. Life-threatening infections due to immunosuppression and second malignancy are other side effects.

Long-term follow-up is required to monitor for tumor recurrence and consequences of therapy. Recurrence if confined to the orbit, requires exenteration and for subclinical metastasis chemotherapy is reintroduced.

Miscellaneous Mesenchymal Tumors

Osteoma is the most common tumor of the bones of the orbit. It may arise from any of the periorbital sinuses with frontal and ethmoidal being the most common. The common presentations are slowly progressive proptosis, acquired Brown's syndrome, compressive optic neuropathy, and nasolacrimal duct obstruction. Osteomas appear hyperdense, rounded or multilobulated on imaging. Complete excision is performed if the tumor is symptomatic.

Fibrous dysplasia (Figs. 10A and B)is a benign developmental disorder of bone that may involve single or multiple bones and is rare after 15 years of age. There may be headaches, proptosis, nasal obstruction or optic canal narrowing with optic nerve compression. In Albright's syndrome, there is involvement of multiple bones on same side of body (polyostotic fibrous dysplasia), cutaneous pigmentation, and endocrine disorders. Fibrous dysplasia is a benign condition, but malignant transformation is possible. Complete local excision is difficult and conservative surgical excision is preferred in patients with compromise of function, progression of deformity, pain, pathological fracture, or development of malignancy.

Fibrous histiocytoma presents as a firm mass that displaces the normal structures. According to WHO, hemangiopericytoma is now classified as a "cellular variant of solitary fibrous tumor" and Fibrous histiocytoma is considered as a variant of solitary fibrous tumor.

TABLE 1: Classification of rhabdomyosarcoma.

Type	prevalence	Site predilection	Microscopic appearance	prognosis
Embryonal	Commonest >80%	Superonasal quadrant of the orbit	Loose fascicles of undifferentiated spindle cells are seen with a minority showing cross striations.	Good (94% survival rate)
Alveolar	About 9%	Inferior orbit	Regular compartments of fibrovascular strands are seen in which rounded rhabdomyoblasts either line up along the connective tissue strands or float freely in alveolar spaces	Most malignant with 10 year survival rate of 10%
Pleomorphic	Least common	None	Most differentiated, cells are strap like or rounded, cross striations are visualized with trichome stain.	Best prognosis (97% survival rate)
Botryoid	Rare	Secondarily invades orbit from paranasal sinuses or conjunctiva	Similar to embryonal variety with presence of cambium level of Nicholson beneath the epithelial layer	Better than classic embryonal

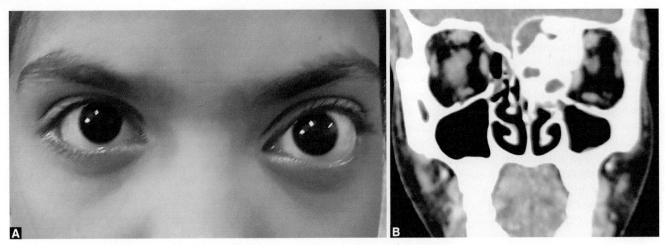

Figs. 10A and B: (A) Fibrous dysplasia of left orbit; (B) Coronal view of CT scan showing left ethmoidal bone expansion due to fibrous dysplasia.

Malignant mesenchymal tumors such as liposarcoma, fibrosarcoma, chondrosarcoma, and osteosarcoma rarely appear in the orbit.

LYMPHOPROLIFERATIVE DISORDERS

Lymphoid Hyperplasia and Lymphoma

Exposure to bioactive solvents, older persons and patients with chronic autoimmune diseases are at increased risk for non-Hodgkin's lymphoma.

Classification of Systemic Lymphomas

The Rappaport classification has been replaced by the Revised European American lymphoma classification as the former did not address the B-cell lymphoma present in the orbit and was not based on phenotypic or genetic studies.[9] Majority of orbital lymphomas are derived from B cells, the T cell lymphomas are rare and lethal.

B-cell lymphomas are divided into Hodgkin's and non-Hodgkin's tumors. Malignant non-Hodgkin's B-cell lymphoma account for more than 90% of orbital lympho-proliferative disease.

The common types of orbital lymphoma (REAL classification):

- Mucosa-associated lymphoid tissue (MALT) lymphoma account for 40–60% of orbital lymphomas. 50% of MALT lymphomas arise from gastrointestinal tract and may be antigen driven. Treatment against *Helicobacter pylori* (antigenic stimulus) may result in regression of early lesions. MALT lymphomas have low-grade malignancy and 50% may develop systemic disease in 10 years or transform to a higher grade lesion.
- Chronic lymphocytic lymphoma (CLL) is a low-grade lesion of small mature appearing lymphocytes.

- Follicular center lymphoma is a low-grade lymphoma with follicular center.
- High grade lymphoma includes large cell lymphoma, lymphoblastic lymphoma, and Burkitt lymphoma.

Clinical Presentation

These arise as painless, gradually progressive masses located in the anterior orbit (Figs. 11A and B) or beneath the conjunctiva (salmon patch appearance). They mold to the surrounding orbital structures rarely causing bony erosion except in high grade malignant lymphomas. 50% orbital lymphomas arise from lacrimal fossa and 17% are bilateral. Plasma cell tumors have the same spectrum of clinical involvement but are composed of mature plasma cells.

Diagnosis and Management

Open biopsy is preferable and tissue should be studied for morphologic, immunologic, cytogenetic, and molecular properties. The risk of developing systemic lesions in non-Hodgkins lymphoma is lowest for conjunctival lesions, greater for orbital, and highest for lesions arising from eyelid.

A thorough general physical examination, complete blood count, bone marrow biopsy, liver and spleen scan, X-ray chest, serum immunoelectrophoresis, CT thorax/abdomen needs to be performed.

Radiotherapy is the treatment of choice for patients with localized ocular adnexal lymphoproliferative disease. The usual dose is 2,000–3,000 cGy. A complete resection is difficult due to infiltrative nature of lymphoid tumors. Additional chemotherapy is required for aggressive lymphomas. Cure is achieved in one third cases.

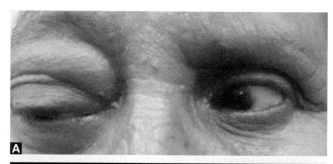

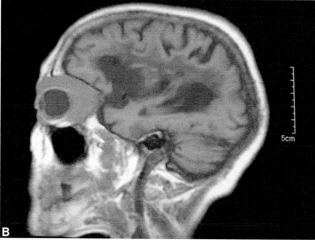

Figs. 11A and B: (A) Right proptosis with periorbital fullness in orbital lymphoma; (B) MRI sagittal scan: The mass molded around the orbital structures.

HISTIOCYTIC DISORDERS

Langerhans cell histiocytosis (histiocytosis X) occurs due to disorder of mononuclear phagocytic system leading to abnormal immune regulation. There is accumulation of proliferating dendritic histiocytes. Children usually between 5 years and 10 years are affected. The severity varies from benign lesion showing spontaneous resolution to death following dissemination. The terms unifocal and multifocal eosinophilic granuloma of bone and diffuse soft tissue histiocytosis are now being used instead of Hand-Schuller-Christian syndrome and Letterer-Siwe disease.

Lytic defects occur in the superotemporal orbit or sphenoid wing causing relapsing episodes of inflammation that may mimic orbital cellulitis. The mass may cause proptosis. Survival rates are 50% in patients presenting before 2 years of age. For those presenting later 87% survival rates are reported.

For localized orbital disease, confirmatory biopsy is followed by debulking and intralesional steroids or low-dose radiation therapy. The bone reossifies completely.

Aggressive chemotherapy is indicated in presence of systemic disease.

TABLE 2: Types of xanthogranuloma.

	Type	Associations
1	Necrobiotic xanthogranuloma (NBX)	Subcutaneous lesions especially in eyelids and anterior orbit that may ulcerate and fibrose; paraproteinemia, multiple myeloma
2	Adult onset asthma with periocular xanthogranuloma (AAPOX)	Periocular xanthogranuloma, asthma, lymphadenopathy, increased IgG levels
3	Erdheim-Chester disease (ECD)	Dense, progressive recalcitrant fibrosclerosis of orbit and internal organs leading to visual loss and death
4	Adult onset xanthogranuloma (AOX)	No systemic involvement

(AAPOX = Adult onset asthma with periocular xanthogranuloma; AOX = Adult onset xanthogranuloma; ECD: Erdheim-Chester disease; MNBX: Necrobiotic xanthogranuloma)

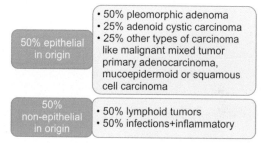

Fig. 12: Classification of lacrimal fossa masses.

Xanthogranuloma.

Occurs in adults and is classified on basis of associated systemic manifestations (Table 2).

LACRIMAL GLAND TUMORS

Classification of Lacrimal Fossa Masses (Fig. 12)[10]

Inflammatory and lymphoid masses expand diffusely and mold around the globe. Epithelial neoplasms appear globular, tend to displace and indent the globe, and remodel the lacrimal fossa bone.

Epithelial Tumors of Lacrimal Gland
Pleomorphic Adenoma (Benign Mixed Tumor)

Occurs usually during fourth and fifth decade with male preponderance. Gradual, progressive, downward, and inward displacement of globe. A firm, lobular mass may be palpable near the superotemporal orbital rim. On CT scan, the lesion appears well circumscribed with slightly nodular configuration (Figs. 13A and B). Microscopically, there is primary proliferation of benign epithelial cells with occasional cartilaginous, mucinous or even osteoid degeneration, thus being called a mixed cell tumor. The mass is circumscribed with a pseudocapsule.

Treatment involves complete removal of the tumor along with its capsule without a preliminary biopsy (Fig. 13C). Initial biopsy may lead to recurrence rate of 32% and risk of malignant transformation.

Adenoid Cystic Carcinoma (Cylindroma)

Highly malignant tumor, that may cause pain due to perineural invasion and bone destruction. Rapid course (usually <1 year) and pain differentiates from benign mixed cell tumor. The tumor tends to infiltrate posteriorly due to lack of true capsule (Figs. 14A to C).

Microscopically, the cells tend to grow in tubules, solid nests or a cribriform Swiss cheese pattern.

Malignant mixed tumor arises from long standing primary benign mixed tumor or from recurred benign mixed tumor following incomplete excision or previous biopsy.

Management of malignant tumor:
Confirmation with biopsy followed by:
- Exenteration
- Radical orbitectomy with removal of roof, lateral wall, floor along with overlying soft tissue, and anterior portion of temporalis muscle
- High dose radiation therapy in conjunction with debulking
- Intracarotid chemotherapy followed by exenteration.

The prognosis is dismal with perineural extension into the cavernous sinus and systemic metastasis ultimately leading to death.

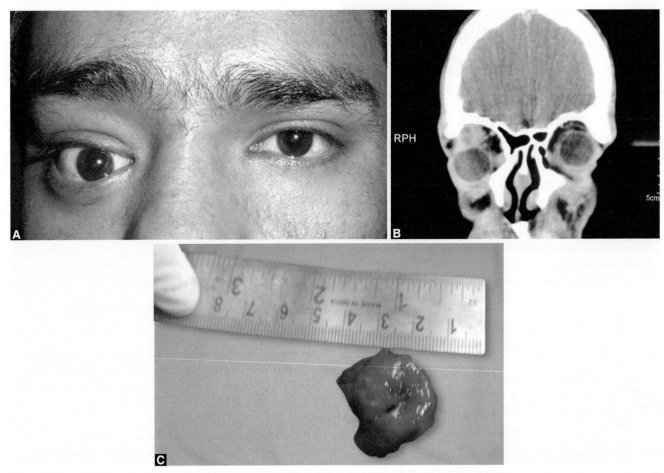

Figs. 13A to C: (A) Left pleomorphic adenoma pushing the globe downwards and medially; (B) CT scan, the lesion appears well circumscribed with slightly nodular configuration; (C) Treatment involves complete removal of the tumor along with its capsule without a preliminary biopsy.

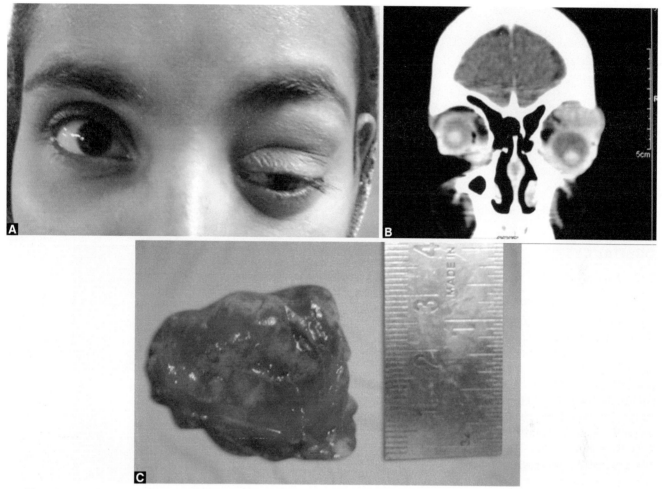

Figs. 14A to C: (A) Left adenoid cystic carcinoma of lacrimal gland pushing the globe downwards; (B) CT scan showing bony destruction; (C) Excised mass showing lack of capsule.

SECONDARY ORBITAL TUMORS

These occur following extension into the orbit from contiguous structures like tumors from within the eye like choroidal melanoma, retinoblastoma; tumors of the eyelid like sebaceous cell carcinoma, squamous cell carcinoma, basal cell carcinoma; squamous cell carcinoma from maxillary sinus; osteomas, and fibrous dysplasia from sinus/nose/facial bones.

METASTATIC TUMORS

Children

Neuroblastoma produces ecchymotic proptosis that may be bilateral. There is bone destruction of lateral wall of the orbit or sphenoid marrow. Primary tumor may be detected in the abdomen, mediastinum or neck. Treatment is by chemotherapy. Radiotherapy is indicated for impending visual loss due to compressive optic neuropathy. Survival rate is 90% for children diagnosed before 1 year of age and 10% for those diagnosed at an older age.

Leukemia may cause unilateral or bilateral proptosis. Acute lymphoblastic leukemia commonly metastasizes to orbit followed by a granulocytic sarcoma or chloroma, a variant of myelogenous leukemia (Figs. 15A and B).

Adults

Breast (49%), prostate (11%), gastrointestinal tumors (9%), thyroid carcinoma (5%), and lung carcinoma (5%) can metastasize to the orbit. Patient presents with pain, proptosis, inflammation, bone destruction and early ophthalmoplegia. Metastatic prostate cancer may present as acute nonspecific orbital inflammation.

Abundant blood supply of extraocular muscles and high volume low flow blood in bone marrow of sphenoid account for their frequent involvement. Elevation of carcinoembryonic antigen indicates a metastatic process.

Treatment is usually palliative.

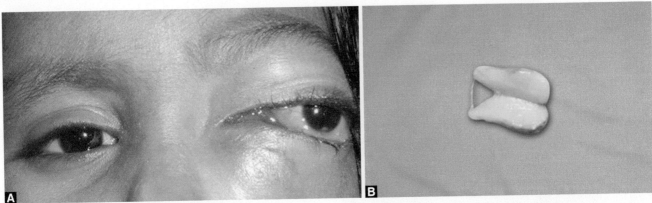

Figs. 15A and B: (A) Orbital involvement in leukemia; (B) Greenish tinge of the chloroma.

ORBITAL CYSTS

Developmental Cysts

Dermoid and Epidermoid Cyst

These are choristomas (origin from aberrant analage). The dermal elements get pinched off along suture lines in course of embryonic development. Histopathologically, there is a fibrous capsule and within the capsule, in epidermoid there is a lining of epithelial cells that is capable of producing keratin. In dermoid cyst in addition, there is a middle layer containing blood vessels, fat globules, sebaceous glands, and follicles. There may be a fibrovascular connection to the adjacent periorbita. The contents of the cyst vary from oily, tan liquid, cheesy white material.

The cyst may appear anytime between 2 years and 50 years with peaks at 3–10 years and then third and fourth decade. The favored location is anterior orbit and is more common in upper portion and presents as painless smooth mass (Fig. 16).

Surgical removal gives complete cure. Deeper cysts require CT scan to assess its extent. Meticulous dissection is warranted to prevent spillage of contents that may induce inflammation and recurrence.

Teratoma

In dermoid and epidermoid analage is derived from one germ layer whereas in teratoma it is derived from one, two, or three germ layers. Teratomas occur at any age but majority are present at birth or appear within first 6 months. There is a dramatic unilateral proptosis at or near time of birth. Teratoma is easier to remove in older patients but in younger age group it may be difficult to salvage the eye.

Cephalocele

Sac-like herniation of brain or its membranes may protrude into the orbit pushing the globe to one side or

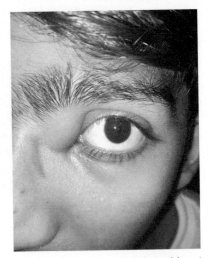

Figs. 16: Internal angular dermoid cyst.

may protrude anteriorly on to the face. Depending on its contents, it may be meningocele, encephalocele, and meningoencephalocele.

Microphthalmos with Cyst

A hiatus in closure of embryonic ocular cleft at about 4th week of embryonic life may continue to expand and result in a small, defective eye (Figs. 17A and B).

Mucocele

Mucocele occurs secondary to obstruction of the ostium of sinus. Continued secretion may lead to erosion of the bone and exit into the orbit. Depending upon the location symptoms may vary from proptosis, eye lid puffiness, ophthalmoplegia, and visual blurring.

Parasitic Cysts

Hydatid cyst, cysticercosis, filariasis, and sparganosis can infest the orbit.

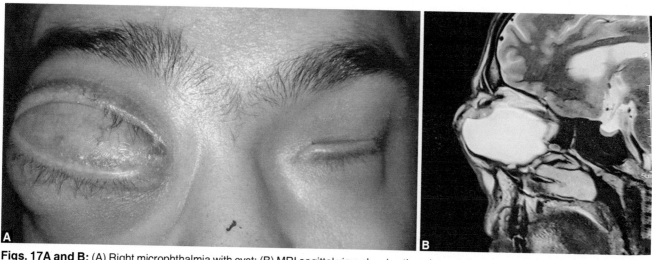

Figs. 17A and B: (A) Right microphthalmia with cyst; (B) MRI sagittal view showing the microoophthalmic eye pushed upward by the cyst.

Echinococcus Cyst

Echinococcus granulosus resides naturally in dog intestine. The eggs are shed in feces and life cycle continues in grazing animals. Human infestation occurs on eating animal tissue containing echinococcal cysts or fondling infected dogs. In human intestine, the embryo enters blood vessels and spreads to other organs.

Treatment is by complete surgical removal. The cyst is aspirated and 10–20% hypertonic saline is injected and left for 5 minutes which causes scolices to detach from the germinal wall. The contents are aspirated and replaced with 1–2% formalin that is kept for 5 minutes. This causes albumin to precipitate on surface of the parasite. Formalin is aspirated and cyst removed.

Cysticercosis

Ocular cysticercosis can involve any part of the eye: approximately 4% involve the eyelid or orbit, 20% involve the subconjunctival space, 8% involve the anterior segment, and 68% involve the posterior segment (subretinal and intravitreal).

On CT scan, the characteristic feature is a hypodense mass with a central hyperdensity suggestive of the scolex. Serial B-scan ocular ultrasonography or CT scanning of the orbit helps to follow the resolution of the cyst, which is recognized by the disappearance of the scolex (Figs. 18A and B). Orbital cysts are best treated conservatively with a 4-week regimen of oral albendazole (15 mg/kg/d) in conjunction with oral steroids (1.5 mg/kg/d) in a tapering dose over a 1-month period.

Hematic Cyst

This may occur following trauma, oral contraceptives, or as a complication of systemic illness like scurvy, hemophilia etc. Unresolving cysts causing proptosis may be aspirated.

Simple Cysts

Serous cysts arise from small bursae between tendon sheaths of ocular muscles like superior rectus and inferior rectus.

Retention Cysts

Obstruction of orifices of glandular appendage like glands of Krause

Implantation Cyst

This occurs following misplacement of surface epithelium into the orbit following trauma.

SYNOPSIS

Orbital tumors may be primary, secondary extending from adjacent structures, or metastatic. The incidence of primary malignant neoplasms of orbit is low; thus, experience over time, pattern recognition based on imaging studies and clinical presenting signs, and familiarity with the full spectrum of histology, anatomic location, and possible extent of the lesion are key in making the correct diagnosis and initiating the appropriate management of orbital tumors. Benign vascular tumors are the most common benign variety and lymphoma is the most common malignant orbital tumor variety. However, the orbit is full of functionally important nerves, muscles, fat, and adnexal structures each of which can develop an abnormal growth pattern and become cancerous. This highlights the importance of experience and familiarity by the orbital oncologist with the full spectrum of histologies and presentations of orbital tumors. The value of imaging studies of the orbit cannot be overemphasized. The orbital surgeon should be familiar with at least the typical radiologic features of each orbital tumor and often will help

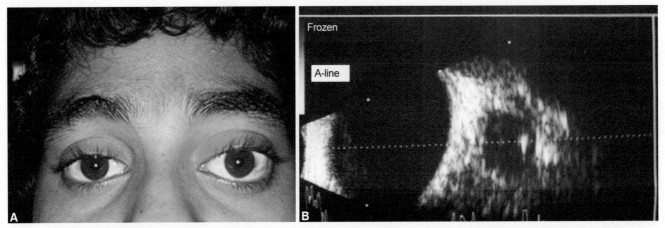

Figs. 18A and B: (A) Left proptosis due to orbit cysticercosis; (B) B-scan showing orbital cyst with scolex.

the radiology colleagues with the accurate diagnosis. Tissue diagnosis is often needed but in order to use the proper biopsy technique (incisional vs. excisional) or to decide whether surgery is even the appropriate next step, there is a need for experience and pattern recognition to allow the orbital surgeon to have a reasonably accurate presumptive diagnosis of tumor prior to any interventions. Prognosis depends on the type of tumor and extent of local or systemic disease at presentation. The extent of surgery is decided based on the expected biology of each tumor and whether or not adjuvant treatments such as radiation or chemotherapy are possible to use as a way to preserve tissue and do less morbid surgery. The goal is always to preserve as much visual and ocular function as possible while eliminating the potentially life-threatening cancer. The extent of surgery also can significantly impact the appearance of the patient. Thus, the orbital oncologic surgeon should take all of these factors into consideration when rendering treatments for malignant tumors of the orbit.

REFERENCES

1. Haik BG, Jakobiec FA, Ellsworth RM, et al. Capillary hemangioma of the lids and orbit: an analysis of the clinical features and therapeutic results in 101 cases. Ophthalmology. 1979;86(5):760-92.
2. Rootman J. Diseases of the Orbit. Philadelphia: JB Lippincott; 1988. p. 231.
3. Awadein A, Fakhry MA. Evaluation of intralesional propranolol for periocular capillary hemangioma. Clin Ophthalmol. 2011;5:1135-40.
4. Ni N, Wagner RS, Langer P, et al. New developments in the management of periocular capillary hemangioma in children. J Pediatr Ophthalmol Strabismus. 2011;48(5):269-76; quiz 268, 277.
5. Calandriello L, Grimaldi G, Petrone G, et al. Cavernous venous malformation (cavernous hemangioma) of the orbit: Current concepts and a review of the literature. Surv Ophthalmol. 2017;62(4):393-403.
6. Harris GJ. Orbital vascular malformations: a consensus statement on terminology and its clinical implications. Orbital Society. Am J Ophthalmol. 1999;127(4):453-5.
7. Kahana A, Bohnsack BL, Cho RI, et al. Subtotal excision with adjunctive sclerosing therapy for the treatment of severe symptomatic orbital lymphangiomas. Arch Ophthalmol. 2011;129(8):1073-6.
8. Kahana A, Levin LA. Peripheral nerve sheath tumors of the orbit. In: Albert DM, Miller JW (Eds). Albert & Jakobiec's Principles and Practice of Ophthalmology. Canada: Elsevier; 2008. pp. 3019-43.
9. Lauer SA. Ocular adnexal lymphoid tumors. Curr Opin Ophthalmol. 2000;11(5):361-6.
10. Tse DT, Hui JI. Epithelial tumors of the lacrimal gland. In: Albert DM, Miller JW (Eds). Albert & Jakobiec's Principles and Practice of Ophthalmology. Canada: Elsevier; 2008. pp. 2977-86.

Malignant Tumors of the Lid

Ruchi Goel

INTRODUCTION

Eyelid and ocular adnexa are in close proximity to the globe, brain, and paranasal sinuses. The tumors may arise de novo from lid structures or from adjacent tissues.

EPIDEMIOLOGY

Approximately 5–10% of all skin cancers arise in periorbital skin.

Basal cell carcinoma (BCC) accounts for nearly 80% of all nonmelanoma skin cancers and 90% of all malignant eyelid tumors.[1,2] Squamous cell carcinoma (SCC) is relatively uncommon in the eyelids, accounting for approximately 9% of all malignant eyelid tumors.[3] Sebaceous gland carcinoma (SGC) and malignant melanoma (MM) of the eyelid are rare lesions accounting for approximately 5% and 1% cases, respectively.[4-6]

PATHOGENESIS

Preexisting lesions, heritable and sporadic genetic mutations, environmental factors, and immunologic factors contribute to carcinogenesis. BCC, SCC, MM, and Merkel cell carcinoma (MCC) share ultraviolet (UV) radiation as one contributing factor, although SCC is less directly related to UV radiation.[7]

CLASSIFICATION BASED ON THE TISSUE OF ORIGIN

- Epithelial tumors—cutaneous BCC, SCC, MCC
- Sebaceous gland—SGC

- Sweat gland—Mucinous, nonmucinous (signet ring and histoid cell), and adenoid cystic carcinoma
- Vascular tumors—Hemangiopericytoma, angiosarcoma, Kaposi sarcoma
- Mesenchymal tumors—Fibrosarcoma, liposarcoma, rhabdomyosarcoma
- Melanocytic—Melanoma (superficial spreading, nodular, lentigo maligna melanoma)
- Lymphoreticular—Non-Hodgkin's lymphoma, Burkitt's lymphoma, Kimura's disease, lymphosarcoma, mycosis fungoides
- Nervous tissue—Neurofibrosarcoma
- Metastatic—Breast (most common), GIT, lungs, skin, genitourinary system.

CLINICAL EVALUATION AND WORK-UP

- Physical characteristics of the suspicious lesion including number, location, size, shape, color, contours, borders (discrete, undefined, regular, irregular, etc.), and (a) symmetry
- Superficial telangiectatic vessels
- Loss of eyelashes and lid architecture and position (ectropion and retraction)
- Fixation to the tarsus and orbital rim
- Examination of the head and neck for premalignant and malignant skin lesions (especially actinic keratosis, lentigo maligna, Bowen's disease, etc.); enlarged lymph nodes; scars from prior biopsies, radiation therapy, surgery, or trauma
- Sensory motor alterations (perineural invasion)—decreased or altered sensation (Vth nerve), pain, ophthalmoplegia, ptosis, or facial weakness

- Complete ophthalmic examination with precise attention to the caruncle and plicae, conjunctiva, inferior and superior conjunctival fornices, extraocular muscles, and nasolacrimal system
- Orbital examination for globe proptosis, dystopia or any palpable masses
- Radiographic evaluation especially for larger tumor or those located near the medial canthus or the lacrimal apparatus
  - CT scan may demonstrate bone alteration or destruction and extension into the nose, sinuses, orbit, or the cranial cavity
  - MRI imaging may show subtle tissue plane invasion or destruction and extension beyond the orbital septum or into the cranial cavity. It may also be useful for assessing perineural spread.

METHODS OF SPREAD

- Local extension into adjacent structures includes intraepithelial spread into epidermis and conjunctival epithelium, lacrimal secretory and excretory system, orbital soft tissues and cranial cavity.

Metastasis

- Lymphatics—preauricular, submandibular or cervical Sentinel lymph node (SLN) is the first node where metastasis occurs. Mapping and biopsy of SLN can be useful for detecting micrometastasis.
- Hematogenous—spread to lung, liver, bone, brain, and gastrointestinal tract
  Serologic workup [e.g. complete blood count, liver function test (LFT), kidney function test (KFT] CT scans of the head, chest, abdomen, and pelvis; upper GI endoscopy and colonoscopy; and positron emission tomography scan (for widespread pathology).
- Perineural spread (PNS)—most commonly in SCC followed by BCC and melanoma. It is responsible for recurrence and can involve contents of superior orbital fissure, foramen rotundum, and foramen spinosum.

BASAL CELL CARCINOMA

Eyelid, periocular or periorbital BCCs grow steadily, rarely metastasize, and are usually not fatal. However, if treatment is delayed they may eventually destroy the eye, orbit, nose, sinuses, nervous system, and the face. Various data support the notion that the hair follicle stem cell is the progenitor of BCC.

Topographic distribution in descending order of frequency is lower eyelid (44%), medial canthus (37%), upper eyelid (9%), lateral canthus (6%), glabella (2%), and more than one eyelid segment (2%).[7] BCC may present with varied clinopathological types (Table 1).

Basosquamous (metatypical) type—characterized by areas within the lesion with squamous differentiation. A superficial biopsy of such a lesion may be difficult to distinguish from SCC.

Inherited Predispositions of BCC

The inherited forms of BCC tend to occur at a younger age group (Table 2).

Histopathology

There is presence of basaloid cells that resemble the basal cells of epidermis but are larger and have high nuclear-cytoplasmic ratio. Nests of well demarcated basaloid cells project in the upper dermis.

Outcome and prognosis: BCCs are usually slow growing with excellent prognosis. They have high cure rates (95–99%) with extremely rare mortality. They rarely metastasize. BCC can locally invade into the orbit necessitating some type of exenteration in about 4% of patients (Fig. 3). Mortality rates from eyelid, periocular or periorbital BCC is less than 3%. Clinical risk factors for recurrence are prior recurrent tumor, large (>2 cm) size, medial canthus or upper eyelid location,

TABLE 1: Clinicopathologic types.[8,9]

Clinical types	Appearance	Metastases
Nodular (Fig. 1) 55–75%	Translucent papule early, Central ulceration, telangiectasia, pearly margin	Rare (0.02–1%)
Infiltrating 15%	Pale, indurated	Rare
Superficial or Multifocal 10%	Multiple erythematous patches, central superficial ulceration	Rare
Micro-nodular 6%	Small nodules, elevated or flat infiltrative	Rare
Sclerosing or Morphoeic 4%	Indurated shiny white pink to yellow plaque, usually intact skin surface, formation of crusts	Rare Local invasion/ Perineural spread
Pigmented 1% (Fig. 2)	Blackish in color	Rare
Cystic	Resembles adnexal cyst	Rare
Linear	Tumor extension from main lesion	Rare

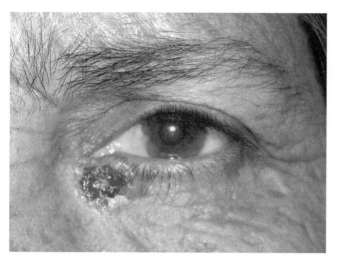

Fig. 1: Nodular basal cell carcinoma with central ulceration.

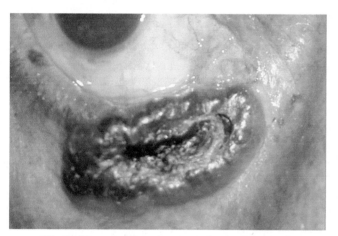

Fig. 2: Pigmented basal cell carcinoma of lower lid.

TABLE 2: Inherited forms of BCC.

1	Basal cell nervous syndrome/Gorlin syndrome	Autosomal dominant; multiple small BCC on face, mandibular cysts, frontal bossing, prominent supraorbital ridge, hypertelorism, congenital cataract, orbital cyst, colobomas, medullated nerve fiber in fundus, male hypogonadism, ovarian tumors.
2	Xeroderma pigmentosum	Autosomal recessive; infancy or childhood; associated with a variety of tumors like BCC, SCC, malignant melanoma; defect in gene responsible for repair
3	Albinism	Autosomal dominant; susceptibility to cutaneous damage bu UV B and cutaneous malignancy
4	Bazex syndrome	X linked; first two decades; atrophoderma with "ice pick" scars, hypotrichosis, hypohydrosis, multiple small BCC on face
5	Rhombo syndrome	Atrophoderma vermiculatum of face, multiple milia, telangiectasia, acral erythema, propensity for BCC

(BCC: basal cell carcinoma; SCC: squamous cell carcinoma)

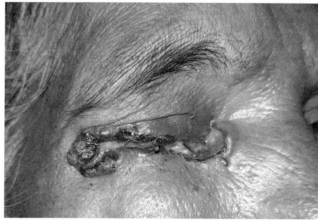

Fig. 3: Pigmented basal cell carcinoma with orbital invasion.

involvement of multiple eyelid segments, clinically ill-defined borders, multicentric tumors, immunosuppression, age less than 35 years, invasion of tarsus, and extension into the orbit, nose, sinuses, or nervous system.

All patents with periocular BCC need to be kept under lifelong follow-up due to the possibility of further primary BCC. Early use of sunscreens, sunglasses, and hats with brims decrease the incidence of BCC.

SQUAMOUS CELL CARCINOMA

Squamous cell carcinoma is an invasive epithelial malignancy derived from epidermal keratinocytes. The wide variation in clinical appearances presents great difficulty in differentiating it from BCC. It can appear de novo or more frequently may arise from a preexisting skin lesion: actinic keratosis (squamous cell dysplasia), intraepidermal carcinoma (IEC, carcinoma in situ), and keratoacanthoma.

Actinic keratosis presents as a rough, scaly, and erythematous patches occurring on chronically sun-exposed skin.

Intraepidermal carcinoma appears as poorly demarcated, erythematous crusted lesion with propensity to involve hair follicle, and simulate chronic blepharitis.

Bowen's disease: It is a specific type or superficial squamous IEC initially described in the trunk and later involving sun-exposed skin of the head and neck. It differs from IEC from having well-defined margins with velvety, scaly erythematous plaque, and moist granular base.

Keratoacanthoma presents as a solitary well-defined nodule with a central keratotic crater surrounded by layers of well-differentiated epithelial cells that may have cytological atypia. Clinically 25% undergo malignant transformation.

Invasive squamous neoplasia: Clinically it appears as roughened scaly plaque, which tends to develop telangiectasia, central ulceration, and/or keratinous crust or fissures over a period of time. If the crust is removed, commonly an ulcer will become apparent, showing a well-defined erythematous base with elevated and firm margins. Lesions may initially resemble blepharitis and a high index of suspicion is required to look for signs such as loss of normal tissue architecture. Biopsy must be performed in all doubtful cases.

For larger lesions an incisional biopsy may be appropriate to allow surgical planning.

Topographic distribution in lower lid, medial canthus, lateral canthus, and upper lid is 60.8%, 17.6%, 11.8%, and 9.8%, respectively.[10]

Histology

Nests, sheets, and strands of malignant epithelial cells showing mitotic figures that arise from keratinocytes located in the spinous layer of the epidermis are seen. The tumor cells have abundant eosinophilic cytoplasm and large vesicular nuclei. Keratinization is evident by the formation of keratinous cyst that are concentric layers of squamous cells. The well-differentiated type has proper keratinized pearls and intracellular bridges (Table 3).

Outcome and prognosis: Lymph node metastasis rates vary between 1% and 21%, whereas perineural spread (PNS) has been found in 4–8%.

Parotid and preauricular lymph nodes are most commonly affected followed by submandibular, submental, and lower cervical lymph nodes. Hematogenous spread is possible but seems much less common than either lymphatic or perineural routes. Predisposing clinical factors to lymph node metastasis include rapidly growing, large (>20 mm), thick (>4 mm), recurrent, or incompletely excised

TABLE 3: Histological variants of SCC.

Clinical Types	Appearance	Metastases
Plaque-like	Roughened, scaly, erythematous, hyperkeratotic	1–21%
Nodular (Fig. 4)	Hyperkeratotic nodule, with crusting and fissures	1–21%
Ulcerating	Indurated, red base	1–21%

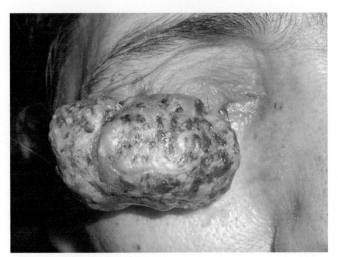

Fig. 4: Nodular squamous cell carcinoma.

tumors. Direct orbital invasion tends to occur with rapidly growing or neglected lesions and is seen in 6% cases. Mohs micrographic surgery, or en face techniques should be planned, as these are associated with low recurrence rates.

Mortality rate of SCC is 15%. Poorly differentiated SCC have worse prognosis with mortality up to 50%. Organ transplant recipients and patients with positive human immunodeficiency virus (HIV) develop SCC at a younger age with a more aggressive behavior. Minimizing sun exposure in childhood and adolescence can reduce the morbidity and mortality of SCC.

SEBACEOUS GLAND CARCINOMA

Sebaceous carcinoma is a malignant neoplasm that originates from cells that comprise sebaceous glands, particularly in the tarsus (meibomian glands), in association with the cilia (Zeis glands), caruncle, and eyebrow. In India, incidence of SGC seems to be higher accounting for 28% and 40–60% in two series. It can exhibit aggressive local behavior and masquerade as benign lesions such as chalazion, blepharitis, keratoconjunctivitis, or ocular pemphigoid, often resulting in delay in diagnosis and misdirected therapy. In a review, 63% occurred in the upper eyelid, 27% in the lower eyelid, and 5% diffusely involved both eyelids.

Sebaceous gland carcinoma can also occur as caruncular, eyebrow or even lacrimal gland mass.

SGC can present as a nodule, diffuse pseudoinflammatory pattern or pedunculated lesion (Table 4).

Histology

Four patterns are recognized—(1) The lobular pattern occurs most frequently and mimics the normal sebaceous gland architecture with less differentiated cells situated

TABLE 4: Clinical features of Sebaceous cell carcinoma.

Clinical types	Appearance	Metastases
Localized or nodular (commonest) (Figs. 5 and 6)	Compact lobules, Tumefaction within the eyelid, Firm to hard texture, yellow colour Minimally infiltrative	17–28%
Diffuse Pseudo-inflammatory pattern	Variably diffuse unilateral eyelid swelling resembling bleparitis, madarosis, moderately to highly infiltrative	17–28%
Pedunculated lesion	Involve margin, shows keratinization	17–28%

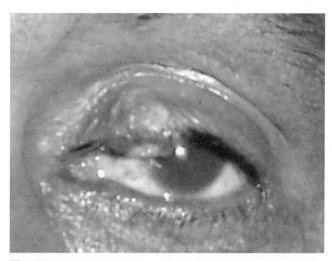

Fig. 5: Nodular sebaceous cell carcinoma of lid involving the lid margin causing loss of eyelid architecture with eyelash loss suggestive of malignancy.

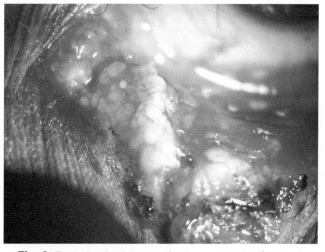

Fig. 6: Typical yellowish cast of sebaceous cell carcinoma.

peripherally, and better differentiated, lipid-producing cells located centrally. (2) In the comedocarcinoma pattern, the lobules show a large necrotic central core surrounded by peripheral viable cells. (3) The papillary pattern occurs frequently in small conjunctival tumors characterized by papillary projections and areas of sebaceous differentiation. (4) The mixed pattern can exhibit any combination of the three patterns. SGC can exhibit intraepithelial spread into the eyelid epidermis and conjunctival epithelium in 44–80% of cases. Incorrect initial histopathologic diagnoses have been reported in 40–75% of cases by an inexperienced pathologist. Pagetoid invasion of the eyelid or conjunctival epithelium can simulate squamous cell carcinoma in situ. The presence of lipid in normal sebaceous glands and in sebaceous neoplasms can be demonstrated with the oilred-O stain by which lipid has a red color.

Immunohistochemical stains help differentiate SGC from SCC and BCC. Epithelial membrane antigen (EMA) strongly stains SGC and SCC but not BCC. Cam 5.2 reactivity is seen in SGC and not SCC.

SGC and Systemic Disease

Association of SGC has been observed in:
- Familial retinoblastoma after radiotherapy
- HIV positive
- *Muir-Torre syndrome:* SGC with visceral malignancy especially colorectal cancer.

Special Diagnostic Tests in SGC

- *Map biopsy:* Due to pagetoid spread, multiple biopsies from bulbar and palpebral conjunctiva are taken to form a map of the extent of tumor spread.

- *Impression cytology:* This is performed in areas of suspicious bulbar conjunctiva.
- Fine needle aspiration cytology of local lymph nodes.

Prognosis and outcome: Sebaceous carcinoma can locally invade the adjacent epithelia or the orbital soft tissues. The most common method of metastasis is to the regional lymph nodes in about 30%. Advanced cases exhibit distant metastasis to lung, liver, bone, and brain. Mortality ranges from 18% to 30%.

Factors that are associated with a worse prognosis in SGC include vascular, lymphatic, and orbital invasion; involvement of both upper and lower eyelids, poor differentiation; multicentric origin; duration of symptoms greater than six months; tumor diameter exceeding 10 mm; a highly infiltrative pattern, and pagetoid invasion. Local recurrence can develop in 18%, death from metastasis in

6%, and exenteration may be necessary in 13%. Caruncular based tumors have 14% mortality rate. With the recently employed treatment methods, there is a tendency to avoid exenteration and to use a more conservative approach.

MALIGNANT MELANOMA OF EYELID

Malignant melanoma results from the malignant proliferation of melanocytes. MM is the cancer with the greatest increase in incidence in recent years. It represents only 5% of malignant skin tumors but is responsible for more than 65% of deaths associated with skin cancer. The majority originate de novo without history of precursor lesions. However, there are three described precursor lesions:

1. Dysplastic nevus clinically is asymmetrical, flat lesions with a slightly raised center. Borders may be irregular or poorly defined. Colors commonly observed are brown, tan, and blue; black is rare. About 28% of melanomas originate in a preexisting dysplastic nevus.

2. Congenital nevus is composed of a collection of melanocytes in the epidermis, dermis, or both and is present at birth or identified by the end of the first year of life. These lesions may be giant, large, small or nevus of Ota.

   The association with MM is uncertain and varies according to study, but in general may be considered to be 5% for giant nevi, 4% for large nevi, 1–2% for small nevi, and 4.6% for those with nevus of Ota.

3. Lentigo maligna is a slowly progressive, usually pigmented, irregularly-shaped lesion. It is usually found on the face in older adults or individuals with actinic damage. It represents melanoma in situ. When there is invasion into dermis, the term "lentigo maligna melanoma" is used.

White and Neil[11] clinically subdivided melanoma as follows:

- Melanoma in situ (atypical melanocytic proliferation)—neoplastic cells are present but have not penetrated the dermal–epidermal junction.

- Superficial spreading melanoma—accounts for about two-thirds of all cutaneous melanoma. In this type of melanoma, radial growth phase predominates during which melanocytic proliferation is intraepidermal. This lesion presents as a dark, flat with well-defined borders. Lesions may be variegated and include tan, black, gray, or pink areas.

- Nodular melanoma—generally originates de novo and has only a vertical growth phase. It tends to arise in the papillary dermis and has a blue-black color (Fig. 7).

- Lentigo maligna melanoma originates as a lentigo maligna that has been present for 10–15 years in skin with severe sun damage. When the surface of the lentigo

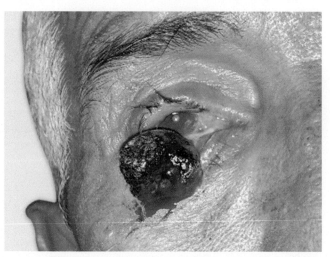

Fig. 7: Lower lid nodular malignant melanoma.

maligna presents an elevation or formation of nodule, it indicates transformation to malignancy.

- Amelanotic melanoma has lost its pigment. It is usually nodular but can be flat and is frequently misdiagnosed.

- Acral lentiginous melanoma—originates on the palms of the hand, soles of the feet, or extremities.

- Desmoplastic melanoma—most frequently located on the head and neck, and frequently subjacent to a lentigo maligna melanoma. It is histologically comprised of melanoma cells between a dense desmoplastic stroma.

In 2009, The American Joint Committee on Cancer published the cutaneous melanoma staging guidelines (Table 5).[12]

Patients with MM should be clinically staged to permit selection of the appropriate type of treatment and follow-up.[13]

Clinical Stage Groupings: Cutaneous Melanoma

- Stage 0 Tis N0 M0
- Stage IA T1a N0 M0
- Stage IB T1b-2a N0 M0
- Stage IIA T2b-3a N0 M0
- Stage IIB T3b-4a N0 M0
- Stage IIC T4b N0 M0
- Stage III Any T N 1-3 M0
- Stage IV Any T Any N M1.

Prognosis and outcome–Prognostic factors for MM are classified into three groups on the basis of the disease extent:[14]

1. *No evidence of metastasis*: Tumor thickness and ulceration are the most important predictors of survival. Other predictors are patient age (elderly patients), site of primary melanoma (trunk or head and neck), level of invasion, mitotic figures, and sex (males).

TABLE 5: TNM staging categories for cutaneous melanoma.

Classification		Thickness (mm)	Ulceration Status/Mitoses
T			
	Tis	NA	NA
	T1	<1.00	a: Without ulceration and mitosis <1/mm²
			b: With ulceration or mitoses >1/mm²
	T2	1.01–2.00	a: Without ulceration
			b: With ulceration
	T3	2.01–4.00	a: Without ulceration
			b: With ulceration
	T4	>4.00	a: Without ulceration
			b: With ulceration
N	No. of metastatic nodes		Nodal metastatic burden
N0	0		NA
N1	1		a: Micrometastasis*
			b: Macrometastasis†
N2	2-3		a: Micrometastasis*
			b: Macrometastasis†
			c: In transit metastases/ satellites metastatic nodes
N3	4+		Metastatic nodes, or matted nodes, or in transit metastases/satellites with metastatic nodes
M	Site		Serum LDH
M0	No distant metastases		NA
M1a	Distant skin, subcutaneous, or nodal metastases		Normal
M1b	Lung metastases		Normal
M1c	All other visceral metastases		Normal
	Any distant metastasis		Elevated

(NA: Not applicable; LDH: Lactate dehydrogenase)
*Micrometastases are diagnosed after sentinel lymph node biopsy.
†Macrometastases are defined as clinically detectable nodal metastases confirmed pathologically.

2. *Regional lymph node metastasis only*: Three most important predictors of survival are number of metastatic lymph nodes (poorer prognosis for higher number), tumor volume [(microscopic (nonpalpable) vs. macroscopic (palpable)], and ulceration. The positivity rate of sentinel lymph node has been reported to be 16%.

3. *Distant metastasis*: Anatomic site of distant metastasis (visceral vs. nonvisceral) is the most important predictor of survival. The Collaborative Eyelid Skin Melanoma Group (CESMG) reported distant metastases in 7%. The local recurrence rate of ~25% has been observed in various studies.

Merkel Cell Carcinoma (Neuroendocrine/ Trabecular Carcinoma)

Merkel cell carcinoma of the eyelid is a rare, highly aggressive skin malignancy.

Merkel cells are found in the basal layer of the epidermis and may play a role in touch sensation. Malignant neoplasms may arise from the Merkel cells.

Clinical appearance: Solitary, asymptomatic, rapidly growing, pink-red to blue-purple "violaceous" vascularized cutaneous nodule with occasional ulceration on a sun-exposed area. The growth is rapid with duration of symptoms less than 6 months.

The National Comprehensive Cancer Network classifies MCC into the following stages: stage I (primary tumor <2 cm), stage II (primary tumor ≥2 cm), stage III (regional nodal involvement), and stage IV (distant metastasis). On the basis of this staging system, the 3-year survival rates for all sites are approximately 90% for stage I, 70% for stage II, 60% for stage III, and 20% for stage IV. A median survival of 9 months is reported for patients with metastatic disease.[15]

Biopsy of Eyelid, Periocular or Periorbital Skin Lesions

Any lesion that may possibly be malignant should be biopsied. It is better to biopsy a benign lesion than to miss or delay the diagnosis of a malignant lesion. It can be either excisional or incisional. An excisional (total) biopsy is reasonable when a lesion is most probably benign, fairly small, easy to remove, or not involving the eyelid margin, canthi, or the lacrimal system. An incisional (partial) biopsy is useful if a malignancy is suspected or is highly likely and for masses on the eyelid margin, canthi, or the lacrimal system. This can be obtained via superficial shave (not in malignant melanoma), full thickness, or punch biopsy.

Sentinel lymph node biopsy is a minimally invasive procedure for identifying microscopic metastasis for additional regional or systemic treatment. It involves injecting a vital blue dye and radio-colloid (usually technetium 99 m) around a tumor or the site of its excision. Lymphatic channels stain blue, and these are mapped using lymphoscintigraphy. A gamma probe aids localization of radioactive sentinel nodes.

Conjunctival map biopsy is used for pagetoid spread of SGC. It includes taking multiple biopsies from bulbar and palpebral conjunctiva to form a map of extent of tumor spread across an ocular surface.

Treatment of Malignant Eyelid Tumors

Surgery is the treatment of choice for eyelid, periocular or periorbital lid tumors. It affords the advantage of total tumor removal and allows for the histopathological examination of the tissue. The two most effective modalities are Mohs' micrographic surgery (MMS) and excision with frozen section control. MMS is extremely useful in BCC and SCC. It has limited use in SGC because of noncontiguous or pagetoid spread and malignant melanoma due to vertical tumor growth (except in melanoma in situ).

Mohs' Micrographic Surgery

The surgeon marks the various margins with either suture or color dye. A diagram explaining the orientation and location of the margins relative to the eyelids is then provided to the pathologist which can guide the surgeon regarding any location(s) of remaining cancer cells or incomplete or unclear ("positive") margins. When all histologic margins are tumor free, the surgeon can begin reconstruction. Advantages of MMS are:

- Highest available cure rate combined with most predictable reconstruction
- Decreased morbidity, mortality, and disability
- Decreased time in the operating room by eliminating potentially long waits for frozen sections
- Objective assessment of complete tumor removal by the micrographic surgeon
  - Conservation of tissues, providing for more simplified reconstruction
  - Minimization of secondary procedures
  - Superior functional and cosmetic results.

MANAGEMENT OF BASAL CELL CARCINOMA AND SQUAMOUS CELL CARCINOMA

Excision with En Face Frozen Section Control of Margins
For well-circumscribed BCC lesions, 2 mm margin is kept. If the tumor is poorly defined, with indistinct margins, recurrent, at least 4 mm margin is used.

Nonsurgical modalities are reserved for patients who are debilitated, fearful or refuse surgery, and who have unrealistic expectations about the cosmetic healing after surgery. Some methods may be beneficial for selected patients. For example, photodynamic therapy, carbon dioxide laser therapy, and therapy with retinoids or α-interferon may benefit patients with multiple tumors. Chemotherapy may be useful for extensive and infiltrative disease as co-adjuvant or for metastasis to distant sites.

For small, superficial BCC on neck, trunk, arms or limbs topical imiquimod is applied once a day for several weeks. Targeted therapy is used in metastatic or locally advanced BCC when surgery or radiation cannot be used. Oral vismodegib and sonidegib are hedgehog pathway inhibitors, administered to stop the growth and spread of cancer cells.

Systemic agents like cisplatin, doxorubicin and Capecitabine have been used for BCC and SCC and topical mitomycin-C 0.4% four times a day for 1 week on therapy and 1 week off therapy been used for SGC.

Radiotherapy is useful for BCC and SCC, as fractioned doses between 5,000 cGy and 7,000 cGy in patients with positive margins, perineural spread, or extensive disease. It is only a palliative treatment and should not be used for canthal lesions because of risk of orbital recurrence. Disadvantages include inability to examine histological margins, occurrence of recurrence after a long time interval, cicatricial changes to eyelids, scarring of lacrimal drainage system, keratitis sicca, radiation induced malignancy, and injury to globe.

Cryotherapy acts by intracellular crystallization of water components resulting in necrosis of both normal and malignant cells. Treatment involves 2–3 rapid freeze cycles at -50°C followed by slow thaw. Due to high recurrence rates, it is used in patients who cannot tolerate surgery.

MANAGEMENT OF SEBACEOUS GLAND CARCINOMA

In SGC, wide local excision, including 5–6 mm normal tissue and frozen section analysis is to be done.

Conjunctival disease: In presence of conjunctival involvement, in addition to surgical excision of eyelid lesion, cryotherapy of the involved conjunctiva is performed. In cases with diffuse conjunctival involvement, mitomycin-C 0.4% four times a day for a week, medication free for a week, repeated till resolution of malignancy. Also MMC 0.2% four times for 2 weeks, off for 2 weeks for three cycles has been used.

Orbital invasion or diffuse conjunctival disease not treatable by above measures is managed by exenteration.

Radiotherapy is reserved for palliative treatment. Systemic chemotherapy has been used for metastatic disease and neoadjuvant therapy (chemotherapy prior to surgery).

TABLE 6: Recommended margin of excision for cutaneous melanomas.

Tumor thickness	Margins (cm)
<1 mm	1 cm
1–2 mm	1–2 cm
2.1–4 mm	2 cm
>4 mm	2 cm

MANAGEMENT OF MALIGNANT MELANOMA

Breslow thickness and Clark's level are important predictors of regional nodal and distant metastasis. Therefore, suspected lesions should not be biopsied by shave or curette technique.

Surgical treatment involves wide excision of margins as shown in Table 6.[16]

Radiation is not used as a definitive therapy and is used only as an adjuvant. Imiquimod cream may be used for treatment of melanoma in situ limited to skin of the eyelid.

If micrometastasis is found in the sentinel lymph node biopsy, complete surgical neck dissection of the lymphnodes followed by external beam radiation therapy/parotidectomy is required.

The common malignant tumors of the eyelid are BCC, SCC, SGC, and melanoma. Histopathology is the mainstay of diagnosis. Immunohistochemistry is especially useful in differentiating BCC, SCC, and SGC. Surgical excision with margin control should be performed as early as possible. BCC has less metastatic potential as compared to SCC, SGC, and melanoma. Sentinal lymph node biopsy is especially indicated in melanoma and SGC. Map dot biopsy is required in SGC due to skip conjunctival lesions. Chemotherapy, radiotherapy, and cryotherapy are used as adjuvants. Exenteration is done in case of orbital invasion. Need for extended follow up in view of recurrence and metastasis should be emphasized to the patient.

REFERENCES

1. Cook BE Jr, Bartley GB. Epidemiologic characteristics and clinical course of patients with malignant eyelid tumors in an incidence cohort in Olmsted County, Minnesota. Ophthalmology. 1999;106(4):746-50.
2. Margo CE, Waltz K. Basal cell carcinoma of the eyelid and periocular skin. Surv Ophthalmol. 1993;38(2):169-92.
3. Font RL. Eyelids and lacrimal drainage system. In: Spencer WH (Ed). Ophthalmic Pathology: An Atlas and Textbook, 4th edition. Philadelphia: W.B. Saunders; 1996. pp. 2270-8.
4. Shields JA, Demirci H, Marr BP, et al. Sebaceous carcinoma of the ocular region: A review. Surv Ophthalmol. 2005;50(2):103-22.
5. Miller SJ. Biology of basal cell carcinoma (Part II). J Am Acad Dermatol. 1991;24(2 Pt 1):161-75.
6. Holds JB. Basic and Clinical Science Course. Orbit, Eyelids, and Lacrimal System. San Francisco: American Academy of Ophthalmology; 2007–2008. pp. 158-76.
7. Mannor GE, Hybarger CP, Meecham WJ. Basal cell carcinoma of the eyelids: An analysis of 841 cases. New Orleans: American Academy of Ophthalmology; 2001.
8. Weber RS, Miller MJ, Goepfert H. Basal and squamous cell skin cancers of the head and neck. Baltimore: Williams & Wilkins; 1996.
9. Spencer WH. Ophthalmic Pathology: An Atlas and Textbook, 3rd edition. Philadelphia: W.B. Saunders; 1986. pp. 2169-78.
10. Donaldson MJ, Sullivan TJ, Whitehead KJ, et al. Squamous cell carcinoma of the eyelids. Br J Ophthalmol. 2002;86(10):1161-5.
11. White GM, Neil HC. Melanocytes, nevi, and melanoma. In: Disease of the Skin. St. Louis: Mosby; 2002. pp. 425-44.
12. Balch CM, Soong SJ, Atkins MB, et al. An evidence-based staging system for cutaneous melanoma. CA Cancer J Clin. 2004;54(3):131-49; quiz 182-4.
13. NCCN Clinical Practice Guidelines in Oncology. (2009). Melanoma V.2.2009. [online] Available from: http://www.nccn.org/professionals/physician_gls/PDF/melanoma.pdf. [Last Accessed January 2019].
14. Balch CM, Soong SJ, Gershenwald JE, et al. Prognostic factors analysis of 17,600 melanoma patients: validation of the American Joint Committee on Cancer melanoma staging system. J Clin Oncol. 2001;19(16):3622-34.
15. Buck CB, Lowy DR. Getting stronger: The relationship between a newly identified virus and Merkel cell carcinoma. J Invest Dermatol. 2009;129(1):9-11.
16. Esmaeli B. Melanocytic lesions of the eyelid and ocular adenexa. In: Albert DM, Miller JW (Eds). Albert & Jakobiec's Principles and Practice of Ophthalmology. Canada: Elsevier; 2008. pp. 3367-78.

Ocular Surface Tumors

Sima Das

INTRODUCTION

Tumors of the ocular surface include a wide range of lesions arising from the epithelium and stroma of the conjunctiva or cornea as well as from the surrounding structures. These tumors can have varied clinical presentation and can be benign or malignant. This chapter aims to discuss the clinical features, diagnosis, and the management of the various ocular surface tumors.

CLASSIFICATION OF OCULAR SURFACE TUMORS

Depending upon the tissue of origin, the tumors of the ocular surface can be classified into various categories (Box 1). The clinical features and the management of the common tumors are described in the following section.

Nonmelanocytic Benign Epithelial Tumors of Ocular Surface

Conjunctival Papilloma

Conjunctival papillomas can occur in children or adults. In children, conjunctival papilloma is associated with HPV 6, 11, and 16 infection.[1] Papillomas can be single or multiple, sessile or pedunculated (Figs. 1A and B). It appears as fleshy, pink, and papillary mass in the bulbar or forniceal conjunctiva. They are usually solitary but can be multiple, confluent, and bilateral. Though most remain asymptomatic, it can cause foreign body sensation, bleeding, and discharge. In adults, conjunctival papillomas are usually unilateral, sessile, and located at the limbus or bulbar conjunctiva. On histopathology, the

---

Box 1: Classification of ocular surface tumors.

Tumors of the epithelium
Melanocytic:
- Benign—conjunctival nevus
  - Racial melanosis
  - Primary acquired melanosis
- Malignant—Conjunctival malignant melanoma
Nonmelanocytic:
- Benign—Conjunctival papilloma
  - Keratoacanthoma
  - Reactive hyperplasia
  - Hereditary intraepithelial dyskeratosis
- Malignant—Ocular surface squamous neoplasia
Conjunctival stromal tumors
- Vascular tumors
- Fibrous
- Neural
- Myogenic
- Histiocytic
- Lipomatous
- Lymphoproliferative
- Metastatic and secondary conjunctival tumors

---

papilloma is composed of epithelial projection covered with nonkeratinized stratified squamous epithelium with a fibrovascular core within.

Though childhood papillomas can regress spontaneously, treatment is indicated in symptomatic lesion and in cases of suspicion of malignancy. "No touch technique" of surgical excision and cryotherapy to the conjunctival margins is preferred to prevent spread of the virus and recurrence of the lesion.[2] Other treatment modalities include topical interferon alpha2b, topical mitomycin C, and oral cimetidine for recurrent lesions.[3-5]

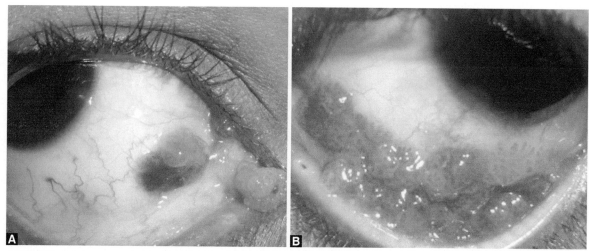

Figs. 1A and B: (A) Conjunctival papilloma involving the medial bulbar conjunctiva and the caruncle in an young adult; (B) Note the presence of brown pigmentation at the base of the lesion. Multiple conjunctival papilloma involving the inferior fornix.

Keratoacanthoma

Keratoacanthoma are rapidly growing lesion of the bulbar conjunctiva and rarely involve the palpebral conjunctiva (Fig. 2). These are benign, solitary lesion with gelatinous or leukoplakic surface and central umbilication in some cases. Keratoacanthoma is a premalignant lesion and is managed with complete surgical excision along with cryotherapy.[6,7]

Pseudoepitheliomatous Hyperplasia

These are raised leukoplakic lesion in the limbal area.[8] The lesions appear secondary to irritation from underlying stroma. Histopathology shows acanthosis, hyperkeratosis, and subepithelial inflammation. These lesions should be excised completely as these are sometimes difficult to differentiate clinically and histopathologically from conjunctival squamous cell carcinoma (SCC).

Nonmelanocytic Malignant Conjunctival Epithelial Tumor

Ocular Surface Squamous Neoplasia

Ocular surface squamous neoplasia (OSSN) is a broad term which includes a spectrum of malignancy ranging from epithelial dysplasia, carcinoma in situ, and invasive squamous cell carcinoma.

Risk factors for development of OSSN: Various risk factors have been proposed for the development of OSSN including chronic exposure to solar radiation and sunlight injury.[9] Systemic immune suppression as in HIV infection and use of immunosuppressives following organ transplant has been associated with OSSN development.[10] Systemic

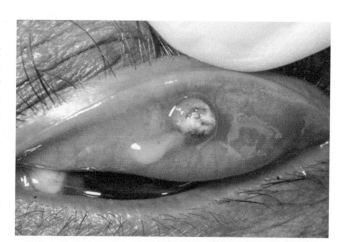

Fig. 2: Keratoacanthoma involving the palpebral conjunctiva.

associations for the development of OSSN include xeroderma pigmentosum and Papillon–Lefèvre syndrome.

Morphological variant: Morphologically, OSSN can be of the following types (Figs. 3A to F):
- Placoid
- Papilliform
- Gelatinous
- Nodular
- Diffuse
- Corneal.

Clinical features: Ocular surface squamous neoplasia arises most commonly from the limbus or the bulbar conjunctiva but can involve predominantly only cornea. It appears as a pink, fleshy, and sessile lesion at the limbus with variable extension on the conjunctiva and corneal surface. Presence of surface keratin, feeder vessels, and

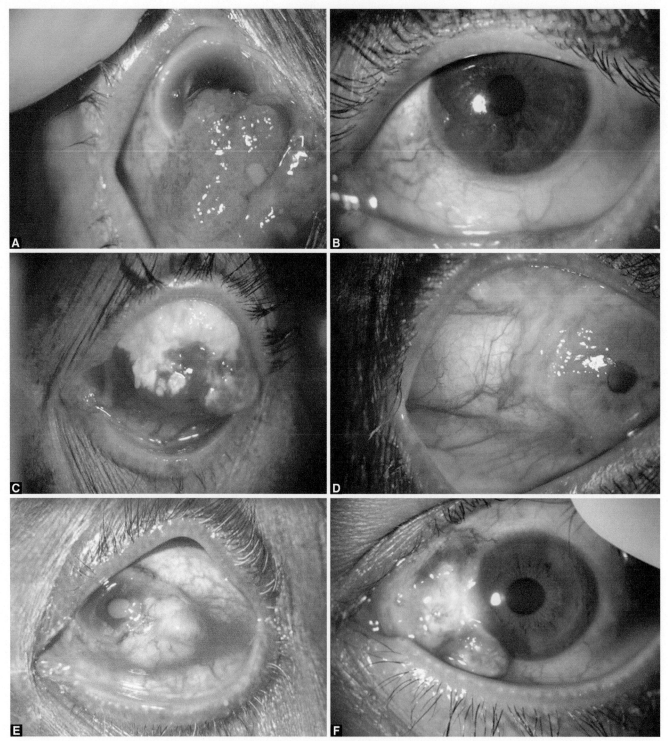

Figs. 3A to F: (A) Morphological variants of ocular surface squamous neoplasia (OSSN). OSSN presenting as papillary mass at the limbus; (B) Corneal OSSN presenting a translucent opacification of cornea with fimbriated edges; (C) Placoid lesion with surface keratin; (D) OSSN presenting as a gelatinous mass along the limbus; (E) Nodular variant of OSSN and; (F) pigmented OSSN.

intrinsic vessels are characteristic features. Rose Bengal staining helps in delineating the complete extent of the lesion and helps in surgical excision. Predominantly corneal involvement can appear as a grayish white opacification of the cornea with wavy margin and can masquerade a corneal scar thus delaying the diagnosis. Other atypical presentations like nodular variant can simulate a nodular scleritis and diffuse involvement of the ocular surface without presence of any nodular mass can be misdiagnosed as blepharoconjunctivitis. OSSN can also be pigmented especially in patients of African origin as part of complexion associated melanosis.[11] Untreated cases can invade the orbit, eyelid, and can have intraocular invasion. Regional lymph node involvement and systemic metastasis can occur in advanced cases. Aggressive variants like mucoepidermoid carcinoma, spindle cell carcinoma, and adenoid squamous cell carcinoma are more likely to be locally invasive and spread systemically.

Classification of conjunctival squamous cell carcinoma: Conjunctival SCC is classified according to the eighth edition of American Joint Committee on Cancer classification (AJCC) which grades the tumor according to the tumor, nodes, and metastasis staging system (Box 2).[12] The clinical classification is based on the tumor size and invasiveness and the pathological classification is based on tumor differentiation. The AJCC classification is predictive of response to treatment.

Box 2: American Joint Committee on Cancer 8th edition classification of conjunctival carcinoma (OSSN).

- *Definition of primary tumor:*
  - **(T)** TX Primary tumor cannot be assessed
  - T0 No evidence of primary tumor
  - Tis Carcinoma in situ
  - T1 Tumor (≤5 mm in greatest dimension) invades through the conjunctival basement membrane without invasion of adjacent structures
  - T2 Tumor (>5 mm in greatest dimension) invades through the conjunctival basement membrane without invasion of adjacent structures
  - T3 Tumor invades adjacent structures* excluding the orbit
  - T4 Tumor invades the orbit with or without further extension
  - T4a Tumor invades orbital soft tissues, without bone invasion
  - T4b Tumor invades bone T4c Tumor invades adjacent paranasal sinuses
  - T4d Tumor invades brain
- *Definition of regional lymph nodes (N):*
  - NX Regional lymph nodes cannot be assessed
  - N0 Regional lymph node metastasis absent
  - N1 Regional lymph node metastasis present
- *Definition of distant metastasis (M):*
  - M0 Distant metastasis absent
  - M1 Distant metastasis present
- *Definition of histopathologic grade (G):*
  - GX Grade cannot be assessed
  - G1 Well differentiated
  - G2 Moderately differentiated
  - G3 Poorly differentiated
  - G4 Undifferentiated

Management: Management of OSSN can be either surgical excision or with topical chemotherapy.

- *Surgical excision:*[13] Surgical excision is done using the "no touch" technique. In no-touch technique the entire dissection and excision of the tumor is done without holding the tumor with instruments at any point during the surgery. The main steps of the surgery are:
  - Conjunctival incision around the clinically visible edge of the lesion is marked taking 4 mm margin.
  - Conjunctival dissection is done at the episcleral plane to reach till the limbus without touching the tumor tissue.
  - A controlled corneal epitheliectomy is done using absolute alcohol taking 2 mm clear margin from the clinically visible corneal edge of the lesion.
  - The remaining adhesion at the limbus is dissected using a beaver knife.
  - Underlying scleral dissection and lamellar sclerectomy is done if fixity of the lesion to the sclera is noted intraoperatively.
  - Double freeze thaw cryotherapy is done to the edges of the conjunctiva from the undersurface. Cryotherapy is also done at the base of the tumor if adhesion to underlying sclera and episclera is noted intraoperatively. Limbal cryotherapy is limited to 6 clock hours.
  - The conjunctival defect is covered either with a sliding conjunctival flap or with amniotic membrane graft secured with sutures or fibrin glue.

Simple epithelial limbal transplantation has been used in conjunction with excision of large OSSN involving more than 6 clock hours of limbus and has been reported to decrease the chances of limbal stem cell deficiency and symblepharon formation.[14]

- *Topical chemotherapy:* Topical chemotherapy can be used as a primary modality of treatment for OSSN or as a neoadjuvant or adjuvant chemotherapy.[15-17] The indications of topical chemotherapy are:
  - Primary treatment modality for predominantly corneal OSSN where surgical excision can cause extensive corneal scarring and affect vision.
  - Diffuse OSSN where surgical excision can cause limbal stem cell loss and ocular surface scarring (Figs. 4A to D).
  - As an adjuvant therapy following surgical excision in cases with positive tumor margin on histopathology.

Topical chemotherapy medications used for OSSN is either topical mitomycin (MMC) or 5-fluorouracil.

Topical MMC: Mitomycin C is used in concentration ranging from 0.02% to 0.04% for treatment of OSSN. Various regimens have been used; a commonly used regimen is

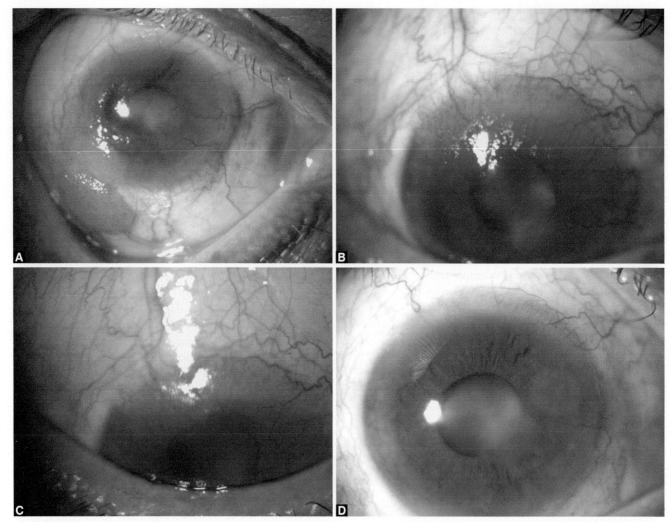

Figs. 4A to D: (A) Diffuse ocular surface squamous neoplasia involving almost 360° of limbus and total corneal involvement; (B and C) Gradual regression of the tumor following treatment with topical interferon; (D) Complete regression of the tumor with minimal corneal scarring.

given in Box 3. The main side effects of mitomycin-C are ocular surface irritation, conjunctival hyperemia, pain on instillation, and punctate corneal epithelial erosions, and usually subside on stopping the treatment.

Topical immunotherapy: Topical interferon alpha 2b is a recently introduced topical treatment modality for OSSN and has shown excellent results in causing tumor regression.[18] It acts by its antiproliferative, antiviral, and immunomodulatory effects and has minimal side effects compared to MMC. For topical therapy it is used at a concentration of 1–3 million IU/mL four times daily. The various methods of use of interferon include immunotherapy as a single agent monotherapy for OSSN, immunoreduction for reducing in the tumor size before anticipated surgery, and immunoprevention to prevent tumor recurrence following excision especially in those with

Box 3: Topical mitomycin C chemotherapy regimen for ocular surface squamous neoplasia.

Mitomycin C eye drops 0.04%
4 times a day
4 days a week for
4 weeks
Followed by a gap of 2 weeks before starting next cycle of treatment.

positive margins on histopathology. For large unresectable diffuse tumor with nodular component, topical therapy can be combined with injection of interferon alpha 2b at concentration of 3–10 million IU. Interferon is injected subconjunctivally around the tumor by ballooning the surrounding conjunctiva. Topical interferon therapy is especially beneficial in immunosuppressed patients with

OSSN who have a high recurrence rate. The systemic side effects include flu-like symptoms and are usually seen more after subconjunctival injection where higher concentration of the drug is used.

Other treatment modalities like plaque brachytherapy are indicated in more extensive tumor with scleral invasion. Brachytherapy is given to the involved scleral bed following excision of the primary tumor. Enucleation or orbital exenteration is indicated in cases with intraocular or orbital invasion.

Histopathology of OSSN: Histopathology of the OSSN reveals cellular atypia and dysplastic changes of the conjunctival epithelium. Based on the thickness of epithelial involvement by the dysplastic cells, the changes can be classified as mild, moderate, and severe dysplasia. Severe dysplasia with full thickness epithelial involvement is also called carcinoma in situ. Breach in the basement membrane and extension of the atypical cell to the conjunctival stroma constitutes an invasive squamous cell carcinoma. Histopathological variants like mucoepidermoid carcinoma, spindle cell squamous carcinoma, and adenoid cystic squamous cell carcinoma are the more aggressive histopathological subtypes and are more likely to have intraocular or orbital extension and are likely to recur following excision and hence needs more aggressive treatment.[19,20]

Melanocytic Conjunctival Epithelial Tumors

Conjunctival Nevi

Nevi are the most common benign melanocytic lesions of the conjunctiva. They are usually congenital or appear within the first few years of life. Acquired nevus in adulthood should raise the suspicion of other pigmented conjunctival lesions like melanosis or melanoma.

Location: The bulbar conjunctiva, caruncle, or plica are the most common location. Nevi at other location should raise suspicion of malignancy.

Clinical features: Nevi are well-defined, placoid, and slightly elevated lesion. They can be variably pigmented and can vary in size, shape, and location. Though most nevi are pigmented, they can be amelanotic at times. The most characteristic feature is the presence of cystic spaces within the lesion which helps to differentiate it from other pigmented conjunctival lesions.[21,22] Feeder vessels, intrinsic vessels, and satellite lesions can be present around the lesion and do not always indicate a malignant transformation (Fig. 5). Nevi can grow in size during adolescence period, pregnancy, and following sun exposure and can have features of inflammation with increased vascularity and thickness. Nevi rarely extend over the cornea. Chances of malignant transformation are less than 1%.

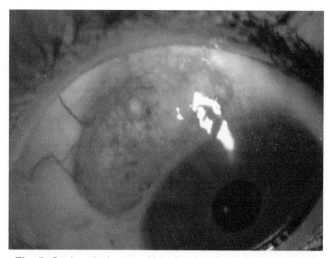

Fig. 5: Conjunctival nevus. Note the presence of characteristic cystic spaces within the lesion.

Histopathology: On histopathology, the conjunctival nevus is composed of nests of benign melanocytes in the basal epithelium. With age, the nevus cells migrate toward the stroma to form compound nevus. Further migration of the nevus cells toward the subepithelial tissues severs the connection with the overlying epithelial cell nest to form a subepithelial nevus.

Treatment: Treatment is usually indicated for cosmesis or in cases of suspected malignant transformation. Large lesions (>10 mm), unusual location like fornices, new onset lesion in adulthood, presence of intrinsic vessels, and feeder vessels, absence of intralesional cysts and episcleral fixity are indications for surgical excision of nevus. Excision with about 2 mm margin is the treatment of choice. Benign nevi can also regrow, hence, the excision should include all pigmented conjunctiva around the lesion to prevent recurrence.

Primary Acquired Melanosis

Primary acquired melanosis (PAM) is acquired, unilateral, flat, diffuse, and variable pigmented lesion of the conjunctiva (Figs. 6A to D). The term PAM was adopted by WHO in 1980 to distinguish this lesion from other congenital and secondary pigmentation of the conjunctiva. It is usually seen in middle aged or elderly person. The most common location is the limbus and the interpalpebral bulbar conjunctiva but extensive lesion can have involvement of the eyelid epidermis also.[23]

Etiology: The following factors have been associated with the development of PAM:
- Sunlight exposure
- Cigarette smoking

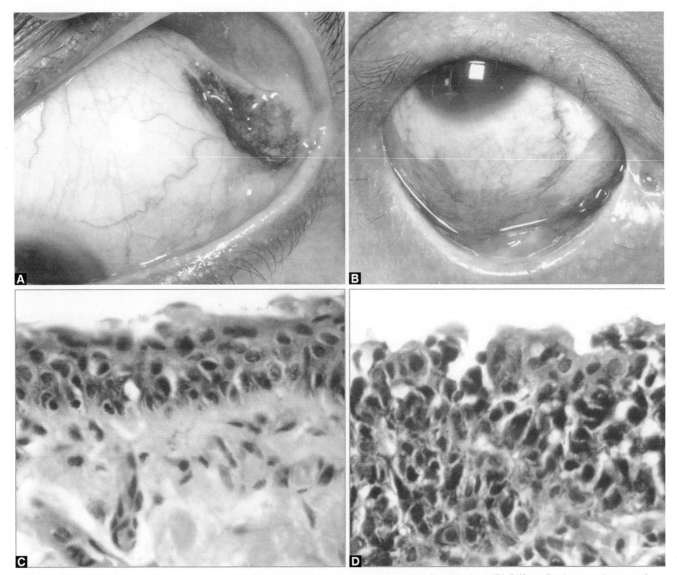

Figs. 6A to D: (A) Primary acquired melanosis of the conjunctiva appearing as a localized lesion; (B) Diffuse flat brown pigmentation; (C) Histopathology showing the appearance of PAM without atypia and; (D) PAM with atypia.

- Relationship with nevi and dysplastic nevus syndrome
- Neurofibromatosis.

Based on histopathology, PAM can be divided into two subtypes, PAM without atypia, and PAM with atypia.

- *PAM without atypia*: These lesions show the presence of conjunctival epithelial pigmentation with or without hyperplasia of melanocytes but without any melanocytic atypia. Presence of atypical melanocytes within the epithelium quantifies the lesion to be designated as PAM with atypia.
- *PAM with atypia*: PAM with atypia is also considered as "melanoma in situ" and about 13% of PAM with atypia can transform to conjunctival melanoma (Fig. 7). Hence, distinguishing the two and complete treatment

of PAM with atypia is essential. Clinically, it is not possible to differentiate the two and a histopathological confirmation is required for the same.

Indications of biopsy of PAM: Excision biopsy is considered for smaller isolated lesion and for large diffuse lesion incision biopsy from multiple conjunctival sites (map biopsy) is the procedure of choice. The following are the indications for biopsy of a pigmented conjunctival lesion suspected to be PAM:

- Large lesion more than 5 mm diameter
- Lesion involving palpebral or forniceal conjunctiva
- Documented growth of a lesion
- Thickness of a lesion

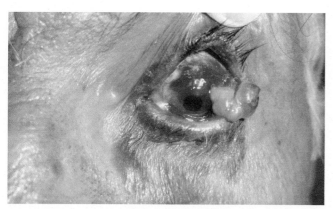

Fig. 7: Conjunctival melanoma appearing as a fleshy, pink conjunctival nodule arising from primary acquired melanosis (PAM) with atypia. Note the involvement of the eyelid skin by PAM with atypia.

- Increased vascularity within lesion
- Appearance of satellite areas around the lesion
- Extension of PAM onto the cornea
- History of other cutaneous melanoma or uveal melanoma.

Treatment of PAM: While PAM without atypia is benign lesions with negligible risk of transformation to malignant melanoma, PAM with atypia can transform to melanoma in about 20% of cases. The following are the management guidelines for a lesion diagnosed as PAM on histopathology:
- Observation alone for PAM without atypia
- Excision with edge cryotherapy for PAM with atypia
- Topical mitomycin-C for diffuse PAM

Conjunctival Malignant Melanoma

Conjunctiva melanoma is more commonly seen in races with lightly pigmented skin.[24] Majority arise from PAM with atypia (75%) but can also arise from preexisting nevus in 20% and de novo in 5%. It is a highly malignant tumor with a mortality rate of 25–30%.

Conjunctival melanoma is usually unilateral and most commonly arises near the limbus and the bulbar conjunctiva. Forniceal, palpebral conjunctiva, and caruncle can also be involved. The tumor is usually solitary but can be multifocal especially if arising in the setting of PAM with atypia. It usually appears as a dark brown, fleshy conjunctival mass but can be amelanotic especially the recurrent tumors. If arising in the context of PAM with atypia, presence of nodularity or increased thickness in an otherwise flat PAM indicates transformation to melanoma (Figs. 8A to C). Palpebral conjunctival lesions can have deeper invasion than evident on clinical evaluation due to fixity of the conjunctival substantia propria to the underlying tarsus.

Staging of conjunctival melanoma: AJCC eighth edition provides a clinical classification of conjunctival melanoma based on the tumor location, tumor extent, and the presence of invasive features (Box 4).[25] The AJCC staging system is predictive of prognosis.

Spread: Conjunctival melanoma can extend contiguously to the eyelid or orbit. Tumor more than 2 mm thickness and orbital extension carries risk of metastasis. Regional lymph node spread can occur in preauricular and submandibular nodes. The risk of local recurrence is 50% and metastasis is 25%.[26]

Differential diagnosis: Conjunctival melanoma needs to be differentiated from other pigmented and nonpigmented lesions of the conjunctiva like:
- *Conjunctival nevus:* Presence of cystic changes within the lesion is characteristic of nevus. In cases where the histopathological diagnosis is doubtful, immunohistochemical staining with HMB-45 or Melan—A may help in confirming the presence or absence of melanocytes
- Staphyloma
- Episcleral extension of uveal melanoma or melanocytoma. Ultrasound biomicroscopy can help in confirming the diagnosis
- Subconjunctival hematoma
- Pigmented conjunctival foreign body
- Pigmented OSSN: Melanoma are smooth surfaced lesion unlike OSSN which have a papillary surface with or without the presence of keratin.

Histopathology: Presence of atypical melanocytes in the conjunctival epithelium and breach in the conjunctival basement membrane with extension of atypical tumor cells to substantia propria is diagnostic of malignant melanoma. The atypical melanocytes can be either spindle, epithelioid, balloon, or small polyhedral type. The histopathological features predictive of poor prognosis include:
- Mixed cell type vs. spindle cell type
- Pagetoid conjunctival spread
- Lymphatic invasion.

Management of conjunctival melanoma: Wide excision by "no touch" technique with 4 mm margin and double freeze thaw cryo to the edges and the involved base remains the treatment of choice for conjunctival melanoma. Delicate removal of the complete tumor without causing any tumor seeding is the key to prevention of recurrence and metastasis. Involvement of the underlying episclera and sclera requires lamellar sclerectomy. Corneal epithelial involvement requires alcohol kerato-epithilectomy or lamellar keratectomy. In melanoma arising from PAM, surrounding PAM also needs to be excised completely

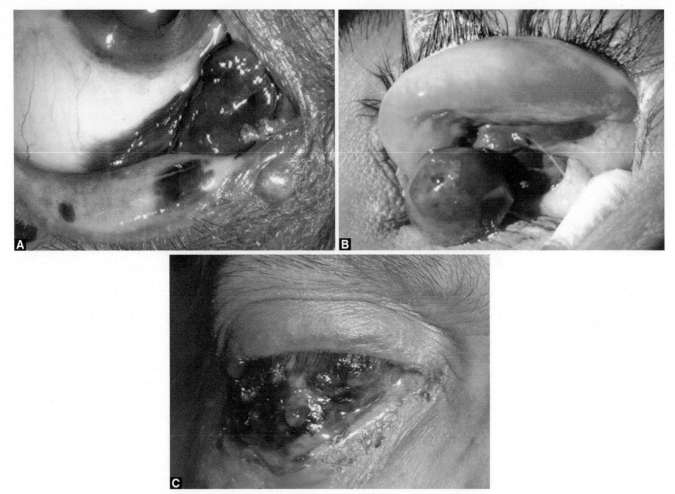

Figs. 8A to C: Conjunctival melanoma, morphological variants. (A) Pigmented lesions involving the medial bulbar conjunctiva and caruncle. Note the presence of primary acquired melanosis over the lower palpebral conjunctiva; (B) Pedunculated conjunctival melanoma arising from superior fornix and; (C) Massive tumor with orbital extension.

or treated with cryotherapy and postoperative topical mitomycin C is given as adjuvant therapy to treat any residual PAM and prevent recurrence. Deep scleral, corneal, or intraocular extension needs extended enucleation. For melanoma with massive orbital extension, orbital exenteration, or external beam radiotherapy is considered as a palliative therapy. In other situations, wide excision is preferred over exenteration as the published data has not found any significant difference in mortality whether a conservative excision or destructive surgery like exenteration has been used as the primary treatment. Regional lymph nodes like preauricular, submandibular, and cervical lymph nodes are involved by lymphatic spread, hence, sentinel lymph node biopsy is indicated in tumors more than 0.8 mm thickness. Local recurrence and metastasis is more likely with tumor in the conjunctival fornix, caruncle, tarsal involvement, or in cases with positive margin on histopathology.[26,27] Tissue biomarkers are finding increasing application in the assessment of melanoma and BRAF mutations have been found to be a factor predictive of metastasis.[28] Systemic chemotherapy with interferon (IFN) and interleukin is indicated in disseminated melanoma as palliative therapy. New evidence suggests that melanoma metastasis could be sensitive to BRAF inhibitors.[29]

Conjunctival Stromal Tumor

Conjunctival stroma contains various tissues like vessels, fibrofatty tissue, nerves, etc. The salient features of the common tumors arising from conjunctival stroma are described here.

Vascular Tumors of the Conjunctiva

Pyogenic granuloma: Pyogenic granuloma commonly arises after any surgical insult to the conjunctiva. It is composed of fibrovascular granulation tissue as an inflammatory

Box 4: American Joint Committee on Cancer 8th edition classification of conjunctival melanoma.

- *Definition of primary clinical tumor (cT):*
  - TX Primary tumor cannot be assessed
  - T0 No evidence of primary tumor
  - T1 Tumor of the bulbar conjunctiva
  - T1a <1 quadrant T1b >1 but <2 quadrants T1c >2 but <3 quadrants T1d >3 quadrants
  - T2 Tumor of nonbulbar conjunctiva (forniceal, palpebral, tarsal, caruncle)
  - T2a Noncaruncular and <1 quadrant nonbulbar conjunctiva T2b noncaruncular and >1 quadrant nonbulbar conjunctiva T2c Caruncular and <1 quadrant nonbulbar conjunctiva T2d caruncular and >1 quadrant nonbulbar conjunctiva
  - T3 Tumor of any size with local invasion
  - T3a Globe T3b Eyelid T3c Orbit T3d Nasolacrimal duct and/or lacrimal sac and/or paranasal sinuses
  - T4 Tumor of any size with invasion of central nervous system
- *Definition of regional lymph nodes (N)*
  - NX Regional lymph nodes cannot be assessed
  - N0 Regional lymph node metastasis absent
  - N1 Regional lymph node metastasis present
- *Definition of distant metastasis (M)*
  - M0 Distant metastasis absent
  - M1 Distant metastasis present
- *Definition of primary pathological tumor (pT)*
  - TX Primary tumor cannot be assessed
  - T0 No evidence or primary tumor
  - Tis Tumor confined to conjunctival epithelium
  - T1 Tumor of bulbar conjunctiva
  - T1a Tumor with <2 mm thickness invasion of substantia propria
  - T1b Tumor with >2 mm thickness invasion of substantia propria
  - T2 Tumor of nonbulbar conjunctiva
  - T2a Tumor with <2 mm thickness invasion of substantia propria T2b Tumor with >2 mm thickness invasion of substantia propria
  - T3 Tumor of any size with local invasion
  - T3a Globe T3b Eyelid T3c Orbit T3d Nasolacrimal duct and/or lacrimal sac and/or paranasal sinuses
  - T4 Tumor of any size with invasion of central nervous system

response to the conjunctival insult. The term is a misnomer as it is neither a granuloma nor pyogenic. It usually arises after chalazion, strabismus, or other conjunctival surgery. Clinically, it appears as a fleshy, red, elevated, sessile, or pedunculated conjunctival mass involving any part of the conjunctiva (Fig. 9A). The surface is friable and can bleed to touch. Treatment is usually with topical steroids. Larger or persistent lesion requires excision with cryotherapy and cauterization of the bleeding base. Underlying inciting factor like foreign body or suture knot needs to be taken care at the same time to prevent recurrence.

Capillary hemangioma: Capillary hemangiomas are usually seen in infancy and can be associated with eyelid or orbital capillary hemangioma of infancy. It appears as diffuse, red, elevated lesion, and tends to regress spontaneously by 4–5 years of age (Fig. 9B). Treatment is indicated for large, unsightly bleeding lesion or if the associated eyelid component is causing amblyogenic ptosis. Intralesional injection of triamcinolone at a dose of 6 mg/kg/body weight can cause regression of the lesion. Injection can be repeated at 6 weekly intervals if indicated. Recently, oral propranolol at a dose of 2 mg/kg/body weight under supervision of a pediatrician has shown excellent response in regression of capillary hemangioma and has replaced intralesional steroid as the first-line treatment.[30] Controlled surgical excision or debulking is indicated in cases where response to medical management is suboptimal and there is need for emergency medical treatment like in a bleeding lesion.

Cavernous hemangioma: Cavernous hemangiomas of the conjunctiva are uncommon and appear as a bluish red conjunctival lesion (Fig.9C). Histopathologically it is composed of large dilated vascular spaces lined by endothelial cells. Treatment is by surgical excision.

Varices: Conjunctival varices are often anterior extension of orbital varices and appear as reddish blue dilated vascular loops. Treatment is often observation alone if cosmesis is a concern.

Lymphangiectasia: Prominent dilated lymphatic vessels of the conjunctiva are called lymphangiectasia (Fig. 9D). They can occur spontaneously or following trauma. These channels can get filled up with blood to form hemorrhagic lymphangiectasia. Associated conjunctival hemorrhage and edema can occur spontaneously and if recurrent is an indication for surgical excision.

Lymphangioma: Conjunctival lymphangioma can be isolated or can be anterior extension of an orbital lymphangioma. It appears as multiloculated dilated cystic conjunctival lesions. The cystic spaces can be filled with straw colored lymphatic fluid or can be blood filled. Histopathology shows dilated lymphatic channels lined by attenuated endothelial cells and filled with blood or lymph or a combination of both. Surgical excision remains the treatment of choice and is indicated in cosmetically unsightly lesions or in cases of recurrent hemorrhage (Figs. 10A and B).

Kaposi sarcoma: This is a malignant conjunctival tumor commonly seen in patients with HIV-AIDS or other causes of immunodeficiency and can be the first sign of HIV-AIDS in some patients.[31] It appears as solitary or multiple red conjunctival lesions which when confluent can mimic hemorrhagic conjunctivitis. Histopathology shows

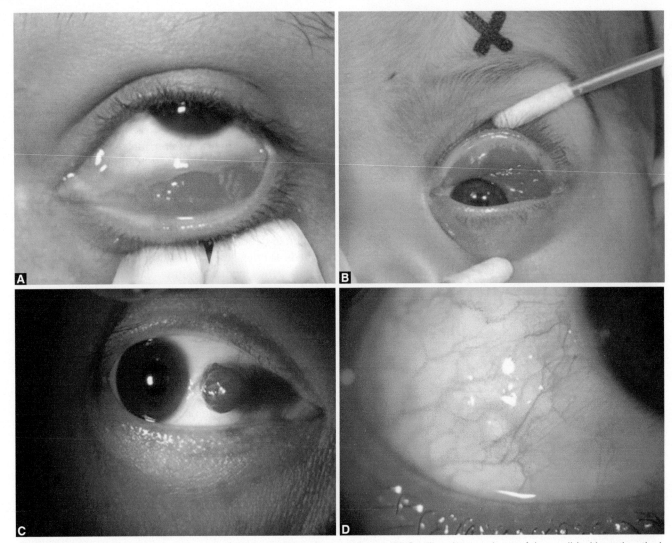

Figs. 9A to D: Vascular tumors of the conjunctiva. (A) Pyogenic granuloma; (B) Capillary hemangioma of the eyelid with conjunctival extension; (C) Cavernous hemangioma; and (D) Conjunctival lymphangiectasia.

malignant spindle cells, capillary channels, and blood-filled vascular slits with no definite endothelial lining. These tumors tend to regress after restoration of immune status following antiretroviral therapy. Response to low-dose radiation therapy is excellent. Surgical excision is reserved for localized tumors. Response to chemotherapy and IFN–alpha 2a is moderate.

Neural Tumors of the Conjunctiva

Neurofibroma

Neurofibroma of the conjunctiva is rare and can be solitary or plexiform (Figs. 11A and B). Plexiform neurofibroma is usually associated with neurofibromatosis type I. On histopathology they show benign proliferation of Schwann cells and axons. Treatment is by surgical excision. For plexiform neurofibroma, debulking is the treatment of choice as complete surgical excision carries considerable morbidity.

Schwannoma

Schwannoma are rare benign neural tumors of the conjunctiva and appear as yellow pink conjunctival mass involving any part of the conjunctiva. Histopathology shows the characteristic spindle cells in Antony A or Antony B arrangement. Treatment is by complete surgical excision with a wide margin as incomplete excision carries a high risk of recurrence.

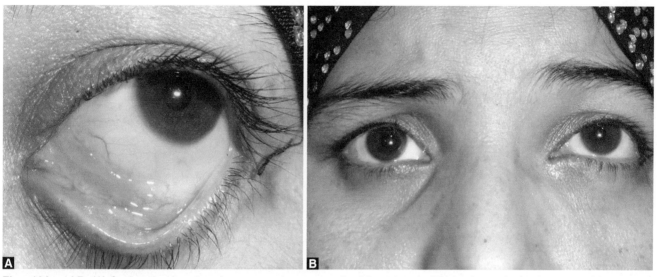

Figs. 10A and B: (A) Conjunctival lymphangioma appearing as an yellowish conjunctival thickening at the fornix as part of the anterior extension of inferior orbital lymphangioma; (B) Note the associated proptosis and superior globe displacement caused by the orbital lymphangioma.

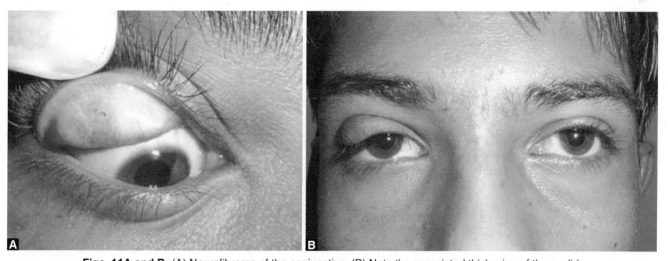

Figs. 11A and B: (A) Neurofibroma of the conjunctiva; (B) Note the associated thickening of the eyelid.

Fibrous Tumor of the Conjunctiva

Fibrous tumors of the conjunctiva are rare. Fibroma and fibrous histiocytoma are the most common fibrous conjunctival tumor. Fibrous histiocytoma can be benign or malignant. Clinically, it appears as a white conjunctival mass which can be well-circumscribed or diffuse. Usually located at the limbus, these lesions are situated deeper in the conjunctiva, usually adherent to the sclera and can extend into the cornea. Treatment is usually by surgical excision.

Lymphoproliferative Tumors of Conjunctiva

Lymphoproliferative tumors of the conjunctiva have a wide spectrum ranging from low grade to high grade. Most of the conjunctival lymphoid tumors are of B cell origin. The lymphoproliferative lesions of the conjunctiva can be divided into three broad categories;

1. Reactive lymphoid hyperplasia
2. Atypical lymphoid hyperplasia
3. Conjunctival lymphoma.

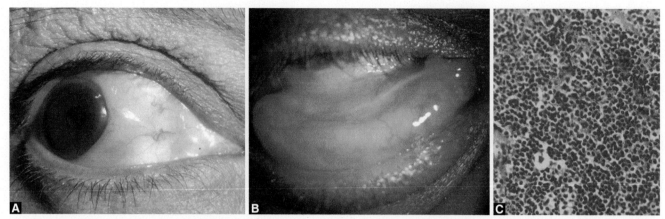

Figs. 12A to C: (A) Conjunctival lymphoma appearing as a pale pink, smooth surfaced mass at the bulbar conjunctiva near the limbus and; (B) At the inferior fornix; (C) Histopathology showing the monomorphic population of lymphocytes.

Clinical appearance of the different types of lymphoproliferative tumors are similar and histopathological evaluation is needed to differentiate them. Conjunctival lymphoma can be isolated or can be part of ocular adnexal lymphoma. In one-third of the patients there can be coexisting systemic lymphoma. Clinically, conjunctival lymphoma appears as a pale pink, salmon colored conjunctival mass which can be located in the fornix, bulbar conjunctiva, caruncle or limbus (Figs. 12A to C). The clinical appearance can resemble follicular or papillary conjunctivitis at times. There can be associated involvement of the orbit, eyelid, and uvea. Systemic association is seen in 47% of bilateral cases and 17% of unilateral cases.[32] Extranodal marginal zone lymphoma (ENMZL) and follicular lymphoma are the common histological subtypes with isolated ocular involvement. Involvement of the conjunctiva by diffuse large B cell and mantle cell lymphoma subtypes (MCL) is commonly seen as part of systemic disease.

The risk factors for development of conjunctival lymphoma include systemic immunodeficiency, autoimmune conditions, immune dysfunction, genetic mutations and infections by *Helicobacter pylori* or *Chlamydia psittaci*, genetic mutation.[33,34]

Classification of Conjunctival Lymphoma

Conjunctival lymphoma can be classified by the Ann Arbor system or the WHO system. The AJJCC clinical and pathological staging system is now used commonly and is provided in Box 5.[35]

Management of Conjunctival Lymphoma

Management of conjunctival lymphoma depends on the extent of the disease. Isolated conjunctival involvement is treated by either complete surgical excision or with external

Box 5: American Joint Committee on Cancer 8th Edition Classification of Ocular Adnexal Lymphoma.

- *Definition of primary tumor (T)*
  - TX Tumor extent not specified
  - T0 Tumor absent
  - T1 Tumor in conjunctiva without eyelid or orbit involvement
  - T2 Tumor in orbit with or without conjunctival involvement
  - T3 Tumor in preseptal eyelid with or without orbital and/or conjunctival involvement
  - T4 Tumor in orbit plus additional bone, maxillofacial sinuses, and brain
- *Definition of regional lymph nodes (N)*
  - NX Regional lymph nodes not assessed
  - N0 Regional lymph node involvement absent
  - N1 Regional lymph node involvement present and superior to mediastinum (preauricular, parotid, submandibular, and cervical nodes)
  - N1a 1 lymph node region involvement superior to mediastinum
  - N1b >2 lymph node regions involvement superior to mediastinum
  - N2 Regional lymph node involvement in mediastinum
  - N3 Regional lymph node involvement in peripheral and central lymph node regions (diffuse or disseminated)
- *Definition of distant metastasis (M)*
  - M0 Distant involvement at other extranodal site absent
  - M1a Distant involvement in noncontiguous tissue (parotid gland, submandibular gland, lung, liver, spleen, kidney, breast)
  - M1b Distant involvement in bone marrow
  - M1c Both M1a and M1b present
- *Definition of histopathologic grade (G)*
  - GX Grade cannot be assessed
  - G1 1–5 centroblasts/10 HPF
  - G2 5–15 centroblasts/10 HPF
  - G3 >15 centroblasts/10 HPF but with admixed centrocytes
  - G4 >15 centroblasts/10 HPF but without centrocytes

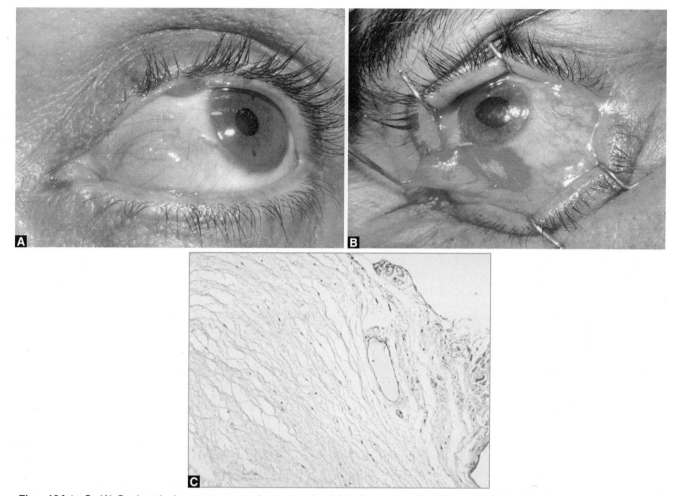

Figs. 13A to C: (A) Conjunctival myxoma appearing as a pale pink bulbar conjunctival lesion; (B) Note the gelatinous appearance of the tumor during excision and; (C) The loose myxoid stroma on histopathology.

beam radiotherapy or rituximab. Associated systemic involvement is treated by either systemic chemotherapy, rituximab, or immunotherapy. The prognosis for survival depends on the histological subtype with ENMZL having a 5-year survival of 97% and MCL having worst prognosis with 5-year survival of 9%.[36]

Myxoid Tumors of the Conjunctiva

Conjunctival myxomas are rare benign conjunctival stromal tumors. They appear as pale pink, solitary, slowly progressive, lesion usually located in the bulbar conjunctiva. On gross examination, it appears as a gelatinous tumor and on histopathology, it is an hypocellular tumor composed of stellate or spindle cells in an acellular stromal matrix. Conjunctival myxoma can be associated with Carney complex which is an association of cardiac myxoma and perioral mucosal pigmentation and can be life–threatening. Treatment is by surgical excision (Figs. 13A to C).

Myogenic Tumors of Conjunctiva

Conjunctival Rhabdomyosarcoma

Though rhabdomyosarcoma is the most common malignant orbital tumor in children, isolated conjunctival involvement is rare. It usually is part of orbital rhabdomyosarcoma. Clinically, it appears as a rapidly growing red conjunctival mass. Treatment is by surgical excision for localized lesion. For extensive tumors where surgical excision carries considerable morbidity, treatment with chemotherapy and radiotherapy is indicated.

Histiocytic Tumor of Conjunctiva

Xanthogranuloma

Conjunctival xanthogranuloma appears as orange pink conjunctival stromal mass usually near the limbus.[37] It can be isolated or can be part of the systemic histiocytic

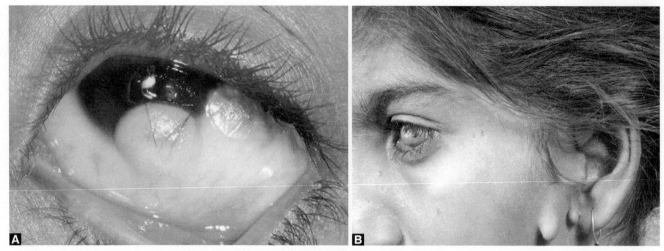

Figs. 14A and B: Conjunctival dermoid. (A) Note the presence of fine hair on the surface of the limbal dermoid; (B) Association of limbal dermoid with Goldenhar syndrome.

disorders or disease. On histopathology, the presence of histiocytes and Touton's giant cell is characteristic. These lesions can resolve spontaneously or with topical or systemic steroid treatment. Surgical excision is usually required for diagnostic purpose.

Conjunctival Choristoma

Choristoma are congenital tumors and involve the presence of normal tissue at an abnormal site. These lesions can be simple choristoma when it consists of tissue derived from one germ layer or complex choristoma when more than one type of tissue is present. Dermoid and dermolipoma are the common tumors in this group. The location is usually at the limbus, bulbar conjunctiva, or fornices. Choristomas can be isolated lesions or can have systemic associations.

Dermoid

Conjunctival dermoid are well circumscribed, yellow-white lesions commonly located at the limbus. Inferotemporal limbus is a common location. They can be small or can involve the cornea and the epibulbar surface extensively causing astigmatism and amblyopia in children. Fine hairs can protrude from the surface in some lesions (Fig. 14A). Conjunctival dermoids can be isolated or associated with Goldenhar syndrome which comprises of epibulbar choristoma, preauricular skin tags, vertebral anomalies, and eyelid coloboma (Fig. 14B). On histopathology, dermoid shows fibrous tissue lined by stratified squamous epithelium and consisting of dermal appendages like hair, sweat, and sebaceous glands. Small lesions can be managed by observation alone. Larger lesions causing astigmatism, obscuration of visual axis, and amblyopia or cosmetic

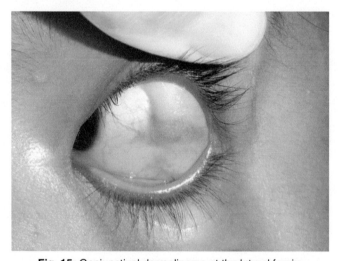

Fig. 15: Conjunctival dermolipoma at the lateral fornix.

disfigurement can be treated by surgical excision with or without lamellar keratoplasty. Residual corneal scar can be a cause for cosmetic concern and needs to be explained to the patient preoperatively.

Dermolipoma

Dermolipoma are soft, yellowish lesions usually located at the temporal and superotemporal fornix (Fig. 15). These lesions can extend posteriorly to involve the lacrimal gland or the orbit. They are congenital lesions but can become apparent later in life when it prolapses through the fornix. Treatment is usually indicated if cosmesis is a concern. Limited excision of the anterior prolapsed portion of the lesion and reconstruction with amniotic membrane grafting or conjunctival autograft is

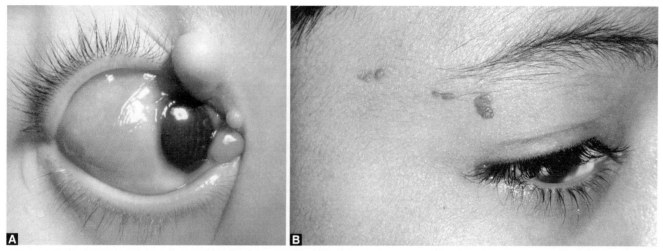

Figs. 16A and B: (A) Epibulbar complex choristoma; (B) Epibulbar choristoma in a patient with linear nevus sebaceous syndrome.

the treatment of choice. Deeper dissection of the orbital portion can cause postoperative scarring and limitation of ocular movements causing bothersome diplopia and is hence avoided.[38] On histopathology, dermolipoma is lined by stratified squamous epithelium with or without keratinization and consists of dense collagenous tissue and large amount of adipose tissue. Adnexal elements can be present occasionally.

Complex Choristoma

Complex choristoma consists of tissues derived from two germ layers. Depending on the type of the tissue predominantly present, these lesions can vary in color from yellow white to pink. The clinical appearance can be variable ranging from a small localized lesion to extensive involvement of the epibulbar surface and cornea (Fig. 16A). Complex choristoma can be associated with basal cell nevus syndrome which in addition to epibulbar choristoma consist of cutaneous sebaceous nevus, eyelid colobomas, optic nerve head coloboma, and central nervous system abnormalities (Fig. 16B).[39] On histopathology, complex choristoma consists of variable combination of tissues like dermal appendages, fat, cartilage, bone, muscle, blood vessel, etc.

Metastatic and Secondary Conjunctival Infiltration

Metastatic tumors of the conjunctiva are uncommon and usually seen in the advanced stages of the malignancy.[40] The common primary sites are the breast or cutaneous melanoma. Breast metastasis appears as a fleshy vascularized conjunctival tumor and can be single or multiple. Metastatic melanoma can be pigmented or

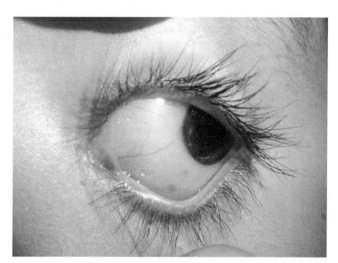

Fig. 17: Acute lymphoblastic lymphoma in a child presenting as a diffuse pale pink conjunctival mass.

amelanotic. Leukemic infiltrates can occasionally involve the conjunctiva and can be the first sign of leukemia in few patients.[41] It can appear as a diffuse or localized pale pink conjunctival thickening and can cause microvascular changes due to the hyperviscosity associated with leukemia (Fig. 17).

In conclusion, conjunctival tumors can be of various types ranging from benign, premalignant, and malignant. The tumors can arise from the various tissue layers of the conjunctiva and the clinical appearance is typical in most cases. Histopathology is essential for confirming the diagnosis and planning the treatment. Management is essentially by surgical excision and medical therapy in the form topical chemotherapy is indicated in few tumors like ocular surface squamous neoplasia.

REFERENCES

1. Lass JH, Jenson AB, Papale JJ, et al. Papillomavirus in human conjunctival papillomas. Am J Ophthalmol 1983;95(3):364-8.

2. Harkey ME, Metz HS. Cryotherapy of conjunctival papillomata. Am J Ophthalmol. 1968;66(5):872-4.

3. Lass JH, Foster CS, Grove AS, et al. Interferon-alpha therapy of recurrent conjunctival papillomas. Am J Ophthalmol. 1987;103(3 Pt 1):294-301.

4. Hawkins AS, Yu J, Hamming NA, et al. Treatment of recurrent conjunctival papillomatosis with mitomycin C. Am J Ophthalmol. 1999;128(5):638-40.

5. Shields CL, Lally MR, Singh AD, et al. Oral cimetidine (Tagamet) for recalcitrant, diffuse conjunctival papillomatosis. Am J Ophthalmol. 1999;128(3):362-4.

6. Munro S, Brownstein S, Liddy B. Conjunctival keratoacanthoma. Am J Ophthalmol. 1993;116(5):654-5.

7. Schellini SA, Marques ME, Milanezi MF, et al. Conjunctival keratoacanthoma. Acta Ophthalmol Scand. 1997;75(3):335-7.

8. Shields CL, Shields JA. Tumors of the conjunctiva and cornea. Surv Ophthalmol. 2004;49(1):3-24.

9. Lee GA, Hirst LW. Ocular surface squamous neoplasia. Surv Ophthalmol. 1995;39(6):429-50.

10. Newton R, Ziegler J, Ateenyi-Agaba C, et al.; Uganda Kaposi's Sarcoma Study Group. The epidemiology of conjunctival squamous cell carcinoma in Uganda. Br J Cancer. 2002;87(3):301-8.

11. Shields CL, Manchandia A, Subbiah R, et al. Pigmented squamous cell carcinoma in situ of the conjunctiva in 5 cases. Ophthalmology. 2008;115(10):1673-8.

12. Amin MB, Edge S, Greene F, Byrd DR, Brookland RK, Washington MK, Gershenwald JE, Compton CC, Hess KR, Sullivan DC, Jessup JM, Brierley JD, Gaspar LE, Schilsky RL, Balch CM, Winchester DP, Asare EA, Madera M, Gress DM, Meyer LR (Eds). AJCC Cancer Staging Manual, 8th edition. Switzerland: Springer; 2017. pp. 787-93.

13. Shields JA, Shields CL, De Potter P. Surgical management of approach to conjunctival tumors. The 1994 Lynn B. McMahan Lecture. Arch Ophthalmol. 1997;115(6):808-15.

14. Mittal V, Narang P, Menon V, et al. Primary simple limbal epithelial transplantation along with excisional biopsy in the management of extensive ocular surface squamous neoplasia. Cornea. 2016;35(12):1650-2.

15. Nanji AA, Moon CS, Galor A, et al. Surgical versus medical treatment of ocular surface squamous neoplasia: A comparison of recurrences and complications. Ophthalmology. 2014;121(5):994-1000.

16. Shields CL, Naseripour M, Shields JA. Topical mitomycin C for extensive, recurrent conjunctival-corneal squamous cell carcinoma. Am J Ophthalmol. 2002;133(5):601-6.

17. Yeatts RP, Engelbrecht NE, Curry CD, et al. 5-fluorouracil for the treatment of intraepithelial neoplasia of the conjunctiva and cornea. Ophthalmology. 2000;107(12):2190-5.

18. Shields CL, Kaliki S, Kim HJ, et al. Interferon for ocular surface squamous neoplasia in 81 cases: Outcomes based on the American Joint Committee on Cancer classification. Cornea. 2013;32(3):248-56.

19. Searl SS, Krigstein HJ, Albert DM, et al. Invasive squamous cell carcinoma with intraocular mucoepidermoid features. Conjunctival carcinoma with intraocular invasion and diphasic morphology. Arch Ophthalmol. 1982;100(1):109-11.

20. Johnson TE, Tabbara KF, Weatherhead RG, et al. Secondary squamous cell carcinoma of the orbit. Arch Ophthalmol. 1997;115(1):75-8.

21. Shields CL, Fasiuddin AF, Mashayekhi A, et al. Conjunctival nevi: Clinical features and natural course in 410 consecutive patients. Arch Ophthalmol. 2004;122(2):167-75.

22. Shields CL, Belinsky I, Romanelli-Gobbi M, et al. Anterior segment optical coherence tomography of conjunctival nevus. Ophthalmology. 2011;118(5):915-9.

23. Jakobiec FA, Folberg R, Iwamoto T. Clinicopathologic characteristics of premalignant and malignant melanocytic lesions of the conjunctiva. Ophthalmology. 1989;96(2):147-66.

24. Seregard S. Conjunctival melanoma. Surv Ophthalmol. 1998;42(4):321-50.

25. Coupland SE, Barnhill R, Conway RM, et al. Conjunctival melanoma. In: Amin MB, Edge SB, Greene FL, et al. (Eds). AJCC Cancer Staging Manual, 8th edition. Switzerland: Springer; 2017. pp. 795-803.

26. Shields CL, Shields JA, Gündüz K, et al. Conjunctival melanoma: Risk factors for recurrence, exenteration, metastasis, and death in 150 consecutive patients. Arch Ophthalmol. 2000;118(11):1497-507.

27. Shields CL, Markowitz JS, Belinsky I, et al. Conjunctival melanoma: Outcomes based on tumor origin in 382 consecutive cases. Ophthalmology. 2011;118(2):389-95.e1-2.

28. Larsen AC, Dahl C, Dahmcke CM, et al. BRAF mutations in conjunctival melanoma: Investigation of incidence, clinicopathological features, prognosis and paired premalignant lesions. Acta Ophthalmol. 2016;94(5):463-70.

29. Dagi Glass LR, Lawrence DP, Jakobiec FA, et al. Conjunctival melanoma responsive to combined systemic BRAF/MEK inhibitors. Ophthalmic Plast Reconstr Surg. 2017;33(5):e114-e116.

30. Vassallo P, Forte R, Di Mezza A, et al. Treatment of infantile capillary hemangioma of the eyelid with systemic propranolol. Am J Ophthalmol. 2013;155(1):165-70.e2.

31. Kurumety UR, Lustbader JM. Kaposi's sarcoma of the bulbar conjunctiva as an initial clinical manifestation of acquired immunodeficiency syndrome. Arch Ophthalmol. 1995;113(8):978.

32. Shields CL, Shields JA, Carvalho C, et al. Conjunctival lymphoid tumors: Clinical analysis of 117 cases and relationship to systemic lymphoma. Ophthalmology. 2001;108(5):979-84.

33. Foster LH, Portell CA. The role of infectious agents, antibiotics, and antiviral therapy in the treatment of extranodal marginal zone lymphoma and other low-grade lymphomas. Curr Treat Options Oncol. 2015;16(6):28.

34. Sjö NC, Foegh P, Juhl BR, et al. Role of Helicobacter pylori in conjunctival mucosa-associated lymphoid tissue lymphoma. Ophthalmology. 2007;114(1):182-6.

35. Sniegowski MC, Roberts D, Bakhoum M, et al. Ocular adnexal lymphoma: validation of American Joint Committee on Cancer seventh edition staging guidelines. Br J Ophthalmol. 2014;98(9):1255-60.

36. Kirkegaard MM, Rasmussen PK, Coupland SE, et al. Conjunctival lymphoma—An international multicenter retrospective study. JAMA Ophthalmol. 2016;134(4):406-14.

37. Chaudhry IA, Al-Jishi Z, Shamsi FA, et al. Juvenile xanthogranuloma of the corneoscleral limbus: Case report and review of the literature. Surv Ophthalmol. 2004;49(6):608-14.

38. Fry CL, Leone CR Jr. Safe management of dermolipomas. Arch Ophthalmol. 1994;112(8):1114-6.

39. Pe'er J, Ilsar M. Epibulbar complex choristoma associated with nevus sebaceous. Arch Ophthalmol. 1995;113 (10):1301-4.

40. Chew R, Potter J, DiMattina A. Conjunctival metastasis as the presenting sign for stage IV lung cancer. Optom Vis Sci. 2014;91(2):e38-42.

41. Lee SS, Robinson MR, Morris JC, et al. Conjunctival involvement with T-cell prolymphocytic leukemia: Report of a case and review of the literature. Surv Ophthalmol. 2004;49(5):525-36.

Intraocular Tumors

Raksha Rao, Santosh G Honavar

INTRODUCTION

Intraocular tumors include benign and malignant tumors arising from the uvea, retinal pigment epithelium, and neurosensory retina (Box 1). Intraocular tumors can generally be distinguished by their clinical characteristics and the presenting symptomatology, location, color, and the imaging characteristics. In the following chapter, the common intraocular tumors are discussed.

Box 1: Classification of intraocular tumors.

A. *Tumors of the uveal tract*
  1. Cystic tumors
  2. Melanocytic tumors
     ◆ Nevus
     ◆ Malignant melanoma
        - Iris melanoma
        - Ciliary body melanoma
        - Choroidal melanoma
     ◆ Melanocytoma
  3. Vascular tumors
     ◆ Circumscribed choroidal hemangioma
     ◆ Diffuse choroidal hemangioma
  4. Osseous, myogenic, neurogenic, fibrous, and histiocytic tumors
     ◆ Choroidal osteoma
  5. Metastatic tumors
B. *Tumors of the retina and optic disk*
  1. Retinoblastoma
  2. Vascular tumors
     ◆ Retinal hemangioblastoma
     ◆ Cavernous hemangioma
     ◆ Racemose hemangioma
     ◆ Vasoproliferative tumor
  3. Glial tumors
C. *Tumors of the pigment epithelium and nonpigmented epithelium*
  1. Congenital hypertrophy of the retinal pigment epithelium
  2. Adenoma and adenocarcinoma
  3. Medulloepithelioma
D. *Intraocular lymphoid tumor*

CYSTS OF THE IRIS

The cysts of the iris can be primary or secondary (Box 2).[1] Primary cysts of the iris can be an iris pigment epithelial (IPE) cyst or a stromal cyst. The IPE cysts are divided into four main types based on their location—pupillary margin, midzonal, peripheral, and dislodged. The dislodged cyst can be freely floating in the anterior chamber or the vitreous.

Box 2: Classification of iris cysts.

I. *Primary cyst*
  1. Iris pigment epithelium cyst
     i. Pupillary
     ii. Mid zonal
     iii. Peripheral
     iv. Free-floating
        a. Anterior chamber
        b. Vitreous chamber
  2. Iris stroma cyst
     i. Congenital
     ii. Acquired
II. *Secondary cyst*
  1. Epithelial
     i. Epithelial downgrowth cyst
        a. Postsurgical
        b. Posttraumatic
  2. Drug-induced cyst
  3. Parasitic cyst
  4. Cyst secondary to intraocular tumors (intralesional cavitation)

The stromal cyst can be congenital or acquired. Secondary cysts are due to epithelial ingrowth, drugs, parasites, or due to cystic cavitation within a tumor in the iris.

Most epithelial cysts remain stable throughout life. Surgical intervention may be necessary in rare cases when a large cyst occludes the pupil or a free-floating cyst is troublesome. Stromal cysts can be managed by simple aspiration followed by cryotherapy or sclerosis of the cyst wall with absolute alcohol.[2]

UVEAL MELANOMA

Uveal melanoma is the most common primary intraocular malignant tumor in adults.[1] It most commonly involves the choroid (90%), followed by ciliary body (6%), or iris (4%).[3] Caucasians are more commonly affected as compared to any other race. The tumor is detected usually in the sixth decade, although a wide variation in age is noted. Uveal melanomas can develop de novo, or from a preexisting nevus and in the region of melanocytosis in congenital ocular/oculodermal melanocytosis. *Oculodermal melanocytosis* manifests as a gray episcleral and cutaneous pigmentation, often with related partial or diffuse uveal hyperpigmentation (Fig. 1). This condition carries a 1 in 400 lifetime risk for uveal melanoma in Caucasians.[4] A choroidal nevus is a flat to slightly elevated, pigmented or nonpigmented lesion that is seen in up to 5% of the Caucasians (Fig. 2). It transforms into a choroidal melanoma in only an estimated 1 in 8,000 of the Caucasians.

An iris nevus can be flat or dome-shaped, circumscribed or diffuse, small or large, pigmented or completely amelanotic. A melanocytoma is a variation of iris nevus that is more deeply pigmented. It can produce secondary glaucoma from necrosis and clogging of the trabecular meshwork by the released pigment and melanophages that contain the pigment.

An iris melanoma arises from the iris stroma. It accounts for only 5% of all uveal melanomas. It is most commonly located in the inferior portion of the iris, and can be well-circumscribed, diffuse, or it can assume a tapioca-like configuration. Circumscribed iris melanomas present as a well-defined mass that can be variably pigmented. A diffuse tumor is less common and is often diagnosed late. It can produce hyperchromic heterochromia, secondary glaucoma, or just irregular pigmented patches.

Iris melanoma can usually be diagnosed clinically. However, ultrasound biomicroscopy (UBM) helps in confirming the solid nature of the lesion and also delineating any extension into the ciliary body. In cases where the presentation is atypical, a needle aspiration biopsy (FNAB) can be performed to obtain a cytological diagnosis. The management of circumscribed iris melanoma depends on the size of the lesion. A well-circumscribed small tumor can be excised with iridectomy or iridocyclectomy. In unresectable larger tumors, plaque radiotherapy is used. Enucleation in iris melanoma is necessary in very large tumors with secondary glaucoma.

A ciliary body melanoma is slightly more common than an iris melanoma. However, it is hardly diagnosed in the early stages, and attains a large size before the patients manifest clinical signs. The most important clinical sign is the presence of dilated, tortuous episcleral blood vessel, known as the sentinel vessel. When there is an epibulbar pigmented lesion, it indicates transcleral extension of the tumor. Less frequently, it can involve the entire ciliary body by diffuse circumferential extension (ring melanoma). A large ciliary body melanoma can cause pressure on the lens and its zonules, leading to subluxation

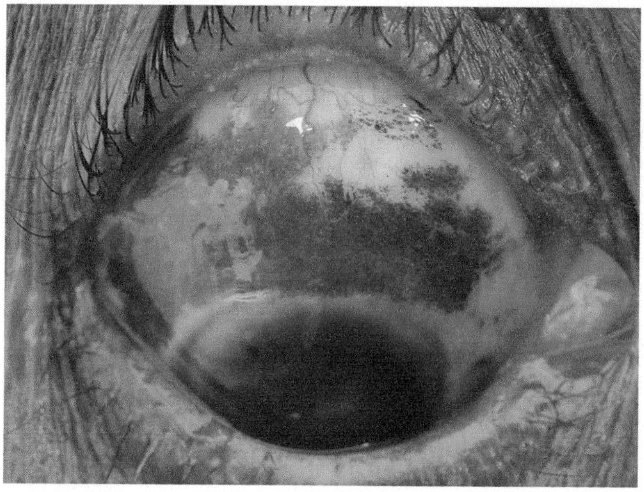

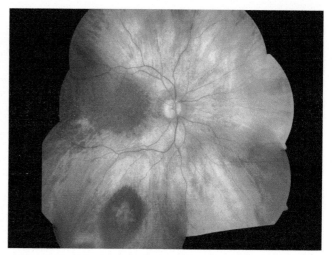

Fig. 1: External photograph revealing scleral melanocytosis in a patient who also had choroidal melanocytosis with choroidal melanoma.

Fig. 2: Fundus photograph showing a choroidal nevus in the inferotemporal quadrant.

and cataract. It can extend either posteriorly into the choroid (ciliochoroidal melanoma) or anteriorly into the iris (iridociliary melanoma). It can infiltrate the anterior chamber angle, causing secondary glaucoma.

A choroidal melanoma generally manifests with symptoms of varying degrees of visual loss, photopsia, floaters, and visual field loss. Choroidal melanoma can present as a pigmented or nonpigmented lesion with a dome, mushroom or diffuse configuration (Fig. 3). The diagnosis of choroidal melanoma can be solely based on ophthalmoscopic examination. It is clinically grouped into three sizes based on the tumor thickness, including small (0–3.0 mm), medium (3.1–8.0 mm), and large (8.1 mm or greater). Medium to large melanomas are more easily distinguished from pseudomelanomas by their characteristic features. Most commonly, they are pigmented mass arising from the choroid with an exudative retinal detachment. Sometimes a choroidal melanoma can break through the Bruch's membrane to assume a mushroom shape. This breakthrough can result in vitreal or subretinal blood. Small to medium melanomas also demonstrate surface orange pigment at the level of the retinal pigment epithelium due to accumulation of lipofuscin pigment. Amelanotic choroidal melanomas are often confused with a metastatic lesion or lymphoma, in which case ultrasound and fine needle aspiration biopsy can help establish the diagnosis. A choroidal melanoma can also assume a horizontal growth with or without any nodular component. This is a diffuse growth pattern and such tumors are frequently larger and carry a higher chance for systemic metastasis.

In small melanomas, the diagnosis may be difficult to establish since they can be easily confused for nevus. To help in recognizing early small choroidal melanomas, a

mnemonic "TFSOM" (To Find Small Ocular Melanoma), by Shields, et al.[4] The mnemonic stands for T = thickness more than 2 mm, F = subretinal fluid, S = symptoms, O = orange pigment and M = margin touching optic disc.[4] Small tumors that do not have any of these features, are unlikely to grow and are more in the favor of being a nevus. Tumors that show at least one of the five features carry a 38% risk of growth, and those with two or more features show growth in over 50% of patients. Tumors that display two or more features are most likely to represent small choroidal melanomas, and intervention may be necessary.

Ancillary testing using transillumination, auto-fluorescence, ultrasonography, fluorescein angiography, and optical coherence tomography (OCT) help in defining the characteristics of the tumor. Fine-needle aspiration biopsy is used in case of an atypical presentation for confirming the diagnosis, or for cytogenetic analysis of the tumor. On histopathology, the tumor develops from the melanocytes of the uvea that are derived from the neural crest cells. Currently, three histopathological uveal melanoma categories are being recognized—spindle, epithelioid, and mixed cell type.

Transillumination involves the use of a bright light placed in the conjunctival fornix in a dark room to obtain a shadow that is cast through the sclera in the area corresponding to the melanoma. On autofluorescence, there are areas of hyperautofluorescence due to the presence of lipofuscin pigment. Fluorescein angiography shows early mottled hyperfluorescence with diffuse late staining of the overlying subretinal fluid. Double circulation (presence of both retinal vessels and the choroidal vessels within the tumor) can be visualized in large melanomas with less pigmentation. A-scan ultrasonography of a choroidal melanoma reveals medium to low internal reflectivity, and B-scan ultrasonography shows a choroidal mass with acoustic hollowness and choroidal excavation. Ultrabiomicroscopy (UBM) can be used to document the iridociliary melanomas. CT and MRI can be used when orbital extension is suspected. OCT can detect secondary changes from choroid melanoma, including subretinal fluid, cystoid retinal edema, and epiretinal membrane.

The management of melanoma depends primarily on the tumor size. For small and medium lesions, transpupillary thermotherapy, plaque radiotherapy, charged particle irradiation or local resection is performed based on the tumor location and accompanying features. Most commonly used plaque radiation worldwide is I-125, followed by Ru-106. For large tumors enucleation is necessary, and for tumors with orbital extension, orbital exenteration is performed. Patients with uveal melanoma are at risk for metastatic disease to the liver, lung, and skin. Systemic monitoring with physical examination and liver

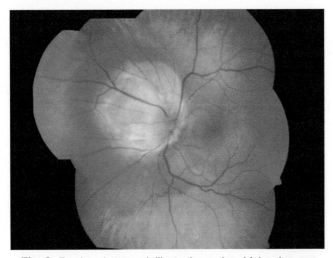

Fig. 3: Fundus photograph illustrating a choroidal melanoma overhanging the optic disk.

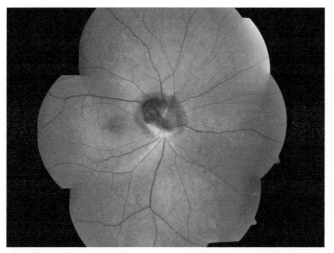

Fig. 4: Fundus photograph showing an optic disk melanocytoma.

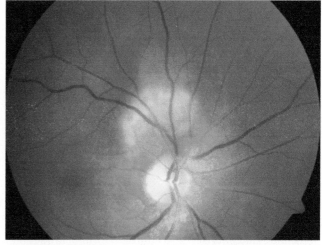

Fig. 5: Fundus photograph showing an orange-colored circumscribed choroidal hemangioma.

function tests twice yearly, and chest radiograph and liver imaging using MRI or ultrasonography annually is advised.

Melanocytoma of the optic disk is a unilateral congenital that is deeply pigmented. It can have a choroidal component or a retinal component (Fig. 4). It can be associated with disk edema, localized subretinal fluid, retinal exudates, disk, and retinal hemorrhages, vitreous pigmentation, and retinal vein obstruction. Malignant transformation into melanoma is very low. Fundus photography and clinical evaluation should be done annually to monitor the size and any retinal changes. Small degrees of growth may not signify malignant change.

CHOROIDAL HEMANGIOMA

Hemangiomas of the choroid occur in two forms—circumscribed and diffuse.[6] Circumscribed choroidal hemangiomas (CCH) are solitary benign vascular tumors which are congenital in origin (Fig. 5). On the other hand, diffuse choroidal hemangiomas (DCH) are usually a part of variable systemic manifestations of Sturge-Weber syndrome (Fig. 6). CCH, although believed to be present since birth, are generally detected in the second or the third decade when they start producing visual symptoms. They can enlarge to involve the fovea, or produce subretinal fluid to cause macular detachment. A DCH most commonly causes an exudative retinal detachment with macular involvement. Long standing fluid in the macular region can result in photoreceptor cell loss and cystoid degeneration of the sensory retina causing permanent visual damage.

The treatment options for a symptomatic choroidal hemangioma include transpupillary thermotherapy, photodynamic therapy, plaque brachytherapy, external

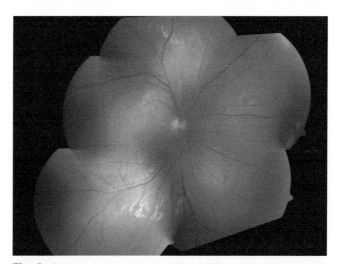

Fig. 6: Fundus photograph revealing a diffuse orange hue to the fundus with exudative retinal detachment due to a diffuse choroidal hemangioma.

beam radiation, and even proton beam radiotherapy. Plaque radiotherapy is the most commonly performed procedure for choroidal hemangioma as it is most effective in retaining a good vision in patients with submacular tumors. Stability in the size of the tumor, regression of the subretinal fluid, and resolution of symptoms can be achieved in a majority of the patients.[6] Low dose external beam radiation therapy can also achieve good results with minimal side-effects.

CHOROIDAL OSTEOMA

Choroidal osteoma is an osseous choristoma in the choroid. It is a benign bony tumor which is mostly unilateral (80%), but can be bilateral (20%). When detected early in its course, the tumor appears as a yellow-orange placoid, juxtapapillary or macular lesion, with small extensions along the otherwise well-defined margins (Fig. 7). With time, choroidal neovascular membrane can develop with retinal hemorrhages and gliosis, leading to loss of typical clinical characteristics of a choroidal osteoma.

B-scan ultrasonography shows a highly reflective echo that persists at lower sensitivity. CT reveals a choroidal plaque with bone density. Choroidal osteoma is generally observed. For subretinal neovascularization, anti-vascular endothelial growth factor (VEGF) therapy and laser photocoagulation can be used.

METASTATIC TUMORS

Metastatic cancer is the most common form of intraocular malignancy. It occurs through the hematogenous route, affecting mainly the choroid. Iris and ciliary body are less frequently involved, and retinal involvement is extremely rare. Most intraocular metastases are carcinomas, with the majority originating from breast cancer in women and lung cancer in men. Other less frequently documented primary malignancies are carcinoma of the gastrointestinal tract, kidney, prostate, thyroid gland, cutaneous melanoma, and bronchial carcinoid tumors.

Iris metastasis appears as unilateral or bilateral, single or multiple tan, yellow, or pink nodules in the stroma (Fig. 8). A ciliary body metastasis is difficult to detect, but may present with anterior segment inflammation. Choroidal metastasis appears as unilateral or bilateral, single or multiple yellow lesions with subretinal fluid.

The diagnosis of metastasis is generally made by taking a history for prior cancers, and by ruling out primary choroidal

tumors with their distinctive clinical characteristics and the use of choroidal imaging. In difficult cases, fine needle aspiration for cytologic confirmation of the tumor is used. Management of uveal metastasis is basically treatment of the primary tumor with chemotherapy. Larger symptomatic tumors that are not responsive to chemotherapy may require plaque radiotherapy.

RETINOBLASTOMA

Retinoblastoma is the most common intraocular malignancy in children. It results from genetic mutation in chromosome 13, and can be hereditary (germline mutation) or nonhereditary (sporadic mutation). Retinoblastoma is usually diagnosed at an average age of 18 months, with 95% of children diagnosed by 5 years of age. Germline retinoblastomas can present as early as first month and sporadic retinoblastomas are detected at an average age of 24 months. Retinoblastoma can be unilateral or bilateral. All bilateral cases are positive for germline mutation, whereas only 10–15% patients with unilateral retinoblastoma carry a germline mutation. The classic symptom is the white reflex, also termed as leukocoria. Strabismus is the second most common symptom. Other symptoms include poor vision, red painful eye, vitreous hemorrhage, phthisis bulbi, sterile orbital cellulitis, and proptosis.

It typically manifests as a unifocal or multifocal, well-circumscribed, dome-shaped retinal mass with dilated retinal vessels. Although initially transparent and difficult to visualize, it grows to become opaque and white. When small, the tumor is entirely intraretinal. As it enlarges, it grows in a three-dimensional plane, extending away from the vitreous cavity (exophytic) or toward it (endophytic) (Figs. 9A and

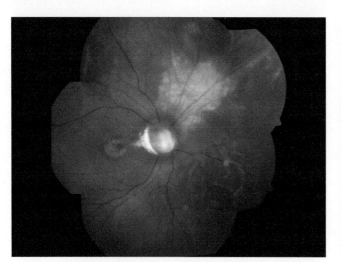

Fig. 7: Fundus photograph showing a peripapillary choroidal osteoma.

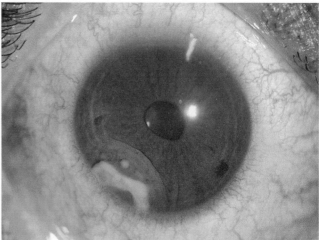

Fig. 8: External photograph of the eye showing a pinkish iris nodule in a patient with breast carcinoma. A fine needle aspiration biopsy confirmed the diagnosis of metastatic tumor of the iris.

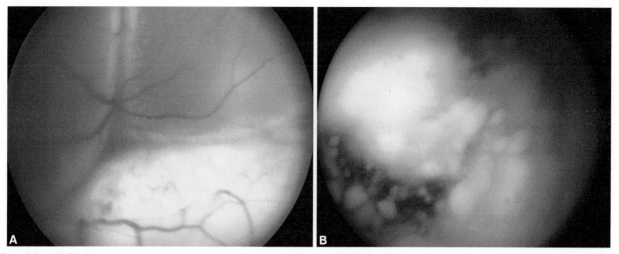

Figs. 9A and B: Clinical presentation of retinoblastoma: (A) Exophytic growth pattern with diffuse subretinal fluid; (B) Endophytic growth pattern with diffuse vitreous seeds.

B). At times, the tumor maybe a combination of these two growth patterns. Diffuse infiltrating retinoblastoma is a rare pattern of presentation where there is no obvious mass, only a flat retinal infiltration, and is acalcific. It is generally seen in older children, and the incidence is less than 2%. Diffuse anterior retinoblastoma, a recent entity, is considered as an anterior variant of diffuse infiltrating retinoblastoma. It is thought to arise from the most peripheral parts of retina with anterior growth, and no retinal focus visible on examination.

Patients with anterior extension of the tumor can present with white fluffy exudates in the anterior chamber resembling a hypopyon, called pseudohypopyon. Neovascularization of iris and glaucoma are other clinical presentations seen in patients with advanced tumor. Orbital cellulitis-like picture occurs when a large tumor undergoes necrosis and induces inflammation in and around the eye. Orbital retinoblastoma, although rare in developed nations, continues to pose a major challenge in the developing nations.

The most important differential diagnosis is Coats' disease. There are several other lesions that can simulate retinoblastoma and are known as pseudoretinoblastomas. These include persistent fetal vasculature, vitreous hemorrhage, toxocariasis, familial exudative vitreoretinopathy, retinal detachment, congenital cataract, coloboma, astrocytic hamartoma, combined hamartoma, endogenous endophthalmitis, retinopathy of prematurity, medulloepithelioma, X-linked retinoschisis, incontinentia pigmenti, juvenile xanthogranuloma, and Norrie's disease.

A child with a suspicious retinoblastoma is best examined under anesthesia for a detailed fundus evaluation. The diagnosis of the tumor and its grading is based on clinical examination, although ocular imaging by

ultrasound is necessary for documentation and computed tomography (CT) or magnetic resonance imaging (MRI) for suspected orbital invasion (Table 1). The grouping system is for retinoblastomas confined to the eye, where eye salvage is the end point, whereas the staging system is for predicting survival in patients with retinoblastoma. International Classification of Retinoblastoma (ICRB) was devised in 2003 and it includes both grouping and staging.[7] The grouping is

TABLE 1: Role of multimodal imaging in retinoblastoma.

RetCam	Wide angle fundus camera that is used in documenting fundus findings at each visit and monitoring the treatment.
Ultrasonography	Detection of calcification, especially useful in establishing diagnosis in an opaque media. Also used in tumor thickness measurement and monitoring the effects of treatment.
Fluorescein angiography (FA)	Performed on the Retcam using a filter. Helps in the visualization of capillary drop-outs, neovascularization, recurrences, and occlusive vasculopathy following IAC.
Hand-held spectral domain OCT (SD-OCT)	Used in documenting early tumors, differentiation from pseudoretinoblastomas like astrocytic hamartomas, detection of small recurrences, and assessment of fovea for visual potential
Computed tomography (CT)	Detects calcification and aids in the identification of orbital and optic nerve extension, although less sensitive than MRI.
Magnetic resonance imaging (MRI)	Delineating the intraocular tumor extent and detection of optic nerve or scleral extension and disease staging

TABLE 2: International classification of retinoblastoma.

Grouping:	
Group A: Small tumor	Retinoblastoma ≤3 mm in size
Group B: Larger tumor	Rb >3 mm, • Macular location (≤3 mm to foveola) • Juxtapapillary location (≤1.5 mm to disk) • Clear subretinal fluid ≤3 mm from margin
Group C: Focal seeds	• Subretinal seeds ≤3 mm from retinal tumor • Vitreous seeds ≤3 mm from retinal tumor • Subretinal and vitreous seeds ≤3 mm from retinal tumor
Group D: Diffuse seeds	• Subretinal seeds >3 mm from retinal tumor • Vitreous seeds > 3 mm from retinal tumor • Subretinal and vitreous seeds >3 mm from retinal tumor
Group E: Extensive retinoblastoma	• Rb occupying 50% globe • Neovascular glaucoma • Opaque media (from hemorrhage in anterior chamber, vitreous, or subretinal space) • Invasion of postlaminar optic nerve, choroid (2 mm), sclera, orbit, anterior chamber • Phthisis or pre-phthisis
Staging:	
Stage 0	Eye has not been enucleated and no dissemination of disease
Stage I	Enucleation with complete histological resection
Stage II	Enucleation with microscopic tumor residual (anterior chamber, choroid, optic nerve, sclera)
Stage III	Regional extension A. Overt orbital disease B. Preauricular or cervical lymph node extension

Stage IV	Metastatic disease
	A. Hematogenous metastasis
	  1. Single lesion
	  2. Multiple lesions
	B. CNS extension
	  1. Prechiasmatic lesion
	  2. CNS mass
	  3. Leptomeningeal disease

based on the tumor size, location, severity, and presence of subretinal and vitreous seeds (Table 2).

Treatment options for retinoblastoma depend on the tumor grade, location, laterality, related tumor seeding, and status of the opposite eye. External beam radiation therapy (EBRT) played a major role in the eye-saving treatment of retinoblastoma before the introduction of chemoreduction in the 1990s. EBRT led to the development of second cancers in and around the treatment site, and also caused orbital hypoplasia. Thus, intravenous chemotherapy (IVC) gained popularity. Although intra-arterial chemotherapy (IAC) is now being widely used, IVC continues to be the primary mode of management in bilateral retinoblastoma. Intravitreal chemotherapy (IVit) is mainly used to achieve regression of extensive vitreous seeds. Enucleation is still performed in advanced retinoblastoma or in eyes with uncontrolled disease.

Intravenous Chemotherapy

Currently, IVC is the most widely used treatment in India (Box 3). Used as a combination triple-drug therapy of vincristine, etoposide, and carboplatin, chemotherapy with focal consolidation achieves excellent success rates in the primary management of retinoblastoma. Chemotherapy alone can achieve an impressive tumor control in less advanced cases, with success rates of 100%, 93% and 90% in ICRB groups A, B and C, respectively (Figs. 10A to D).[8-10] Rates of regression of retinoblastoma and eye salvage with standard triple-drug chemotherapy have been suboptimal for ICRB group D and E tumors. In group D eyes, approximately half of the eyes require either EBRT or enucleation for tumor control.[8] A combination of chemotherapy and radiation in eyes with vitreous seeds has yielded globe salvage rates varying from 22% to 70%. Periocular carboplatin and topotecan injection also resulted in higher intravitreal drug level. Transscleral penetration of posterior sub-Tenon carboplatin leads to augmented vitreous concentration. High-dose chemotherapy with concurrent periocular carboplatin has been tried as a primary management strategy, specifically in eyes with diffuse vitreous seeds. This has led to better tumor control in advanced cases, with 95% eye salvage rate in eyes with focal vitreous seeds and a 70% eye salvage rate in those with diffuse vitreous seeds.

Intra-arterial Chemotherapy

Intra-arterial chemotherapy (IAC) for the treatment of intraocular retinoblastoma was first performed by Algernon Reese with direct internal carotid artery injection of the alkylating agent triethylene melamine in 1954. Suzuki and Kaneko described the technique of "selective ophthalmic artery infusion" (SOAI) in 2004 by the balloon technique, where a micro-balloon catheter is positioned by a transfemoral artery approach at the cervical segment of

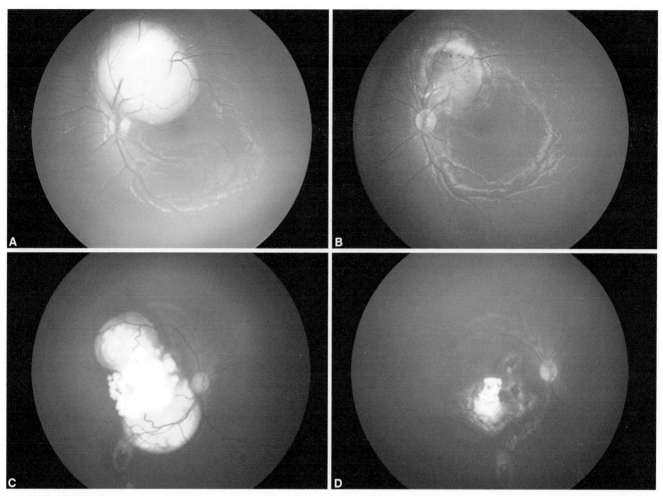

Figs. 10A to D: Standard-dose chemotherapy in retinoblastoma: (A) A group B eye; (B) After 6 cycles of standard-dose chemotherapy; (C) A group C eye with focal vitreous seeds; (D) After 6 cycles of standard-dose chemotherapy.

the internal carotid artery just distal to the orifice for the ophthalmic artery.[11] At this point, the balloon catheter is inflated, and chemotherapy is injected with flow thereby directed into the ophthalmic artery. The authors noted there are several small, but nevertheless important, branches proximal to the origin of the ophthalmic artery (i.e. cavernous branches of the ICA) into which infused chemotherapy could flow, and concluded that this infusion method is not truly selective. In 2006, Abramson and Gobin pioneered direct intra-arterial (ophthalmic artery) infusion or superselective intra-arterial chemotherapy or "chemosurgery".[12]

Patient is examined under anesthesia by the treating ocular oncologist. Documentation of each affected eye is performed by wide-angle fundus photography, fundus fluorescein angiography (FFA), and B-scan ultrasonography. The decision to treat with IAC is undertaken in consultation with an ocular oncology team, an endovascular neurosurgeon, and a pediatric oncologist.

The procedure is performed under general anesthesia using a sterile technique (Figs. 11A to D). Nasal decongestion is achieved by topical decongestant drops or spray. Anticoagulation with intravenous infusion of heparin is delivered to a target activated clotting time of 2–3 times baseline. Through a transfemoral approach, the ipsilateral internal carotid artery is catheterized with a 4F pediatric guide catheter. The arterial anatomy is visualized with serial angiography runs, and the ostium of the ophthalmic artery is superselectively catheterized with a Prowler 10 microcatheter by the peep-in technique. A superselective injection through the microcatheter is performed to check adequate positioning and assessing the amount of reflux, if any, into the internal carotid artery before chemotherapy is injected. Each chemotherapy dose is diluted in 30 mL of saline and administered in a pulsatile fashion over 30 minutes to prevent lamination of medication and loss of dose to peripheral tributaries. Repeat angiography is performed immediately after the procedure to ensure

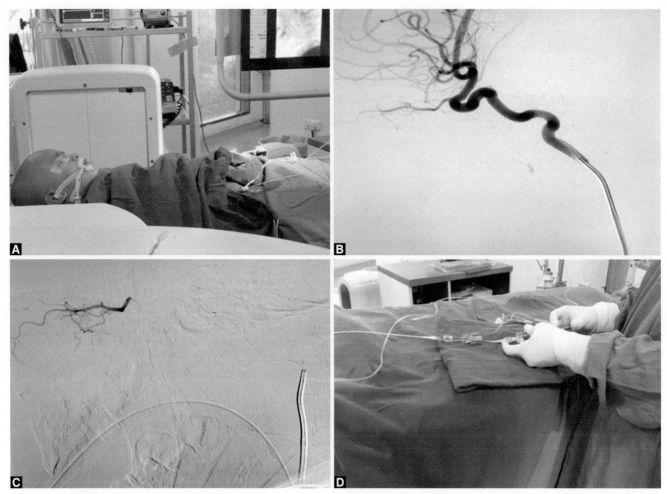

Figs. 11A to D: Intra-arterial chemotherapy: Procedure in the cath lab: (A) Patient under general anesthesia with a transfemoral catheter; (B) An angiography performed at the beginning of the procedure, showing a patent internal carotid artery; (C) An angiography performed with the microcatheter at the ostium of the ophthalmic artery, showing a patent ophthalmic artery; (D) Infusion of the chemotherapeutic drug through the transfemoral catheter.

patency of the vessels, and the catheter removed. At the end of the procedure, the heparin is reversed with intravenous protamine and hemostasis achieved with manual compression of the femoral artery upon removal of the catheter. The child is monitored for 6 hours before discharge.

Intra-arterial chemotherapy has emerged as an effective treatment for advanced retinoblastoma. It is increasingly being used in tumors as a primary treatment, especially in unilateral retinoblastoma. It can be used as a secondary therapy for those cases which have recurred or have not responded adequately to IVC. Shields et al. observed 94% globe salvage in group D eyes, and 91% vitreous seed regression, when IAC was used as a primary therapy.[13-15] In a study comparing 2-year ocular survival rate between naïve eyes with vitreous seeds (IAC as a primary therapy)

and previously treated eyes with vitreous seeds (IAC as a secondary therapy), Abramson et al. observed that IAC seemed to be more effective in eyes that have failed to respond to previous therapies. In an overall study on IAC in retinoblastoma, Abramson, et al. observed that eyes with vitreous seeds tend to require higher treatment sessions and doses, and multiple agents, as compared to eyes without vitreous seeds.

Intravitreal Chemotherapy

Vitreous seeds are aggregates of tumor cells found in the avascular vitreous, which are relatively resistant to the effect of intravenous chemotherapy due to lack of blood supply. These appear due to the disruption of the apical tumor either spontaneously (primary) or treatment-induced necrosis (secondary). Suboptimal concentration of chemotherapeutic agents in the vitreous results in persistence of vitreous seeds. Refractory vitreous seeds are the persistent or recurrent vitreous seeds which do not respond to the standard treatment modalities. Persistent seeds are those which are present during chemoreduction, and continue to persist after the completion of chemoreduction. Recurrent seeds are those which appear after the completion of chemoreduction. IVitC achieves higher drug concentration within the vitreous and effectively causes regression of vitreous seeds, without associated systemic side effects.

Intravitreal chemotherapy in retinoblastoma was first introduced by Ericson and Rosengren using thiotepa in 1960. Methotrexate has also been tried as an intravitreal drug for retinoblastoma. In 1987, Inomata and Kaneko investigated the sensitivity of retinoblastoma to 12 anticancer drugs and found that the retinoblastoma cells were most sensitive to melphalan in vitro. Melphalan is now the most extensively used drug to control the vitreous disease in retinoblastoma. Munier, et al. discussed a potentially safe technique to perform intravitreal injections to prevent extraocular extension of the tumor. They advocated the application of triple freeze-thaw cryotherapy at the injection site to prevent egress of the tumor cells in the needle track.

With melphalan, vitreous seed regression ranging from 85% to 100% of eyes and globe salvage in 80–100% of eyes have been reported.[16-18] Intravitreal melphalan is given as a weekly injection until regression. The disadvantage of melphalan is that it is not stable in solutions, and has to be used within an hour of reconstitution of the drug. A combination of intravitreal melphalan and topotecan has also been used to achieve excellent regression in refractory vitreous seeds. The authors use intravitreal topotecan for achieving vitreous seed regression in all recurrent and refractory cases. Topotecan is a very safe drug for intraocular use, is stable in solution, and can be given as a 3-weekly injection.[19]

Radiation Therapy

Retinoblastoma is a highly radiosensitive tumor, and radiation therapy can be curative. Radiation in the form of EBRT was the most popular globe-salvage therapy in retinoblastoma before the introduction of chemotherapy in 1990s. Although it is no longer the primary modality of treatment for retinoblastoma due to the associated complications, it has its own therapeutic indications. Episcleral plaque radiotherapy is a form of brachytherapy wherein the source of radiation is placed on the episclera adjacent to the tumor, and the tumor absorbs radiation, sparing other healthy ocular tissues from the ill effects of radiation.

Box 3: Intravenous chemotherapy.

Procedure:
IVC when given as a primary treatment for retinoblastoma causes reduction in tumor volume, and this is known as chemoreduction (CRD). Most commonly, a combination of three drugs of standard dose (SD) is used, although high dose (HD) may be necessary in advanced cases or tumors not responding to SD.

Drugs:
Triple drug combination therapy of vincristine, etoposide, and carboplatin (VEC) is employed, generally given 4 weekly for 6 cycles.
Day 1: Vincristine + etoposide + carboplatin
Day 2: Etoposide

Drug	SD-VEC (≥ 3 years of age)	SD-VEC (<3 years of age)	HD-VEC
Vincristine*	1.5 mg/m^2	0.05 mg/kg	0.025 mg/Kg
Etoposide	150 mg/m^2	5 mg/kg	12 mg/Kg
Carboplatin	560 mg/m^2	18.6 mg/kg	28 mg/Kg

*Maximum dose <2 mg

Indications:
(1) Primary tumor; (2) Recurrent tumor; (3) Recurrent subretinal seeds; (4) As adjuvant therapy in postenucleation patients with high-risk features (discussed elsewhere); (5) Orbital retinoblastoma; (6) As palliative therapy in metastatic retinoblastoma

Advantages:
(1) Long-term tumor control; (2) Reduces incidence of pinealoblastoma; (3) Reduces incidence of second cancers; (4) Reduces incidence of systemic metastasis

Disadvantages:
(1) Systemic side-effects including thrombocytopenia, leukopenia and anemia; (2) Allergic reactions to carboplatin and etoposide; (3) Long-term effects include hearing loss, renal toxicity and secondary leukemia

Focal Therapy

Although episcleral plaque therapy may also be considered as a form of focal therapy, the term generally refers to the use of cryotherapy, transpupillary thermotherapy (TTT), and laser therapy in the treatment of retinoblastoma. These are generally used for consolidation once the tumor has attained a considerably lower volume with chemoreduction, usually after two or three cycles, or for the treatment or small recurrent tumors of subretinal seeds. However, they can also be used as the sole therapy for small retinoblastomas.

Enucleation

Enucleation is the oldest form of treatment for retinoblastoma, and is still indicated in advanced cases.[11] Unilateral disease with no salvageable vision is best treated by enucleation and the patient can be rid of the disease for life. Enucleation is a simple procedure, although special precautions need to be taken when handling an eye with retinoblastoma. These are necessary to avoid accidental perforation that can potentially cause orbital seeding of the tumor. Use of a primary silicone or polymethylmethacrylate implant by the myoconjunctival technique provides adequate static and dynamic cosmesis. Porous polyethylene or hydroxyapatite implants do not offer additional advantage unless pegged, and these are best avoided if a child is likely to need adjuvant chemotherapy or EBRT following enucleation since fibrovascular integration of these implants would be impeded.

An enucleated eyeball is always submitted for pathology to assess for pathological high-risk factors (HRF). In a landmark paper by Honavar et al., the need for adjuvant chemotherapy has been emphasized to reduce the risk of secondary orbital recurrence and systemic metastasis.[20] The incidence of metastasis was 4% in those who received adjuvant therapy, compared with 24% in those who did not. Hence, when HRF is positive, adjuvant treatment with chemotherapy and/or EBRT is indicated. Adjuvant chemotherapy consists of a combination of vincristine, etoposide and carboplatin given 4 weekly for 6 cycles (Box 4).[20]

Orbital Retinoblastoma

Orbital retinoblastoma is an advanced form of retinoblastoma seen mostly in developing countries of Asia and Africa. The incidence varies among different countries, and is in the range of 18–40%.[21] Primary orbital retinoblastoma is the orbital extension of the disease which is evident at presentation either clinically or radiologically. Most of the patients present with proptosis, or a large fungating mass which bleeds on touch. Tumor necrosis

Box 4: High-risk features in retinoblastoma.

High-risk features on pathology where adjuvant chemotherapy is indicated:
- Anterior segment invasion
- Ciliary body infiltration
- Massive choroidal invasion (invasion ≥ 3 mm in basal diameter or thickness)
- Full thickness scleral extension
- Extrascleral extension
- Retrolaminar optic nerve invasion
- Optic nerve invasion at line of transection
- Combination of optic nerve infiltration till any level (prelaminar/ laminar/ retrolaminar) and choroidal infiltration (any thickness)

High-risk features on pathology where adjuvant radiotherapy is indicated (in addition to chemotherapy):
- Full thickness scleral extension
- Extrascleral extension
- Optic nerve invasion at line of transection

causes inflammation of the surrounding tissues and the patient may present with sterile orbital cellulitis. Secondary orbital retinoblastoma occurs in an enucleated socket after an uncomplicated surgery. It may present as an orbital mass with an unexplained displacement of the implant, or a palpable orbital mass. Accidental retinoblastoma occurs in the event of an inadvertent perforation of the eye harboring retinoblastoma. This can occur due to improper enucleation technique, or various intraocular surgeries in an eye with unsuspected intraocular retinoblastoma. Overt orbital retinoblastoma refers to previously unrecognized extrascleral or optic nerve extension discovered during enucleation as an episcleral nodule, or an enlarged and inelastic optic nerve with or without nodular optic nerve sheath. Microscopic orbital retinoblastoma is identified on histopathological examination of the enucleated eyeball as full thickness scleral infiltration, extrascleral extension or invasion of the optic nerve.

The presence of orbital disease is generally known to carry a poor prognosis. Orbital disease increases the risk of systemic metastasis by 10–27 times and the mortality rates range from 25% to 100%.[21] However, with an intensive multimodal management and careful monitoring, patients with orbital disease are known to do well (Figs. 12A to D).

Metastatic Retinoblastoma

With an incidence of less than 5% of all retinoblastoma cases, metastatic retinoblastoma is most often seen in developing countries. It usually occurs as a relapse following enucleation for intraocular retinoblastoma, especially in those who had high risk pathologic features. Most commonly, metastasis occurs to the central nervous system (CNS), bone and bone marrow. The metastasis occurs in one of the three ways—by direct dissemination into the CNS

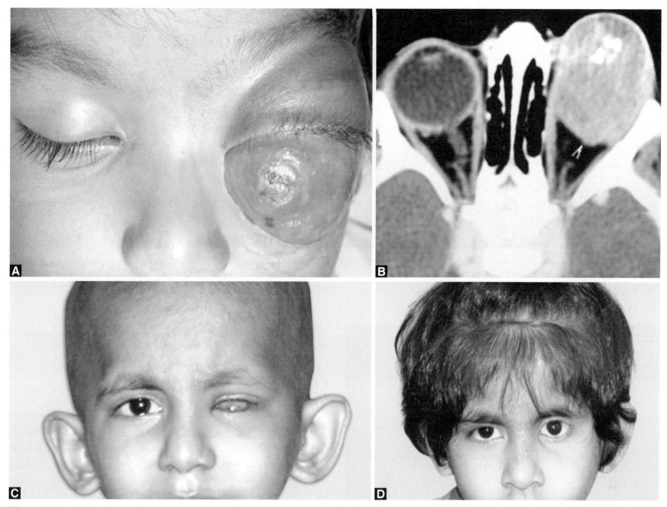

Figs. 12A to D: Multimodal management in orbital retinoblastoma: (A) External photograph of primary orbital retinoblastoma taken during examination under anesthesia; (B) Axial computed tomography image displaying extraocular extension of the intraocular tumor; (C) After 12 cycles of high-dose chemotherapy, external beam radiotherapy, and enucleation; (D) Healthy child cured of orbital retinoblastoma, with a well-fitting prosthesis.

via the optic nerve, choroidal invasion, and hematogenous spread, or orbital extension with lymph node involvement. Bony metastasis, usually involving the long bones or the craniofacial bones, causes nontender palpable mass.

RETINAL HEMANGIOBLASTOMA

Retinal vascular tumors include retinal hemangioblastoma, cavernous hemangioma, racemose hemangioma, and vasoproliferative tumor. Only retinal hemangioblastoma will be discussed in detail here. Retinal hemangioblastoma (capillary hemangioma) can either be a solitary condition, or associated with von Hippel-Lindau (VHL) syndrome. VHL syndrome is an autosomal dominant condition with the locus for VHL gene located on chromosome 3. It presents with a myriad of systemic manifestations including cerebellar hemangioblastoma, hypernephroma,

pheochromocytoma, pancreatic cysts, and several other tumors and cysts in different organs. A patient diagnosed with a solitary hemangioblastoma has a risk of 45% for developing VHL when diagnosed at the age of 10 years and 1% at the age of 60 years. Retinal hemangioblastoma classically presents as a reddish tumor in the peripheral retina or on the optic disk with dilated, tortuous, parallel leash of feeding and draining blood vessels (Fig. 13).

Management of retinal hemangioblastoma depends on the tumor size, location, complications, and whether the patient has VHL syndrome. Those associated with VHL syndrome generally appear at an earlier age, are more aggressive, and require active treatment. Small tumors with limited retinal exudation can be managed by laser photocoagulation, photodynamic therapy, or cryotherapy. More advanced lesions may require vitreoretinal surgery.

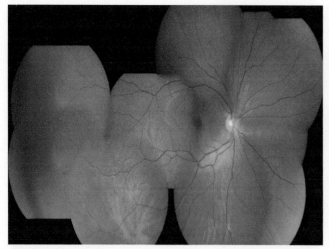

Fig. 13: Fundus photograph showing a reddish tumor in the temporal periphery with paired dilated vessels suggestive of a retinal hemangioblastoma.

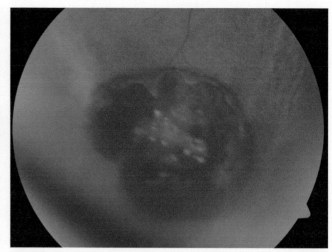

Fig. 15: Fundus photograph showing a slightly elevated pigmented lesion suggestive of congenital hypertrophy of retinal pigmented epithelium.

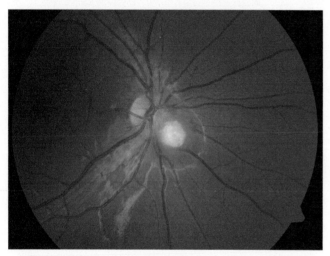

Fig. 14: Fundus photograph showing a calcified astrocytic hamartoma.

ASTROCYTIC HAMARTOMA

Astrocytic hamartoma is composed of glial cells, with the majority being astrocytes. It is a congenital lesion that may be seen in association with tuberous sclerosis complex. Tuberous sclerosis is a syndrome with a variety of manifestations including intracranial astrocytoma, adenoma sebaceum, cardiac rhabdomyoma, and other hamartomas. Retinal astrocytic hamartoma can be calcified, noncalcified, or mixed (Fig. 14). The calcified tumors may be partially or fully calcified. They appear as glistening yellow clusters of calcification, which is distinct from the dull, chalky-white calcification of retinoblastoma. The

noncalcified tumor appears as a gray-yellow or transparent lesion. Management of these lesions is periodic follow-up.

CONGENITAL HYPERTROPHY OF RETINAL PIGMENT EPITHELIUM

Congenital hypertrophy of the retinal pigment epithelium (CHRPE) can be solitary or multifocal. Solitary CHRPE is located in the midperiphery or periphery fundus and does not cause any symptoms. It is usually detected on routine fundus examination. It appears as a well-delineated minimally raised placoid lesion that is frequently homogenous black in color (Fig. 15). When not homogenously black, it is due to several small depigmented patches within the lesion, called lacunae. Very rarely, a nodular growth can develop within the lesion, with a feeder vessel and retinal exudation. In such cases, a low-grade RPE adenocarcinoma must be ruled out by fine needle aspiration biopsy.

The multifocal variant of CHRPE or grouped CHRPE appears as "bear tracks". These are characterized by multiple groups of well-defined lesions in a sectoral distribution. The lesions can sometimes be nonpigmented, appearing as "polar bear tracks". There is no association of these lesions with any systemic cancer, unlike the RPE hamartomas which are associated with familial adenomatous polyposis (FAP) and Gardner syndrome. These RPE hamartomas are typically multiple and bilateral, and unlike CHRPE, have no well-defined margins, no sectoral distribution, have irregularly depigmented margins, and a pointed, fish-tail configuration.

The management of solitary and multifocal CHRPE is periodic observation. If RPE adenocarcinoma is suspected, observation is recommended unless there is subretinal fluid or large amount of exudation. In such cases, laser photocoagulation, cryotherapy, or plaque brachytherapy can be considered. For those with the RPE hamartomas, periodic observation is recommended. However, regular screening for FAP and colon cancer is advised.

MEDULLOEPITHELIOMA

Medulloepithelioma is a rare tumor of the nonpigmented ciliary epithelium. It is an embryonal neoplasm arising from the inner layer of the optic cup prior to its differentiation into mature elements. The most common site is the ciliary body. The tumor can be classified histopathologically into nonteratoid (immature elements) and teratoid (mature elements) types, and both can be either benign or malignant.

The diagnosis of medulloepithelioma is generally in the first decade of life. One of the frequent clinical features is a notch in the lens due to congenital absence of zonules in the region of the tumor. The tumor is typically a fleshy, pinkish mass (Fig. 16). The tumor can be frequently cystic and rarely pigmented. A prominent feature is the development of a neoplastic cyclitic membrane and traction on the zonules. In delayed diagnosis, retinal detachment is a frequent complication. In addition, secondary glaucoma may develop due to iris neovascularization and secondary angle closure. Ultrasonography reveals a mass pattern with acoustic solidity and high internal reflectivity. Most eyes are enucleated due to associated complications. However, in cases where the diagnosis has been made early and the tumor is small with minimal secondary complications, it can be managed by iridocyclectomy. The role of plaque radiotherapy is yet to be established.

INTRAOCULAR LYMPHOMA

Intraocular lymphomas are a form of extranodal lymphomas and are classically of two types—vitreoretinal and uveal. Both of them are primarily non-Hodgkin's lymphoma (NHL) of B-cell type. The most common intraocular lymphoma is the primary vitreoretinal lymphoma (PVRL) (Fig. 17). It can also be an extension of primary CNS lymphoma (PCNSL), involving the brain and the cerebrospinal fluid.[22] Most commonly it presents as uveitis, and is frequently bilateral. Multiple subretinal yellow infiltrates are typically seen in this form. It usually belongs to the subtype diffuse large B-cell lymphoma (DLBCL), which is a high-grade lymphoma. In contrast, the primary uveal lymphomas are low-grade B-cell lymphomas. Uveal lymphomas are characterized by amelanotic, solitary or multifocal,

unilateral or bilateral uveal lesions (Fig. 18). Secondary vitreoretinal and choroidal lymphomas occur in patients with disseminated disease.

The management of suspected uveal lymphoma begins with a systemic evaluation to exclude systemic lymphoma and myeloma. In the presence of systemic lymphoma, systemic chemotherapy generally causes resolution of the uveal lesions. A larger lesion with extensive retinal detachment or other complications is managed by external beam radiotherapy, usually 2,000–2,500 cGy, in divided doses. For PVRL without CNS lymphoma, external beam radiotherapy, 3,500–4,000 cGy in divided doses is the preferred treatment. For CNS lymphoma, concurrent cranial radiation is generally recommended.

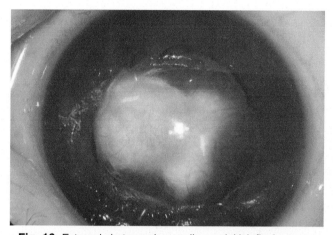

Fig. 16: External photograph revealing a pinkish fleshy tumor with a cyclitic membrane suggestive of a medulloepithelioma.

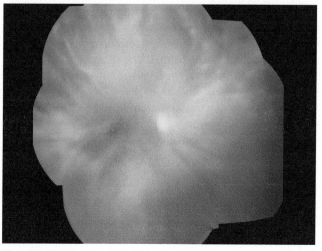

Fig. 17: Fundus photograph revealing extensive vitreous cells which on biopsy revealed lymphomatous cells, suggestive of vitreoretinal lymphoma.

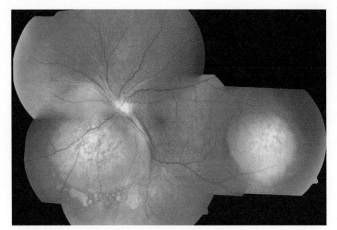

Fig. 18: Fundus photograph revealing two large yellowish choroidal lesions with surrounding subretinal fluid which on biopsy proved to be choroidal lymphoma.

PARANEOPLASTIC RETINOPATHY

Paraneoplastic syndromes of the retina are a diverse group of disorders occurring in the setting of a systemic malignancy. The timely recognition of these entities is important as they can lead to an early detection and treatment of an unsuspected, underlying malignancy, giving the patient a lead time in cancer survival.

Cancer associated retinopathy (CAR) is the most common of the intraocular paraneoplastic syndromes. Patients with CAR generally present in the seventh decade. The most common symptom is visual loss, which is painless and occurs gradually over months. The diagnosis of CAR precedes the diagnosis of an underlying malignancy in about one-half of the patients. Other visual complaints include photopsia, photosensitivity, color vision abnormalities, impaired dark adaptation, and nyctalopia. On examination, the fundus reveals optic nerve pallor, constricted retinal arterioles, and retinal pigment epithelial (RPE) hyperplasia and atrophy. The diagnosis of CAR can be established by testing the levels of anti-retinal antibody (anti-recovering and anti-alpha enolase antibodies) and with the aid of an electroretinogram (ERG). The ERG in CAR depicts global reduction in retinal function, which occurs even in the presence of an entirely normal-looking fundus.

Melanoma associated retinopathy (MAR) often occurs in patients who have a previously diagnosed cutaneous melanoma, and the development of visual symptoms generally coincides with a recurrence or metastasis. Patients presenting with MAR are generally in their sixth decade. Clinical features of MAR classically represent rod dysfunction, with nyctalopia as one of the initial manifestations. Fundus examination may be normal, or in advanced cases there may be optic disk pallor, retinal vessel attenuation, and areas of RPE mottling. Autoantibodies against the bipolar cells of the retina have been identified in patients with MAR. The ERG in CAR depicts reduction in rod activity, which occurs even in the presence of an entirely normal-looking fundus.

REFERENCES

1. Shields JA, Shields CL. Cysts of the iris pigment epithelium. What is new and interesting? The 2016 Jose Rizal international medal lecture. Asia Pac J Ophthalmol (Phila). 2017;6(1):64-9.
2. Shields CL, Arepalli S, Lally SE, et al. Iris stromal cyst management with absolute alcohol-induced sclerosis in 16 patients. JAMA Ophthalmol. 2014;132(6):703-8.
3. Shields J, Shields C. Posterior uveal melanoma: Clinical features. In: Shields J, Shields C (Eds). Atlas of Intraocular Tumors, 3rd edition. Philadelphia, PA: Lippincott, Wolters Kluwer; 2016. pp. 45-59.
4. Shields CL, Demirci H, Materin MA, et al. Clinical factors in the identification of small choroidal melanoma. Can J Ophthalmol. 2004;39(4):351-7.
5. Shields CL, Furuta M, Berman EL, et al. Choroidal nevus transformation into melanoma: Analysis of 2514 consecutive cases. Arch Ophthalmol. 2009;127(8):981-7.
6. Shields J, Shields C. Vascular tumors and malformations of the uvea. In: Shields J, Shields C (Eds). Atlas of Intraocular Tumors, 3rd edition. Philadelphia, PA: Lippincott, Wolters Kluwer; 2016. pp. 248-63.
7. Chantada G, Doz F, Antoneli CB, et al. A proposal for an international retinoblastoma staging system. Pediatr Blood Cancer. 2006;47(6):801-5.
8. Shields CL, Mashayekhi A, Au AK, et al. The international classification of retinoblastoma predicts chemoreduction success. Ophthalmology. 2006;113(12):2276-80.
9. Shields CL, Fulco EM, Arias JD, et al. Retinoblastoma frontiers with intravenous, intra-arterial, periocular, and intravitreal chemotherapy. Eye (Lond). 2013;27(2):253-64.
10. Shields CL, Shields JA. Retinoblastoma management: Advances in enucleation, intravenous chemoreduction, and intra-arterial chemotherapy. Curr Opin Ophthalmol. 2010;21(3):203-12.
11. Suzuki S, Yamane T, Mohri M, et al. Selective ophthalmic arterial injection therapy for intraocular retinoblastoma: The long-term prognosis. Ophthalmology. 2011;118(10):2081-7.
12. Abramson DH, Marr BP, Dunkel IJ, et al. Intra-arterial chemotherapy for retinoblastoma in eyes with vitreous and/or subretinal seeding: 2-year results. Br J Ophthalmol. 2012;96(4):499-502.
13. Shields CL, Manjandavida FP, Lally SE, et al. Intra-arterial chemotherapy for retinoblastoma in 70 eyes: Outcomes based on the international classification of retinoblastoma. Ophthalmology. 2014;121(7):1453-60.
14. Shields CL, Jorge R, Say EA, et al. Unilateral retinoblastoma managed with intravenous chemotherapy versus intra-arterial chemotherapy: Outcomes based on the international classification of retinoblastoma. Asia Pac J Ophthalmol (Phila). 2016;5(2):97-103.

15. Shields CL, Kaliki S, Al-Dahmash S, et al. Management of advanced retinoblastoma with intravenous chemotherapy then intra-arterial chemotherapy as alternative to enucleation. Retina. 2013;33(10):2103-9.

16. Ghassemi F, Shields CL. Intravitreal melphalan for refractory or recurrent vitreous seeding from retinoblastoma. Arch Ophthalmol. 2012;130(10):1268-71.

17. Francis JH, Abramson DH, Gaillard MC, et al. The classification of vitreous seeds in retinoblastoma and response to intravitreal melphalan. Ophthalmology. 2015;122(6):1173-9.

18. Shields CL, Manjandavida FP, Arepalli S, et al. Intravitreal melphalan for persistent or recurrent retinoblastoma vitreous seeds: Preliminary results. JAMA Ophthalmol. 2014;132(3):319-25.

19. Rao R, Honavar SG, Sharma V, et al. Intravitreal topotecan in the management of refractory and recurrent vitreous seeds in retinoblastoma. Br J Ophthalmol. 2017;102(4):490-5.

20. Honavar SG, Singh AD, Shields CL, et al. Postenucleation adjuvant therapy in high-risk retinoblastoma. Arch Ophthalmol. 2002;120(7):923-31.

21. Honavar SG. Orbital retinoblastoma. In: Singh AD, Murphee LA, Damato BE (Eds). Clinical Ophthalmic Oncology-Retinoblastoma, 2nd edition. NY: Springer; 2015.

22. Jahnke K, Korfel A, Komm J, et al. Intraocular lymphoma 2000-2005: Results of a retrospective multicenter trial. Graefes Arch Clin Exp Ophthalmol. 2006;244(6):663-9.

Histopathology Slides

⟫ **Histopathology Slides**

31

Histopathology Slides

RK Saran, Shweta Raghav

DERMOID

- Thick-walled with greasy pilosebaceous content
- Fibrous wall lined by keratinizing squamous epithelium with skin adnexa; cyst contains squames, hair, and sebum.
- Hair shafts highlighted with polarized light
- Hair matrix differentiation (shadow cells)
- Rupture may cause granulomatous inflammation with foreign body giant cell reaction
- Positive stains
- Epithelium-keratin, EMA (Fig. 1).

SQUAMOUS PAPILLOMA (ACROCHORDON)

Papilloma and nevus are the most common benign tumor of eyelid skin.

They show acanthotic epithelium with hyperkeratosis and papillary projections with inner fibrovascular core (Fig. 2).

HIDROCYSTOMA (SUDORIFEROUS CYST)

They arise from sweat glands and are thin-walled. Transparent vesicles are lined by flattened epithelial cells having watery fluid or empty cavity (Fig. 3).

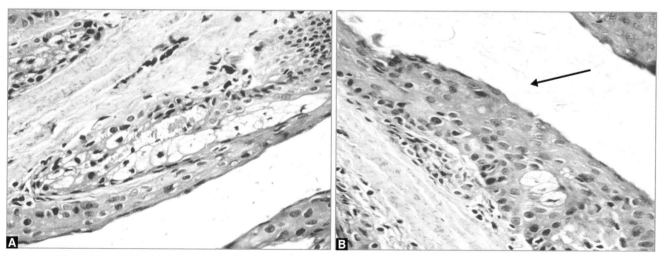

Figs. 1A and B: (A) Cyst wall showing sebaceous gland (vacuolated cells) below the stratified squamous lining; (B) Showing cyst lining having exfoliated squamous cells.

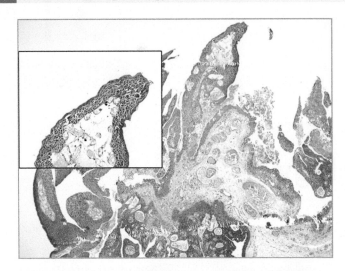

Fig. 2: Squamous papilloma x 10 HE section showing various frond of papilla of squamous cells with fibrovascular core. Inset x20 showing benign squamous cells.

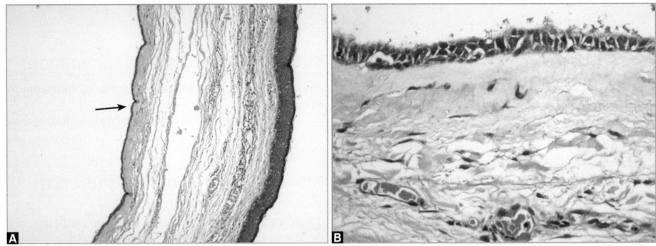

Figs. 3A and B: (A, Arrow) showing flattened epithelium; (B) Showing apocrine snouts and pseudo-stratification of epithelium.

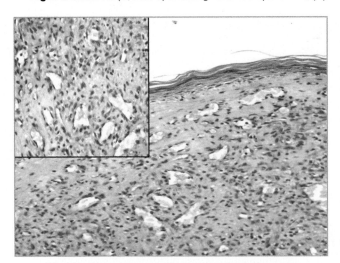

Fig. 4: Haemangioma showing spindle looking cells (endothelium) with slit spaces having RBCs .

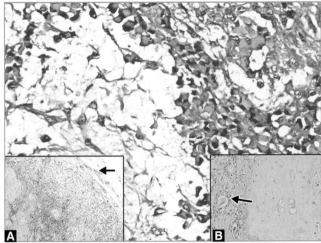

Fig. 5: Pleomorphic adenoma of lacrimal gland. Inset A: Admixed are myxoid matrix bluish color with spindling of cells. Inset B: Showing chondromyxoid tissue and focal ductal differentiation (arrow).

HAEMANGIOMA

- Capillary hemangioma—closely packed spindle cells with spaces containing blood
- Scant fibrous stroma
- Lumens may be thrombosed or organized
- May contain hemosiderin
- Cavernous hemangioma—intravascular calcification and thrombosis is common
- Shows large cystically dilated vessels with thin walls (Fig. 4).

PLEOMORPHIC ADENOMA OF LACRIMAL GLAND

- Composed of benign epithelial and myxoid mesenchymal elements

- Usually encapsulated
- May have squamous metaplasia, fat, bone or cartilage
- Often prominent component of S100+ hyaline cells with diffuse eosinophilic staining (Fig. 5).

BASAL CELL CARCINOMA

- Large solid lobules of predominant basaloid cells with peripheral palisading and cystic areas
- Clefting between the stroma and edges of tumor nodules that can be extensive or focal
- Can be associated with a characterstic myxoinflammatory stroma that shows variable proportion of mucin, lymphocytic inflammation, prominent fibroblasts and collagen thickening

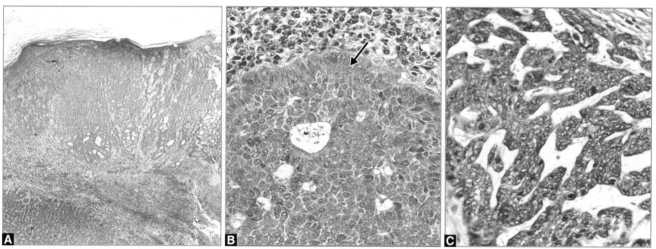

Figs. 6A to C: (A) X2 HE Basal cell carcinoma branching cords of basaloid cells arising from skin; (B) Periphral palisading of basaloid cells (arrow); (C) Branching cords on high power x 20.

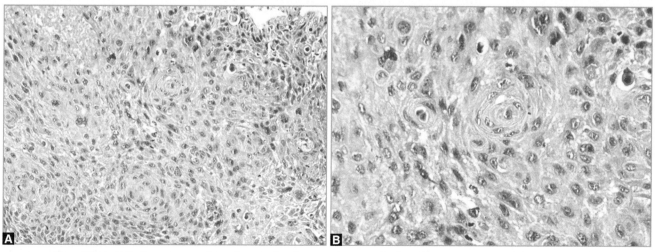

Figs. 7A and B: Squamous cell carcinoma showing prominent nucleoli and squamous pearls (A) 20X & (B) 40X.

- Infiltrative BCC—trabecular pattern of invading neoplastic cells (Fig. 6).

SQUAMOUS CELL CARCINOMA

- Invasion of malignant squamous cells into dermis
- Abnormal deep keratinization may have keratin pearls
- Cells are large and eosinophillic with marked atypia
- Well-differentiated tumor cells are polygonal with abundant acidophilic cytoplasm and hyperchromatic nuclei with various size and thinning properties, dyskeratotic cells, and intercellular bridges
- Poorly differentiated SCC shows pleomorphism with anaplastic cells, abnormal mitotic figures, little or no evidence of keratinization and loss of intercellular bridges (Fig. 7).

SEBACEOUS CELL CARCINOMA

- Exhibit intraepithelial spread into conjuctival, eyelid, and corneal epithelium
- Individual cells have finely vacuolated and frothy cytoplasm
- Lipid deposition may induce a foreign body granulomatous reaction that may resemble a chalazion clinically
- Pleomorphism and high nuclear mitotic rate
- Lobular pattern—resembles a normal sebaceous gland with well-differentiated lipid-producing cells centrally and undifferentiated cells in periphery
- Comedocarcinoma—large necrotic central core with peripheral viable cells
- Papillary—papillary projections and sebaceous differentiation
- Mixed—combination of all three patterns (Fig. 8).

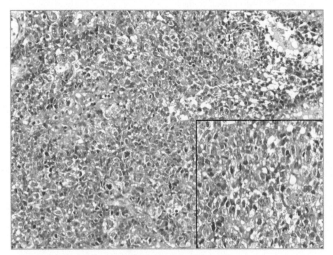

Fig. 8: Sebaceous cell carcinoma- cells - foam cells with vacuolated cytoplasm between basophilic cells inset 60X.

ADENOID CYSTIC CARCINOMA OF LACRIMAL GLAND

- Most common malignant tumor of lacrimal gland
- Aggressive, may infiltrate eyelid or brain
- Basaloid growth with cribriform change
- Prerineural invasion with focal tumor necrosis (Fig. 9).

MALIGNANT MELANOMA

This shows radial and vertical growth pattern. In radial pattern it grows horizontally within the epidermal and superficial dermal layer like lentigo maligna, superficial spreading and acral/mucosal lentiginous. It does not metastasize during this stage.

Vertical growth is heralded clinically by development of nodule in the relatively flat surface and correlates with the emergence of a clone of cells with true metastatic potential. It determines the biologic behavior of malignant melanoma.

Stains

S100: It is a calcium-binding protein in nucleus and cytoplasm of melanocytes. Its sensitivity is 97–100% but specificity is limited (75–87%) as this protein is also identified in Langerhan cells, chondrocytes, adipocytes, and myoeithelial cells.

MelanA/MART-1: Sensitivity is 75–92% and specificity is 95–100%.

HMB-45: Marker for cytoplasmic premelanosomal glycoprotein gp 100. Sensitivity is 69–93% and specificity is nearly 97% (Fig. 10).

RETINOBLASTOMA

- Trabeculae, sheets, and nests of small blue cells with scanty cytoplasm, hyperchromatic nuclei, and scanty stroma
- *Flexner*-Wintersteiner rosettes (cells line up around empty lumen delineated by a distinct eosinophillic circle composed of terminal bars analogous to outer limiting membrane of normal retina)
- *Homer*-Wright rosettes (nuclei are displaced away from lumen) and fluerettes (tumor cells arranged side by side which show differentiation towards photoreceptors)
- Azzopardi phenomena (basophilic deposits around blood vessels, also seen in small cell carcinomas), frequent mitotic figures, and variable apoptotic cells
- Frequent necrosis of tumor cells away from vessels and calcification
- It is important to look for any presence of tumor in the optic nerve

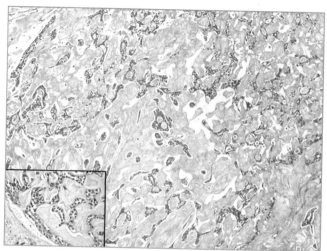

Fig. 9: Adenoid cystic carcinoma of lacrimal gland x 10 hyaline basement membrane like material is seen secreted by tumor cells showing basaloid morphology. Inset x20 showing better basaloid cells.

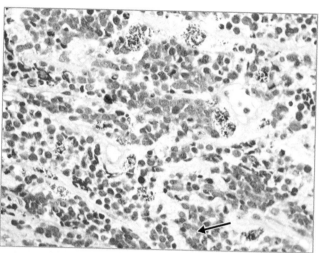

Fig. 11: Arrow (retinoblastoma rosette) x 20 blastimal like sheets of malignant round cells, with scattered choroid cell layer pigments.

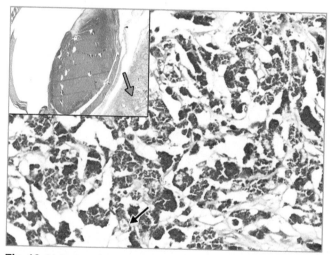

Fig. 10: Melanoma iris involving posterior chamber of eye x 2 (inset blue arrow). HE x 20 numerous tumor cells having vesicular nuclei and prominent nucleoli and brown coarse granules of melanin in cytoplasm.

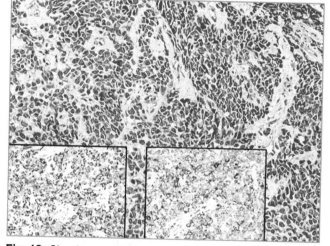

Fig. 12: Showing small blue round cell tumour with IHC positivity for Desmin and SMA. Left desmin x 20 inset. Right SMA x20 background HE x 10 Malignant round cells, high cellular High N/C ratio, inconspicuious nucleoli.

- Retinocytoma—marked photoreceptor differentiation, cells have abundant cytoplasm, less hyperchromatic nuclei, benign, with calcification but without necrosis, or mitotic activity
- Differentiated retinoblastoma: bipolar–like cells are present
- Undifferentiated retinoblastoma—large, anaplastic cells without rosette formation (Fig. 11).

RHABDOMYOSARCOMA

- Most common orbital sarcoma in childhood

- Usually embryonal and alveolar subtypes (alveolar more aggressive) less commonly pleiomorphic
- Syncytium of strap cells with abundant eosinophillic cytoplasm
- Can have minimal rhabdomyoblastic differentiation except in occasional mature strap cells with cross striations
- Can have closely packed small round cells with coarse nuclear chromatin and scanty cytoplasm and increased mitotic activity
- Alveolar pattern shows fibrovascular-septa that resembles lung alveoli (Fig. 12).

Instruments and Suture Materials

⇒ **Oculoplastic Instruments**

Oculoplastic Instruments

Smriti Nagpal Gupta, Ruchi Goel

INTRODUCTION

Ophthalmology is predominantly a microsurgical field. Hence, ophthalmic instruments need to be small, precise, and light weight. Ideally, these should also be corrosion resistant, have an antireflective coating, and be easy to sterilize and re-use. Titanium alloys and stainless steel are the commonly used metals for most instruments.

TISSUE FORCEPS (FIGS. 1A TO F)

- *Pierce Hoskin forceps*: These are fine-toothed forceps. These provide a firm hold with minimal tissue damage and are used to stabilize the globe while passing sutures, hold the intraocular lens (IOL), perform forced duction test, to hold the tissue flap while suturing, etc. (Fig. 1A)

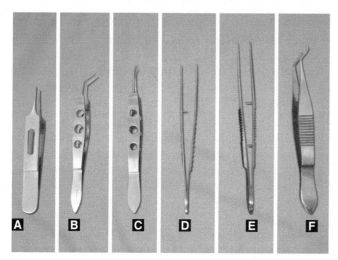

Fig. 1: Tissue forceps.

- *Kelman McPherson forceps*: These are fine, nontoothed forceps with bent tips, used to hold IOL haptics, for suture tying, and during suture removal, for removing lens capsule tags, etc. (Fig. 1B)
- *Castroviejo Suture-tying forceps*: These are fine, nontoothed forceps with curved ends and are used to hold delicate structures like fine sutures, scleral flap, amniotic membrane, etc. (Fig. 1C)
- *Plain forceps*: These are simple forceps without any teeth. These have serrations near the tip for better grip and are used to hold delicate tissue like conjunctiva, mucosa, or lacrimal sac flaps, without causing tissue damage (Fig. 1D)
- *Toothed forceps/tissue forceps (1X2)*: These forceps have 1X2 teeth at their tip and are used when firm grip over tough tissue is needed, such as periosteum, scar tissue or rarely, skin (Fig. 1E)
- *Superior Rectus Forceps (Dastoor)*: These are toothed forceps with an "S"-shaped curve near the tip. These are used to hold superior rectus muscle while passing the bridle suture, or when passing sutures to hold and identify the muscles during orbitotomy surgery (Fig. 1F).

SCISSORS (FIGS. 2A TO F)

- *Enucleation scissors*: These are large, strong scissors with sharp edges and blunt ends, used for cutting optic nerve during enucleation. The blunt ends avoid any accidental damage to the globe (Fig. 2A)
- *Orbitotomy scissors*: These are large stout scissors used for deep orbital dissection during orbitotomy and may also be used during harvesting of fascia lata in ptosis surgery (Fig. 2B)

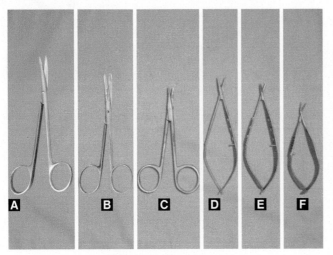

Figs. 2A to F: Scissors.

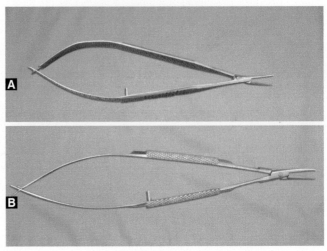

Figs. 3A and B: Needle holder.

- *Steven's Tenotomy scissors*: These are sharp scissors which may be straight or curved. These are used to cut tissues like skin and extraocular muscles and for blunt dissection and undermining of tissues in oculoplastic surgeries (Fig. 2C)
- *Westcott scissors*: These are stout, spring action scissors with sharp blades and blunt tips, useful for cutting delicate tissues and for dissection. These may be used as an alternative to plain scissors or tenotomy scissors. Blades maybe straight or curved (Fig. 2D)
- *Spring scissors/corneoscleral scissors*: These are fine, curved, sharp, spring-action scissors for cutting delicate tissues like conjunctiva, cornea, sclera, and for cutting sutures (Fig. 2E)
- *Vanna's scissors*: These are very fine, delicate spring scissors. The blades may be straight, curved or angled. These are rarely used for oculoplastic surgery, more commonly used for intra-ocular procedures (Fig. 2F).

NEEDLE HOLDER

It may be straight or curved, available in few different sizes. This is used for holding and passing needles while suturing. Handle is serrated for a firmer grip (Figs. 3A and B).

- *Fine (Barraquer's)*—Mostly used for intraocular surgeries
- *Large (Castroviejo)*—Mostly used in extraocular procedures.

RETRACTORS

These are not self-retaining and must be held by an assistant (Figs. 4A to D).

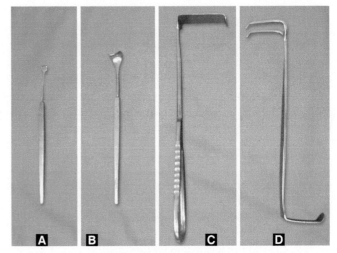

Figs. 4A to D: Retractors.

- *Cat's paw/Knapp's lacrimal sac retractor*: It is a multi-pronged fork like instrument, curved at the tip. It is used to retract tissue like periosteum and skin, during dacryocystorhinostomy (DCR) surgery, orbitotomy, and biopsies (Fig. 4A)
- *Desmarre's retractor*: It has broad spatula-like end which is folded over itself. It is available in adult and pediatric sizes. It is used to retract eyelids during examination in uncooperative patients or in presence of excessive ecchymosis or edema, used to retract orbital tissue and fat while performing LPS resection, and may be used to perform double eversion for examining the fornix and lid eversion during lid surgeries. This is also useful for exposure during squint and retinal surgeries, especially when postequatorial exposure is needed (Fig. 4B)

- *Langenbeck retractor*: This is a large retractor with a hollow handle and a steel blade at right angles to the handle. This is used to retract skin and subcutaneous tissue (Fig. 4C)
- *Czerny's retractor*: This is a large Z-shaped retractor with two spikes on one end and a broad steel plate like surface on the other. This is typically used while harvesting fascia lata for ptosis correction. It helps to retract the wound edges and provide adequate exposure and working space (Fig. 4D).

CHALAZION CLAMP AND MEYERHOEFER CURETTE (FIGS. 5A AND B)

The chalazion clamp (Fig. 5A) has one solid disk-shaped end and one hollow ring-like end with an adjusting screw. The hollow end is usually applied on the conjunctival side, over the chalazion and the screw tightened. This also helps to achieve hemostasis. The curette (Fig. 5B) is used to curette out all the contents of the chalazion and to break all adhesions. It has a small shallow cup-shaped tip with sharp margins.

Towel Clamps (Figs. 6A and B)

Used to hold drapes in position; may even be used to hold traction sutures, tubings, wires of probes, etc.
- Backhaus clamp (Fig. 6A)
- Bulldog clamp (Fig. 6B).

Nettleship's Punctum Dilator (Fig. 7A)

It is a rod-shaped instrument with narrow pointed end, used to dilate puncta and distal end of the canaliculus. It is

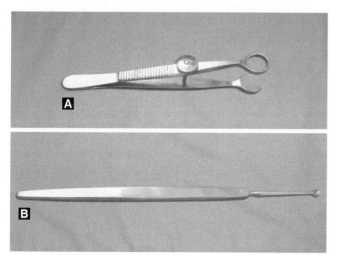

Figs. 5A and B: Chalazion clamp and curette.

useful in punctal stenosis, while performing syringing and probing, and during DCR and DCT surgeries.

Bowman's Lacrimal Probe (Fig. 7B)

These are fine wire-like, blunt-ended cylindrical probes, available in varying diameters size 0000 (0.45 mm) to 08, with a flat plate in the center for grip. These are used for probing in congenital nasolacrimal duct obstruction (NLDO), to identify site of block in cases of epiphora and during DCR and dacryocystectomy (DCT) surgeries. The ends are rounded to avoid canalicular damage.

Periosteal Elevator/Rollet Lacrimal Sac Rugine (Fig. 8)

This instrument has a sharp, tapering edge which is used to dissect off and peel the periosteum. It is used during DCR surgery, orbitotomy, and exenteration.

Lacrimal Cannula (Fig. 9)

It is a hollow curved cannula with blunt end to avoid canalicular trauma. It is available in varying sizes and used for syringing and for scraping and flushing the canaliculus with antibiotics in cases of canaliculitis.

Nasal Packing Forceps and Hartmann Nasal Speculum (Figs. 10A and B)

Used for nasal packing for DCR surgery.

Lacrimal Sac Dissector and Curette (Fig. 11)

It has a sharp and a blunt end. The sharp tip is used to create the initial bony opening during DCR surgery and to curette out the thin bone. The blunt end is used for soft tissue dissection in the sac fossa region, to avoid damage to the lacrimal sac.

Lacrimal Trephine (Sisler) (Figs. 12A and B)

It has a plastic hub affixed to the shaft, by which it can be grasped and rotated. An intraluminal stylet, provided with it, is removable. While the trephine itself has a sharp edge at the tip, the stylet is blunt tipped to avoid trauma to the surrounding canalicular tissue. The hub is fashioned for a Luer lock, whereby it can be attached to a syringe. It is long enough to span the normal length of the canaliculus. It is used to trephine and open distal canalicular blocks. It may rarely be used for biopsy of conjunctiva or sclera. Different gauges are available.

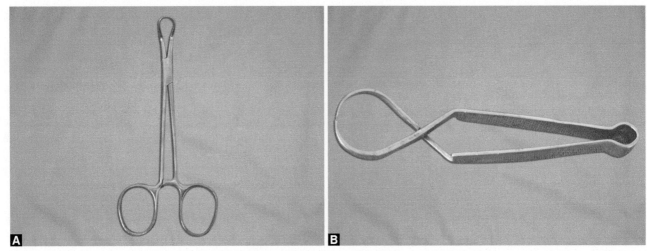

Figs. 6A and B: Towel clamps.

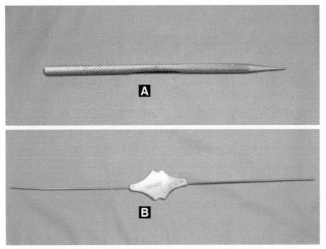

Figs. 7A and B: (A) Nettleship's punctum dilator; (B) Bowman's lacrimal probe.

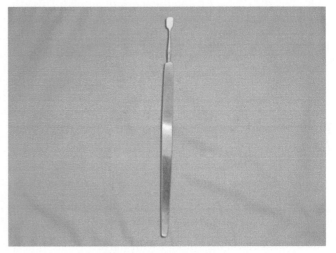

Fig. 8: Periosteal elevator.

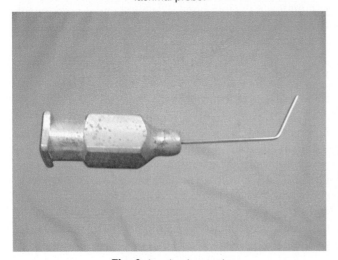

Fig. 9: Lacrimal cannula

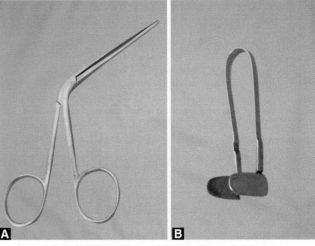

Figs. 10A and B: (A) Nasal packing forceps; (B) Hartmann nasal speculum.

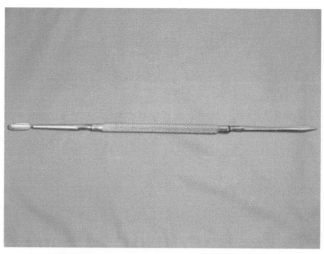

Fig. 11: Lacrimal sac dissector and curette.

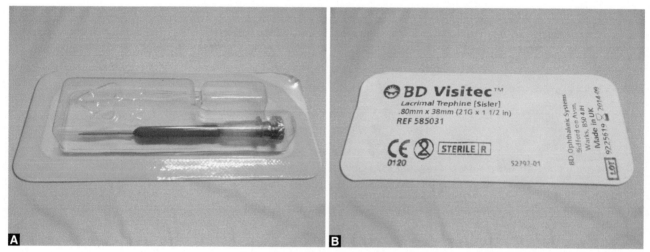

Figs. 12A and B: Lacrimal trephine.

Castroviejo's Calipers (Fig. 13A)

These have one fixed and one adjustable arm, with a screw for adjustment and a millimeter scale attached to the fixed arm. Total length of the scale is 20 mm. It is used to take measurements during lid surgeries, during conjunctival or squint surgeries, to measure size of biopsy specimen.

Steel Ruler (Fig. 13B)

Used to make intraoperative measurements, for instance during telecanthus repair, levator palpebrae superioris (LPS) resection, etc.

Chisel and Hammer (Figs. 14A and B)

Chisel has a sharp edge which rests against the bone to be cut and hammer is hit on it from behind. Chisel and

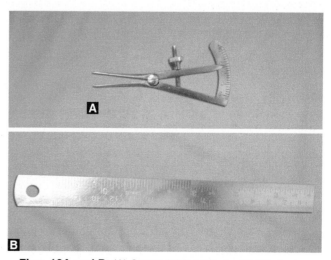

Figs. 13A and B: (A) Castroviejo's calipers; (B) Steel ruler.

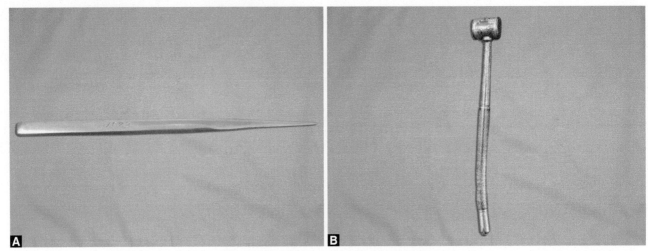

Figs. 14A and B: (A) Chisel; (B) Hammer.

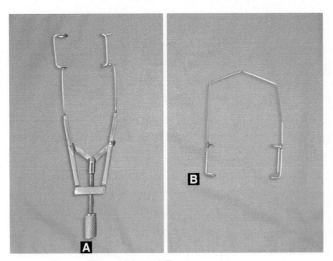

Figs. 15A and B: Lid speculum.

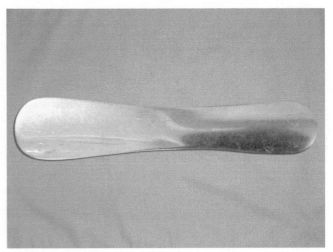

Fig. 16: Jaeger lid plate.

hammer are used to break hard bone, especially in DCR surgery in cases of posttraumatic NLDO.

Lid Speculum (Figs. 15A and B)

This is used to open up the eyelids and expose the ocular surface. This may be used during various intraocular and extraocular surgeries, as well as for examination and during removal of foreign bodies.

- *Lieberman eye speculum*: This is larger and heavier than the wire speculum; mostly used for extraocular surgeries and is universal (Fig. 15A)
- *Barraquer wire speculum*: This is universal, i.e. can be used for either eye; is light and exerts minimum pressure on the eyeball. This is available in adult and pediatric sizes (Fig. 15B).

Jaeger Lid Plate (Fig. 16)

It is a flat plate-like instrument with slightly curved ends which conform to the contour of the globe. It is used to protect the globe during lid surgeries like LPS resection, sling surgery, and during lid incisions. It may also be used as a blunt retractor during orbital surgeries.

Wells Enucleation Spoon with Optic Nerve Guide (Fig. 17)

It is a spoon-like instrument with a groove at its tip, which encases the optic nerve. It is used to support, stabilize, apply traction, and protect the globe during enucleation. While performing enucleation, the enucleation scissors are inserted under the spoon, thereby avoiding globe perforation.

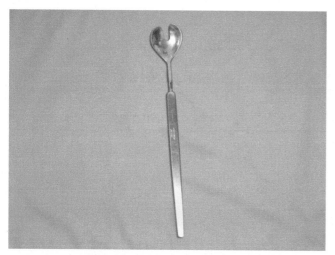

Fig. 17: Wells enucleation spoon.

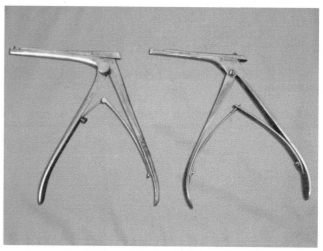

Fig. 19: Kerrison bone punch.

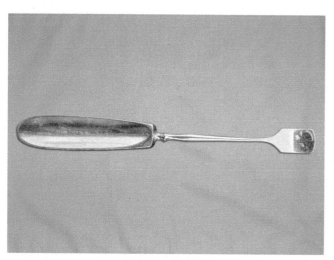

Fig. 18: Evisceration scoop.

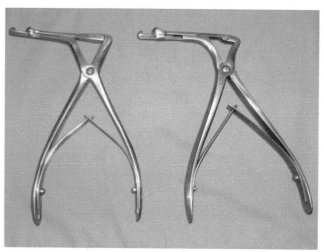

Fig. 20: Citelli's bone punch.

Evisceration Scoop (Fig. 18)

It has a handle with a small rectangular blade at its end which is slightly curved and with blunt edges. It is used to scoop out the intraocular contents during evisceration.

Bone Punch/Rongeur

- *Kerrison's bone punch* (Fig. 19): It has a spring between its handles and blades which slide over one another. The punch has sharp cutting edges that oppose and punch the tissue in between. The tip is blunt to push away and avoid damage to the surrounding tissues and mucosa. Variable sizes of blade length and width are available. Longer ones are generally used for endonasal DCR surgery. Though classically used to create the osteotomy in external DCR, these punches are also used to nibble

at and remove bone in orbital surgeries like orbitotomy, orbital decompression, and orbital fracture repair

- *Citelli's bone punch* (Fig. 20): This is similar to Kerrison's punch and has a C-shaped loop near its end.

Bard-Parker Handle (Fig. 21A)

This may be flat or rounded, with a groove to attach disposable surgical blades which are loaded onto it; commonly used in oculoplastic surgery to make surgical incisions.

Stainless Steel Disposable Blades (Fig. 21B)

These blades are available in different sizes. Commonly used are number 11 and number 15 blades.

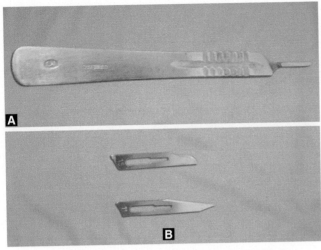

Figs. 21A and B: (A) Bard-Parker handle; (B) Blades.

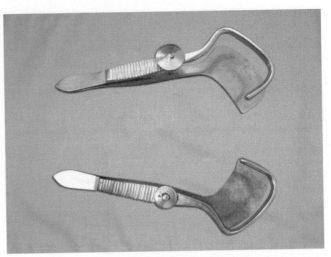

Fig. 23: Entropion clamp.

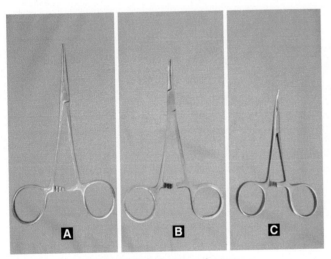

Figs. 22A to C: Artery forceps.

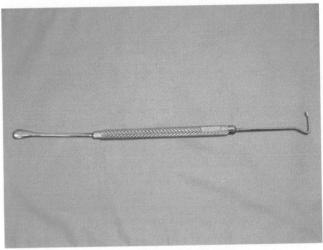

Fig. 24: Jameson muscle hook.

Artery Forceps (Figs. 22A to C)

These are available in different sizes. They are locking forceps with serrated tips for a tight grip. These are used for hemostasis, to crush muscles and other tissues prior to excision, and as a clamp to hold traction sutures, towels, i.v. sets, wires, etc.
- Straight (Fig. 22A)
- Curved (Fig. 22B)
- *Halstead's mosquito artery forceps*: These are smaller and more precise. Especially useful for hemostasis (Fig. 22C).

Entropion Clamp (Fig. 23)

It has two arms and an adjustment screw in between. One arm has a solid plate like end, which is kept on the conjunctival side. The other arm has a hollow curved rim like end, which is applied on the skin side, and the screw is tightened. The instrument is self-retaining. The clamp helps to protect the globe while giving incision on the lid, maintains the lid in position, and also helps in hemostasis. When applied over the lid, the handle is kept temporally. Hence, the same instrument is used for right upper and left lower lid, while the opposite one is for right lower and left upper lid. The instrument is used for lid surgeries like entropion and ectropion repair.

Jameson Muscle Hook (Fig. 24)

This is a slender instrument with curved end. This is used to hook and isolate muscles during squint surgery, during enucleation and during orbital procedures and may also be used to stabilize lacrimal sac and nasal mucosal flaps during DCR surgery.

Wright's Fascia Needle (Fig. 25)

It is a sturdy, long, curved, needle-like instrument with a sharp tip, an eyelet for threading the fascia through it, and a round ring-shaped handle. It is used during fascia lata sling surgery for ptosis repair. The slight curve helps in easy passage of the instrument and avoids damage to the globe.

Suction Tip with Stylet (Fig. 26)

In ophthalmology we prefer using bent suction tips for better grip and ease of use. Tips of different internal diameters are available, of which 2 mm, 3 mm, and 4 mm ones are commonly used. Suction tip is attached to a pliable sterilized tubing, which in turn is attached to the suction machine or wall outlet. During oculoplastic surgery, the tip is held by an assistant, and suction of fluids and blood away from the field helps to improve visualization of the surgical site. The edges of the tip are blunt to avoid damage to surrounding tissue.

Cheatle's Forceps (Fig. 27)

These are large forceps, typically used for picking and transferring various things, like other instruments, gauze pieces, sterile towels, etc.

Rampley's Sponge Holding Forceps (Fig. 28)

These are used to hold the gauze piece or sponge to clean the surgical field.

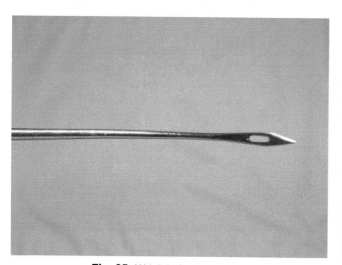

Fig. 25: Wright's fascia needle.

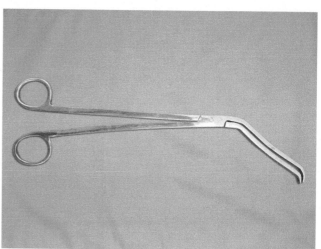

Fig. 27: Cheatle's forceps.

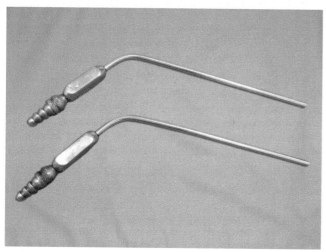

Fig. 26: Suction tip.

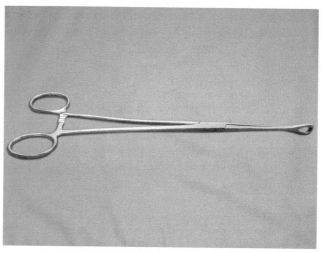

Fig. 28: Rampley's sponge holding forceps.

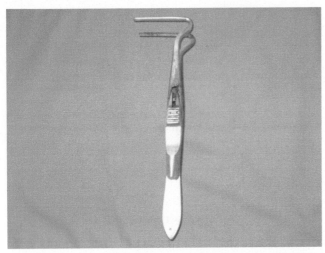

Fig. 29: Ptosis clamp.

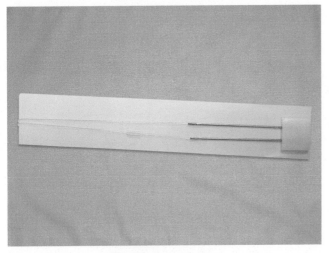

Fig. 30: Silicone sling.

Ptosis Clamp (Fig. 29)

It has two arms with curved ends and with a locking mechanism. It is used to grasp the LPS muscle during ptosis (levator excision) surgery and provide traction.

Silicone Sling (Fig. 30)

It is an artificial sling used for ptosis surgery. It is composed of a flexible silicon rod, about 40 cm in length, with straight sharp malleable metallic needles attached at each end and a silicon sleeve to tighten the sling and hold it in position. The silicon is flexible allowing for lid closure and adjustments and the sling has excellent biocompatibility.

STENTS

Various stents are used in DCR surgery or after repair/reconstruction of the lacrimal drainage system, to maintain patency of the passage just created. These help to mechanically dilate the lumen of the passage they traverse and also help in conduit of fluid through the passage by capillary action. These include:

- *Bicanalicular stents* (Fig. 31A): These are of various designs. Crawford's stent is a commonly used one

  The silicone stent is swaged onto malleable steel bodkins at each end, with olive-shaped bulbous tips. These tips help to dilate the puncta and help in easier passage of the stent through the canaliculus. Once in the nasal cavity, they are retrieved using the Crawford's hook. Various modifications have been designed with differences in the length, shape, and diameters of the metallic bodkins. Retrieval is often done either under direct endoscopic visualization or using artery forceps. The metallic arms are passed through each canaliculus. Once in the nasal cavity, the metallic bodkins are cut and the silicone arms are tied to prevent extrusion.

- *Monocanalicular (Minimonoka) stent* (Fig. 31B): It is a 30 mm long silicon tubing with a "punctal fixation device" at its proximal end, which makes it self-retaining. This punctal fixation device is composed of a collarette, with a vertical tube followed by a small bulb at the junction of the vertical and horizontal parts of the stent. This bulb fits into the ampulla and prevents displacement of the stent once in position. The collarette sits on top of the punctum. It is the only visible part of the stent once it is fit snugly, prevents intracanalicular migration of the stent, and is used to pull out the stent during removal. Monocanalicular stent is used mainly for proximal lacrimal system (punctum and canaliculus) intubation, in cases of punctual stenosis or following canalicular repair

- *Jone's tube* (Fig. 31C): These are glass or pyrex tubes used in cases of conjunctivo-DCR, to maintain patency of the newly created tract, from the conjunctival sac in the medial canthal area to the nasal cavity. Since every patient's anatomy is different, a range of sizes is available. The required length is measured in each patient by passing a probe from the medial canthal area till the nasal septum, and a tube 2 mm shorter than this is used. The tube has a flange at one end and the other end which goes into the nasal cavity is bevelled. Over the years, various modifications have been tried to prevent tube extrusion. These include medpor coating, frosted surface, introducing angles and curves and recently, adding silicone flanges to the tube (StopLoss Jones Tube).

ORBITAL IMPLANTS (FIG. 32)

Orbital implants are used postenucleation or evisceration surgery, to replace the lost volume of the natural eye. In

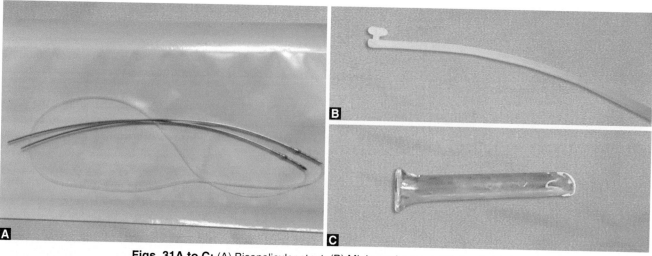

Figs. 31A to C: (A) Bicanalicular stent; (B) Minimonoka stent; (C) Jone's tube.

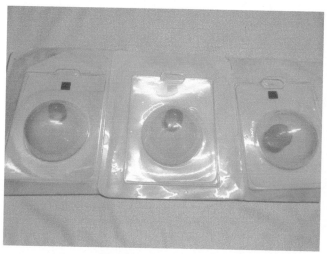

Fig. 32: Orbital implants.

1885, Mules was the first to report use of a glass implant postevisceration. Since then, various different materials and types of implants have been used. They are classified into nonintegrated, semi-integrated, and integrated implants. The nonintegrated ones are simple spheres with no mechanism for attaching the extraocular muscles to it or for fibrovascular ingrowth. Commonly available ones include glass, poly methyl methacrylate (PMMA), and silicone spheres. Integrated implants are of porous materials, which allow fibrovascular ingrowth into the implant, and also insertion of pegs or posts, to directly anchor the extraocular muscles to the implant. These may be made up of hydroxyapatite, alumina or porous polyethylene.

Different sizes of implants are available. The size required maybe determined preoperatively using the axial length of the globe as a guide, or per-operatively using implant sizers.

Conformer (Fig. 33)

Conformers made of PMMA are used after enucleation or evisceration surgery, to maintain the shape and volume of the conjunctival fornices. These also help to maintain socket volume and limit postoperative tissue edema. Often these have holes for drainage of secretions. Different sizes are available. The conformer is normally kept in place for 6 weeks while the socket heals and then a suitable prosthesis can be fitted.

BONE SAW (FIGS. 34A TO D)

This is a hand-held electrically powered bone saw, with an oscillating removable blade. The blade can be detached from the hand-piece and sterilized for re-use. The frequency of vibration can be altered depending on hardness of the bone to be cut. This saw is commonly used during lateral orbitotomy, to cut the lateral orbital rim. Action of the handpiece is controlled using a foot-switch.

ELECTROCAUTERY (FIGS. 35A AND B)

Wet field bipolar electrocautery is commonly used to cauterize small blood vessels. Electric current flows between the tips of the handpiece, over a moist field, and cauterizes the tissue in between the tips. Bipolar cautery allows for a relatively precise delivery of energy with minimal collateral tissue damage. Cauterization is also used for inducing scarring, e.g. for punctal occlusion and to induce conjunctival scarring.

CRYO-PROBE (FIGS. 36A AND B)

It has an insulated handle with a round ball-like metallic tip. The tip is cooled using compressed nitrous oxide (N_2O) gas.

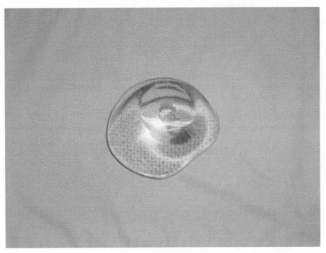

Fig. 33: Conformer.

Temperatures as low as –89°C may be achieved at the tip. Different diameters are available. Generally a probe of size 2.5 mm is used in oculoplasty. The tissue, on which the probe is to be applied to, is dried, the probe is applied and cooling started. The cool probe adheres to the tissue and helps to provide traction. This is especially useful during orbitotomy surgeries for excision biopsies, particularly for cavernous hemangioma, glioma, schwannoma, etc. Cryotherapy is also used for destruction of aberrant/misdirected cilia, and to destroy tumor tissue in malignancies like basal cell carcinoma (BCC), squamous cell carcinoma (SCC), melanoma, etc. and for obtaining margin control.

SUTURES AND NEEDLES

Effective wound closure is important for the final success of any surgical procedure. Closure of the wound using

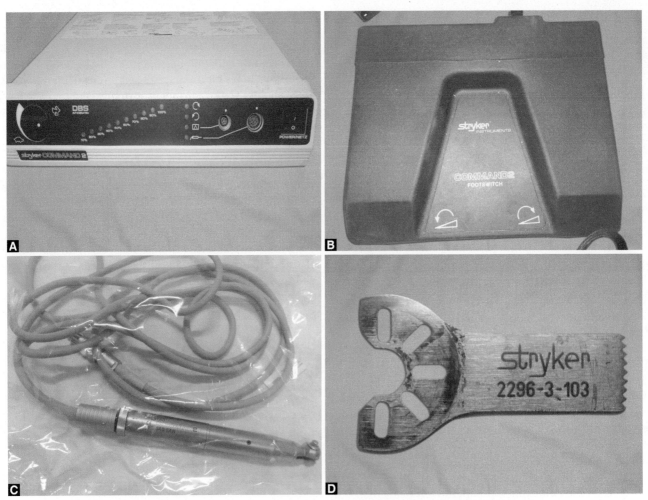

Figs. 34A to D: Bone saw. (A) Console; (B) Foot pedal; (C) Handpiece; (D) Blade of bone saw.

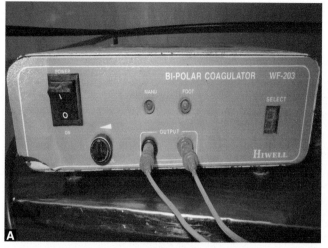
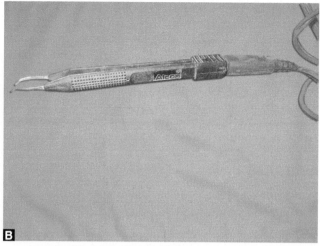

Figs. 35A amd B: Bipolar coagulator. (A) Console; (B) Tip with handpiece.

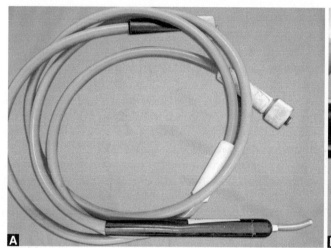
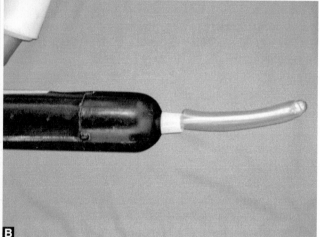

Figs. 36A and B: Cryo-probe

sutures permits wound healing by primary intention, since the sutures help to appose the wound edges until healing occurs. Appropriate wound closure requires knowledge of both, the proper surgical technique as well as the properties of the suture and needle.

Suture selection depends on the anatomic site, surgeon's preference, and the required suture characteristics. The main consideration in needle selection is to minimize tissue trauma.

Sutures

An ideal suture should have the following properties:

- Easy to handle
- Easy to sterilize
- Cause minimal tissue injury or reaction (i.e. no allergenic, electrolytic, or carcinogenic properties)

- Hold securely when knotted, does not fray
- High tensile strength
- Should get absorbed once healing occurs
- Resistant to infection
- Universal (i.e. can be used in any surgical procedure)
- Low cost, easy availability.

However, at present, no single suture possesses all these properties. Hence, different sutures are required depending on the biological interaction of the materials employed, the tissue configuration, and the biomechanical properties of the wound. The sutures are available in different colors, which helps in differentiating them, and may also improve suture visibility (e.g. when there is excessive bleeding).

The various properties of a suture material may be described as follows:

Elasticity: The ability of a material to regain its initial length after stretching.

Suture glide: The capacity of the suture thread to pass smoothly through the tissue during placement. It is a function of its coefficient of friction. Threads with a high coefficient of friction can have a saw effect as they pass through the tissues. On the other hand, a very low coefficient of friction may lead to suture slippage. Monofilament threads usually glide very well, whereas braided threads have a higher coefficient of friction. Hence they are often coated, to minimize tissue trauma.

Suture properties

Tensile strength: The ability of a material or tissue to resist deformation and breakage.

Memory: Tendency of a suture to retain its original shape. High memory makes it difficult to tie using that suture.

Breaking strength: Limit of tensile strength at which suture breaks.

Knot strength: Amount of force necessary to cause a knot to slip (related to the coefficient of static friction and plasticity of a given material).

Plasticity: Measure of the ability to deform without breaking.

Wound breaking strength: Limit of tensile strength of a healing wound at which separation of the wound edges occurs.

Tissue biocompatibility: Relates to the degree of tissue reaction evoked.

Absorbability: Relates to the degradation of suture and decrease in its tensile strength.

Absorption may occur by enzymatic degradation (in natural materials) or by hydrolysis (in synthetic materials). Hydrolysis causes less tissue reaction. Sutures that undergo rapid degradation lose their tensile strength early, are considered absorbable. Half-life is defined as the time required for the tensile strength of a material to be reduced to half its original value. Dissolution time is the time that elapses before a thread is completely dissolved. These times are influenced by a large number of factors including thread thickness, type of tissue, and the general condition of the patient. Absorption is generally faster in inflamed tissues.

Absorbable sutures maybe used to repair tissues that heal rapidly, with minimal support, like conjunctiva, subcutaneous tissue, muscles, or mucosal closure.

Nonabsorbable sutures may be used for skin closure, corneo-scleral suturing, or even as a sling material for frontalis suspension.

Filament configuration: Monofilament and multifilament. Multifilament sutures are generally braided; hence have an increased tissue drag, increased chances of tissue reaction, and an increased risk of infection. However, these also generally hold better due to the increased friction, have a better tensile strength, better pliability, and increased flexibility. Monofilament sutures pass smoothly, but there is risk of loosening of the knots. These are generally stiff and difficult to handle.

Suture material/source: Natural or synthetic.

Suture size: Suture size refers to the diameter of the suture strand and is denoted using the "United States Pharmacopeia (USP)" classification system. The size is characterized by zeroes. The more the zeroes, the smaller the resultant strand diameter. Another system which is used extensively in Europe is the European Pharmacopoeia (EP) decimal classification system, which defines the diameter of the suture strand in millimeter.

Surgical sutures are sterilized using ethylene oxide (ETO) and packaged in two layers, with all the suture information written on the package.

Some of the commonly used sutures include:

Nonabsorbable Sutures

Silk: Natural suture; silk sutures are made from threads of cocoon of silkworm. It may be virgin or braided and is relatively inelastic. It produces tissue necrosis resulting in early release of the wound, hence, it induces less with the rule astigmatism when used in cataract surgery. The braided silk is prepared by degumming process that removes the extraneous material amounting to 30% of the original volume of the raw silk. This is essential for compactness. The advantage is that neither the suture soaks up fluid nor becomes limp or brittle. On the other hand the virgin silk is not processed to remove the gums within the fiber. This allows twisted filaments of silk-worm fiber to stick together forming strong fine suture material used in cataract surgery. Although it is nonabsorbable, it loses much of its tensile strength in 1 year. Also, silk causes moderate to high tissue reaction.

Nylon (polyamide): Synthetic suture; it is extremely inert but elastic, causes minimal tissue reaction, and has a biodegradation rate of 20% per year. Due to its late absorption it induces with the wound astigmatism in cataract surgery. It is stiff and fractures easily; may cause corneal vascularization and follicular reaction in the upper lid. Nylon is available as both monofilament and multifilament sutures. This is the suture of choice for wound closure of corneal incisions.

Polypropylene (prolene): Synthetic suture; it is stiff, produces little tissue reaction, resists infection, and stretches less than nylon of comparable size. Monofilament polypropylene ties securely and handles well. Its smoothness allows easy placement and its release characteristics allow early removal. Since it is largely unaffected by body tissues, it is used for scleral fixation of intraocular lens, fixation of Cionni's ring, iridodialysis repair, brow lift, and correction of involutional ectropion.

TABLE 1: Characteristics of commonly used absorbable sutures.

Suture	Material	Duration	Characteristics
Collagen	Homogenous dispersion of bovine tendon	16–25 days with decrease in tensile strength from 5th day	Loses strength like catgut, but is less irritating
Plain catgut	Submucosal layer of sheep intestine or serosal layer of beef intestine	Half life is 5–7 days and loses all its effective strength by 15 days	Pale straw colored
Chromic catgut	Plain catgut tanned in chromic salts	Half life is 17–21 days and loses all its effective strength by 30 days	Dark brown in color. Causes lesser reaction then plain catgut
Vicryl	Polyglactin 910 (copolymer of glycolide and lactide)	60–90 days and tensile strength remains for 30 days	Extremely high initial tensile strength. Can be used in all situations where absorbable suture needs to be used. It is commonly used for suturing nasal mucosal flaps in dacryocystorhinostomy, muscle reinsertion in squint surgery and lid margin repair.
Dexon	Polyglycolic acid	2–3 weeks	Mild reaction, high tensile strength; Green in color, braided, multifilament

Polyester (Dacron): These are types of synthetic sutures. Maybe uncoated (Merselene) or coated (Ethibond); are extremely strong, with good handling properties and cause minimal tissue reaction.

Polybutylate coated braided polyester (Ethibond): Synthetic suture made by fine filaments of polyester and a special braiding process, which produces a firm, strong suture which remains soft and pliable. Braiding is followed by polybutylate coating to impart lubrication and smooth passage through scleral tissues during retinal surgery and sling surgery. It is used in scleral buckling surgery for securing the buckle.

Steel: It is a synthetic suture. Metallic steel sutures (30 μ) have no elasticity. It was used earlier for corneoscleral suturing. Nowadays steel wires maybe used for transnasal wiring for correction of telecanthus.

Absorbable Sutures

The commonly used absorbable sutures are vicryl, plain catgut, chromic catgut, dexon, and collagen. Suture characteristics of some of the sutures are given in Table 1.

Needles

Surgical needles may be eyed or swaged. Although eyed needles can be sterilized and re-used with different types of sutures, swaged needles help to save time and cause less tissue damage.

An ideal needle should have the following properties:
- Sufficiently rigid to prevent easy bending
- Enough length so that it can be grasped with needle holder and pulled from tissues with ease

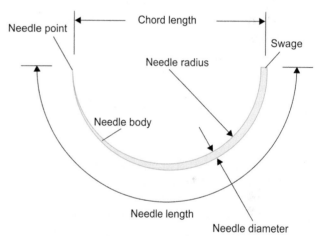

Fig. 37: Parts of surgical needle

- Should be as atraumatic as possible
- Should have sufficient diameter so as to create a tract for the suture knot to be buried.

Nowadays, needles are made of stainless steel alloys, which resist corrosion. These may be coated with silicone to facilitate smooth passage through tissues.

Parts of a Needle (Fig. 37)

1. *Swage:* It is the end of the needle where the suture attaches.
2. *Body:* May have variable diameter, length, curvature, and shape profile.
3. *Point:* It is the sharp tip of the needle. It may be (Fig. 38):
   - *Cutting:* Triangular configuration with cutting edge at the top/inner edge. It cuts at the tip and edge of the needle. Hence, the suture tract is superficial to the needle tip and it may pull out tissue during passage.

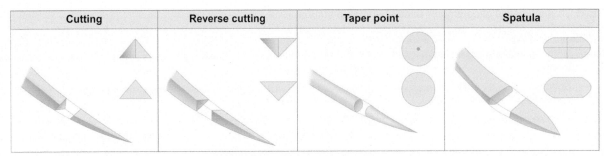

Fig. 38: Types of needle point.

- *Reverse cutting*: Triangular configuration with cutting edge at the bottom/outer edge. Cuts at tip and edge of needle. Suture tract is deeper to passage of needle tip, hence, risk of accidental perforation is there while passing partial thickness sutures. This type of needle is ideal for oculoplastic surgery as it passes easily through the epidermis
- *Taper point*: The needle is round bodied and gradually tapers to a point. Hence, cuts only at the tip. It is atraumatic since it stretches and separates tissue to pass through rather than cutting it. It produces the smallest hole of all needles and minimizes potential tearing. Thus it is used for suturing delicate tissues or where a watertight closure is required. E.g. Iris repair, conjunctival closure in trabeculectomy, etc.
- *Spatulated*: The needle has a thin flat trapezoid profile, which cuts at the tip and at edges parallel to tissue plane. Such a profile helps the needle to split the tissue and avoid accidental perforation. Most commonly used for anterior segment surgeries
- *Taper cut:* Combines a reverse cutting tip with a round body. Hence, it has advantages of both, with better tissue penetration with less trauma, and may be used even for tough tissues like fascia.

Characteristics of a Needle
- *Length*—distance of the circumference from the swage to the point
- *Chord length*—distance of the straight line from the swage to the point (which determines the width of the bite)

- *Radius*—length of the line from the center of the circle of which needle is a part
- *Needle diameter*—measured in mils (1/1000 of an inch). 1 mil is about 25 μm. A smaller diameter needle requires less force and cause less trauma during passage through the tissue
- *Curvature*—a needle is often described as a segment or fraction of the total circle of which it is a part Common ones are:
  - 1/4 circle, 3/8 circle: These provide large, shallow bites. Commonly used in ophthalmology
  - 1/2 circle, 5/8 circle: These provide short and deep bites. The sharp curve is more useful for oculoplastic surgeries
  - *Bicurve needle*: One which has two radii. The radius near the point is usually shorter than the radius of the body near the swage
  - *Straight*: Straight needle is used to pass sling suture for correction of entropion/ectropion
- *Strength*—resistance to deformation during repeated passes through tissue
- *Ductility*—resistance to breakage
- *Sharpness*—Measure of the ability of the needle to penetrate tissue (affected by the angle of the point and the taper ratio (i.e. ratio of taper length to needle diameter))
- *Clamping moment*—stability of a needle in a needle holder.

Choice of a needle depends on all of its properties, including length, curvature, and sharpness and varies with the type of tissue which is to be sutured.

Question Bank

◆ Question Bank Oculoplasty (Previous University Questions)

Question Bank Oculoplasty
(Previous University Questions)

Abhilasha Sanoria

ANATOMY AND PHYSIOLOGY

- Orbital spaces and their significance
- Pictorial demonstration and structure of upper eyelid
- Cavernous sinus and its tributaries with diagram and explanation
- Description of the periosteum of the orbit
- Relations of the nasolacrimal duct and its development
- Sensory nerves of both upper and lower eyelid
- Lacrimal sac
- Lacrimal pump
- Tear film and its role
- Anatomy of orbit
- Levator palpebrae superioris
- Structures passing through the superior orbital fissure.

THYROID

- Thyroid related ophthalmopathy—pathogenesis
- Ocular features of thyrotoxicosis
- Ocular manifestations and management of dysthyroid ophthalmopathy
- Management of lid retraction in thyroid-associated orbitopathy (TAO) and etiopathogenesis.

TUMORS

- Pathology of basal cell carcinoma
- Basal cell carcinoma clinical features
- Glioma
- Differential diagnosis of malignant tumors of lid
- Meningioma
- Glioma

- Cavernous hemangioma of orbit
- Retinoblastoma clinical features, genetics and management
- Choroidal melanoma management
- Rhabdomyosarcoma.

PSEUDOTUMOR

- Clinical features, differential diagnosis of a 55-year-old man with pseudotumor right orbit.

PTOSIS

- Congenital ptosis with surgical and medical management
- Acquired ptosis
- Management of unilateral ptosis in a 3-year-old child
- Clinical features and management of complicated congenital ptosis
- Classification of blepharoptosis and its relevance to management and complications
- Surgical management of ptosis
- Principles of ptosis surgery.

CONTRACTED SOCKET

- Morphological classification of contracted socket and discuss strategies of management of anophthalmic socket.

FRACTURES OF ORBIT

- Blow-out fracture of orbit
- Discuss orbital fractures in relation to structural anatomy.

CYSTICERCOSIS

- Ocular and orbital cysticercosis.

ENTROPION AND ECTROPION

- Etiopathogenesis of cicatricial entropion
- Surgical correction of spastic entropion
- Entropion surgery.

LACRIMAL APPARATUS

- Nasolacrimal duct obstruction and management
- Lacrimal gland lesions, differential diagnosis, and management
- Pathology, clinical features, differential diagnosis, and management of lacrimal gland tumors
- Causes of failure of dacryocystorhinostomy (DCR) and management of failed DCR
- Dacryocystorhinostomy
- Tumors of lacrimal gland
- Landmarks and complications of DCR surgery
- Clinical picture and management of congenital epiphora. Indication for surgical intervention.

PROPTOSIS

- Management of a case of unilateral axial proptosis in an adult
- Differential diagnosis of acute proptosis in children
- Painful proptosis
- Indications, procedures, and complications of lateral orbitotomy
- Various approaches to the orbit
- Indications and method of trans frontal orbitotomy
- Discuss the management and differential diagnosis of orbital cellulitis.

MISCELLANEOUS

- Discuss the various surgical procedures for the management of defects in eyelids
- Role of radiologists for diagnosis of tumors of eye
- Botulinum toxin in ophthalmology
- Ultrasonography B-scan indications and utility
- Orbital mucormycosis
- Causes of orbital hemorrhage.

INDEX

Page numbers followed by *b* refer to box, *f* refer to figure, *fc* refer to flow chart, and *t* refer to table.